Table of Contents   PDR® Pharmacopoeia Pocket Dosing Guide 2013

FOREWORD 2

ABBREVIATIONS; CONVERSION TABLES 4

FOOTNOTE KEY 8

ANALGESICS 16

Arthritis Therapy, Narcotics, NSAIDs, Miscellaneous

ANTI-INFECTIVES (SYSTEMIC) 32

AIDS Therapy, Antiviral Agents, Bone and Joint Infection, Fungal Infection, LRI, Bacterial Meningitis, MAC, Otitis Media, PCP, Bacterial Septicemia, Skin/Skin Structure, URI, UTI, Miscellaneous

ANTINEOPLASTICS 92

CARDIOVASCULAR AGENTS 101

Angina, Antiarrhythmics, Antilipidemics, Coagulation Modifiers, Heart Failure, Antihypertensives

DERMATOLOGY 145

Acne Preparations, Anti-Infectives, Antipruritics, Antipsoriatics, Miscellaneous

EENT 154

EENT/Nasal Preps (Anticholinergics, Corticosteroids); EENT/Optho Preps (Antibiotics, Antibiotic/Corticosteroid Combinations, Corticosteroids, Antifungals, Glaucoma Therapy, NSAIDs, Ocular Decongestants/Allergic Conjunctivitis)

ENDOCRINE/METABOLIC 163

Androgens, Antidiabetic Agents, Antithyroid Agents, Gout Agents, Osteoporosis Therapy, Thyroid Agents, Miscellaneous

GASTROINTESTINAL AGENTS 185

Antidiarrheals, Antiemetics, Antispasmodics, Antiulcer Agents, GERD Therapy, Laxatives, Ulcerative Colitis, Zollinger-Ellison Agents, Miscellaneous

GYNECOLOGY 207

Anti-Infectives, Contraceptives, Dysmenorrhea, Hormone Therapy, Premenstrual Dysphoric Disorder, Miscellaneous

HEMATOLOGY

Anemia, Hema
Toxoids/Immu

NEUROLOGY/PS

ADHD/Narcole
Therapy, Antian
Anticonvulsant
Antiparkinson's
Bipolar Agents,
Relaxants, OCD

PULMONARY/RES

Asthma/COPD P

UROLOGY

BPH Therapy, Er
Antispasmodics

REFERENCE CHAR

Antihistamines, C
Combinations, Im
Insulin Formulatio
Systemic Corticos
Corticosteroids

INDEX

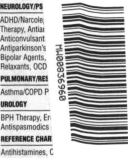

Foreword

Welcome to the *PDR Pharmacopoeia Pocket Dosing Guide*, now in its 13th edition. This convenient little book is designed to be at your fingertips whenever you need to double-check dosage recommendations, review available forms and strengths, or confirm a pregnancy rating. The 2013 edition has been completely updated to include the newest drugs, forms, strengths, and indications.

To aid quick lookups and comparisons, *PDR Pharmacopoeia* is organized by major drug category and specific indication. Under each indication, you'll find applicable drugs sorted by class and listed alphabetically by generic name. For combination products, generic ingredients are listed alphabetically, with the strengths of the ingredients presented in the same order.

The book's major sections are listed on the Table of Contents page. The location of entries for specific brands, generics, and indications can be found in the index at the end of the book. For drugs with multiple uses, the index lists the page of each indication separately. Headings under a generic drug entry include listings for both single and combination forms of the generic product.

The *PDR Pharmacopoeia* also offers you a variety of quick-reference tables listing frequently used formulas and comparative prescribing information. For the exact location of these convenient resources, check the index at the end of the book.

The *PDR Pharmacopoeia* is drawn exclusively from FDA-approved drug labeling published in *Physicians' Desk Reference®* or supplied by the manufacturer. Although diligent efforts have been made to ensure the accuracy of this information, please remember that this book is supplied without warranties, express or implied, and that the publisher and editors disclaim all liability in connection with its use.

Remember, too, that this book deals only with dosage for the typical patient, and includes little information on usage in special populations and circumstances. The need for dosage adjustments/warnings in the presence of hepatic or renal insufficiency is signaled in the Comments column of the entries. For details regarding these adjustments, as well as complete pediatric and geriatric dosage guidelines, consult the latest edition of *PDR®* or the manufacturer. Be sure to check these sources, too, whenever contraindications, warnings, or precautions may be an issue.

Throughout the book, you will find a drug's Controlled Substances Category (if any) immediately following its name. The drug's pregnancy rating and breastfeeding status appear in the Comments column of the entry. Keys to the symbols can be found below:

CONTROLLED SUBSTANCES CATEGORIES
CII. High potential for abuse, leading to severe psychological or physical dependence. **CIII.** Abuse may lead to moderate or low physical dependence or high psychological dependence. **CIV.** Abuse may lead to limited physical dependence or psychological dependence relative to those in CIII. **CV.** Abuse may lead to limited physical or psychological dependence relative to those in CIV.

🄔 USE-IN-PREGNANCY RATINGS
A. Controlled studies show no risk. **B.** No evidence of risk in humans. **C.** Risk cannot be ruled out. **D.** Positive evidence of risk: Use only when no safer alternative exists for a serious problem. **X.** Contraindicated in pregnancy. **N.** Not rated.

❁ Breastfeeding Safety
^ May be used in breastfeeding. > Caution advised or effect undetermined. v Contraindicated or not recommended.

H Dosage adjustment required for hepatic insufficiency.
R Dosage adjustment required for renal insufficiency.
W See Footnotes section.

DOSAGE FORMS
A key to the abbreviations begins on page 4.

FOOTNOTES
A key to the footnotes begins on page 8.

PDR® PHARMACOPOEIA POCKET DOSING GUIDE 2013
PHYSICIANS' DESK REFERENCE

Director, Clinical Services: Sylvia Nashed, PharmD
Senior Manager, Clinical Services: Nermin Shenouda-Kerolous, PharmD
Clinical Database Manager: Christine Sunwoo, PharmD
Senior Drug Information Specialist: Anila Patel, PharmD
Drug Information Specialists: Demyana Farag, PharmD; Pauline Lee, PharmD; Kristine Mecca, PharmD
Clinical Editor: Julia Tonelli, MD
Manager, Art Department: Livio Udina
Managing Editor: J. Harris Fleming, Jr.
Editor: Sharon Stompf
Project Manager: Gary Lew

CEO: Edward Fotsch, MD
President: Richard C. Altus
Senior Vice President, Publishing & Operations: Valerie Berger
Senior Director, Operations & Client Services: Stephanie Struble
Senior Director, Content Operations and Manufacturing: Jeffrey D. Schaefer
Associate Director, Manufacturing & Distribution: Thomas Westburgh

Printed in Canada   2013

ABBREVIATIONS

ABBREVIATIONS & DESCRIPTIONS	
bid	twice daily
biw	twice a week
CAP	community-acquired pneumonia
Cap	capsule
Cap, ER	extended-release capsule
CI	contraindicated
Cnt	concentrate
conc	concentration
Cre	cream
d	day
D/C	discontinue
Eli	elixir
Foa	foam
Gel	gel/jelly
gm	gram
gtt	drop
gtts	drops
h	hour
hs	at bedtime

ABBREVIATIONS & DESCRIPTIONS	
min	minute
mIU	million international units
ml	milliliter
mth	month
NTE	not to exceed
N/V	nausea and vomiting
Oint	ointment
Pkt	packet
PO	by mouth
Pow	powder
prn	as needed
q	every
qd	once daily
qid	four times daily
qod	every other day
qow	every other week
SC	subcutaneous
SL	sublingual
Sol	solution

IM	intramuscular	**Sol,Neb**	solution, nebulized
inh	inhalation	**Spr**	spray(s)
inj	injection	**Sup**	suppository
Tab,IR	immediate-release tablet	**Susp**	suspension
IU	international units	**Syr**	syrup
IV	intravenous	**Tab**	tablet
kg	kilogram	**Tab,ER**	extended-release tablet
Liq	liquid	**tid**	3 times daily
Lot	lotion	**tiw**	3 times weekly
Loz	lozenge	**U**	units
mcg	microgram	**w/a**	while awake
MDI	metered-dose inhaler	**wk**	week
mEq	milli-equivalent	**yo**	years old
mg	milligram		

WEIGHTS & MEASURES; CONVERSIONS & FORMULAS

METRIC WEIGHT

1 kilogram (kg)	= 1000 gram
1 gram (gm)	= 1000 mg
1 milligram (mg)	= 0.001 gm

U.S. FLUID MEASURE

1 fluidrachm	= 60 minim (min)
1 fluidounce	= 8 fld drachm
	= 480 min

METRIC WEIGHT

1 microgram (mcg)	= 0.001 mg
1 gamma	= 1 mcg

U.S. FLUID MEASURE

1 pint (pt)	= 16 fl oz
	= 7680 min
1 quart (qt)	= 2 pt
	= 32 fl oz
1 gallon (gal)	= 4 qts
	= 128 fl oz

APOTHECARY WEIGHT

1 scruple	= 20 grains (gr)
1 drachm	= 3 scruples
	= 60 gr
1 ounce (oz)	= 8 drachms
	= 24 scruples
	= 480 gr
1 pound (lb)	= 12 oz
	= 96 drachms
	= 288 scruples
	= 5760 gr

AVOIRDUPOIS WEIGHT

1 ounce	= 437.5 gr
1 pound	= 16 oz

CONVERSION FACTORS

1 gram	= 15.4 gr
1 grain	= 64.8 mg
1 ounce (Av)	= 28.35 gm
	= 437.5 gr
1 ounce (Ap)	= 31.1 gm
	= 480 gr

COMMON MEASURES

1 teaspoonful	= 5 ml
	= 1/6 fl oz
1 tablespoonful	= 15 ml
	= 1/2 fl oz
1 wineglassful	= 60 ml
	= 2 fl oz

1 pound (Av)	= 453.6 gm	1 teacupful	= 120 ml
			= 4 fl oz
1 kilogram	= 2.68 pound Ap		
	= 2.2 lbs Av		
1 fluidounce	= 29.57 ml		
1 fluidrachm	= 3.697 ml		
1 minim	= 0.06 ml		

TEMPERATURE

For °F to °C, the formula is: 5/9 (°F minus 32) = °C
For °C to °F, the formula is: 9/5 (°C plus 32) = °F
Kelvin = Celcius+273.15; Kelvin = (Fahrenheit-32) x 5/9 + 273.15

COCKCROFT/GAULT CREATININE CLEARANCE FORMULA

$$CrCl \text{ (males* ml/min)} = \frac{(140 - Age)(Body Weight in kg)}{(SrCr)(72 kg)}$$

*For females multiply result by 0.85

BODY SURFACE AREA [BSA (M²)]

BSA = ([Ht (cm) • Wt (kg)]/ 3600) ½

ANION GAP (AG)

$AG = (Na^+ + K^+) - (Cl^- + HCO_3^-)$ or $AG = Na^+ - (Cl^- + HCO_3^-)$

NEUTROPENIA CALCULATION

ANC = (% segs + % bands) X total WBC

FOOTNOTES

1 Potential neurotoxicity, ototoxicity & neuromuscular blockade. Avoid concurrent use w/ neurotoxic/nephrotoxic agents & diuretics.

2 Contraindicated in pregnant patients at term & nursing mothers.

3 Give only under supervision of a physician experienced w/ antineoplastics.

4 Contraindicated in pregnancy. Increased risk of endometrial carcinoma.

5 Proarrhythmic properties/drug should only be used in life-threatening arrhythmias.

6 Risk of paralysis by spinal/epidural hematoma w/ neuraxial anesthesia/lumbar puncture. Increased risk w/ concomitant anticoagulation, NSAIDs, or traumatic/repeated lumbar puncture.

7 ACE Inhibitors can cause injury & death to developing fetus in 2nd & 3rd trimesters.

8 Excess amounts may lead to water & electrolyte depletion.

9 Drugs that act directly on the renin-angiotensin system can cause injury & even death to developing fetus. D/C if pregnancy detected.

10 Initiate/reinitiate only in hospitalized patients. Rapid correction of hyponatremia (>12mEq/L/24h) can cause osmotic demyelination. Slower rates of correction advised in severe malnutrition, alcoholism, or advanced liver disease.

11 Should only be used by physicians experienced w/ immunosuppression therapy.

12 Granulocytopenia, anemia, thrombocytopenia, carcinogenic, teratogenic & aspermatogenic in animal studies.

13 May cause or aggravate neuropsychiatric, autoimmune, ischemic & infectious disorders; monitor closely.

14 INH associated w/ hepatitis. Avoid in acute hepatic diseases.

15 Neutropenia, agranulocytosis. TTP, aplastic anemia.

16 Tumorigenic in chronic toxicity studies. Avoid unnecessary use.

17 Abrupt cessation may induce arrhythmia or MI.

18 Abrupt cessation may exacerbate angina.

19 Monitor for bone marrow, lung, liver & kidney toxicities. Serious toxic reactions.

20 Risk of ocular damage, aging skin & skin cancer. Do not interchange w/ Oxsoralen-Ultra without retitration.

21 Risk of ocular damage, aging skin & skin cancer. Do not interchange w/ regular Oxsoralen or 8-Mop. Determine minimum phototoxic dose & phototoxic peak time.

22 Overdose in children can cause death.

23 Chromosomal aberrations. Severe bone marrow suppression.

24 Avoid if CrCl <30 ml/min.

25 CI during pregnancy. Thromboembolism, thrombotic & thrombophlebitic events reported. Peliosis hepatitis & benign hepatic carcinoma observed w/ long-term use. Associated w/ benign intracranial HTN.

26 Risk of agranulocytosis, seizures, myocarditis, other cardiovascular/respiratory effects. Increased mortality in elderly patients w/ dementia-related psychosis.

27 See Immunization chart for details.

28 Not for prevention of CV disease or dementia. Increased risks of MI, stroke, invasive breast cancer, pulmonary emboli, DVT & probable dementia in postmenopausal women. Prescribe at lowest effective doses for shortest duration.

29 May increase risk of suicidality in children, adolescents & young adults.

30 Increased risk of death in elderly patients w/ dementia-related psychosis.

31 Lactic acidosis & severe hepatomegaly w/ steatosis reported.

32 Severe acute exacerbations of hepatitis B reported in patients who have discontinued anti-hepatitis B therapy; monitor hepatic function closely.

33 Fatal hypersensitivity reactions reported.

34 Associated w/ hematologic toxicity. Prolonged use associated w/ myopathy.

35 Fatal & nonfatal pancreatitis reported.

36 May cause severe peripheral neuropathy.

37 Chronic administration may result in nephrotoxicity; monitor renal function w/, or if at risk of, renal dysfunction.

38 HIV resistance may emerge.

39 May cause severe hypersensitivity reactions including anaphylaxis. May cause severe hemolysis w/ G6PD deficiency. Use associated w/ methemoglobinemia. May interfere w/ uric acid measurements.

40 Potential for severe, life-threatening human birth defects. Only available under a restricted distribution program called "S.T.E.P.S."

41 Severe liver injury & liver failure reported; may be fatal or require transplantation. Reserve for patients intolerant to metronidazole and in whom surgery/radioactive iodine is not appropriate.

42 Hepatotoxicity associated with use of APAP at doses that exceed 4000 milligrams/day.

43 Serious GI adverse events reported, d/c if constipation or symptoms of ischemic colitis develop.

44 Caution w/ auditory or renal impairment. Avoid/caution w/ other ototoxic or nephrotoxic agents.

45 Intracranial hemorrhage, hepatitis & hepatic decompensation reported w/ ritonavir coadministration. Monitor closely w/ chronic hepatitis B or C coinfection.

46 Serious & sometimes fatal infections & bleeding occur very rarely.

49 High potential for abuse; avoid prolonged use. Misuse may cause sudden death & serious CV adverse events.

50 CI w/ phosphodiesterase type 5 (PDE5) inhibitors (eg, sildenafil, vardenafil & tadalafil).

51 Swallow caps whole or sprinkle contents on applesauce. Do not crush, chew, or dissolve cap beads. Avoid alcohol or any alcohol-containing medications; may result in rapid absorption of potentially fatal dose of morphine.

52 Not for use by females who are or may become pregnant or are breastfeeding. Birth defects documented. Approved for marketing only under iPLEDGE. Prescriber & patient must be registered w/ iPLEDGE.

53 Increased susceptibility to infection & possible development of lymphoma & other neoplasms may result from immunosuppression.

54 Sodium oxybate is a GHB (gamma hydroxybutyrate), a known drug of abuse. Do not use w/ alcohol or other CNS depressants. Only available through Xyrem Success Program®.

55 Severe neurologic events reported.

56 Potential for human birth defects, hematologic toxicity (neutropenia & thrombocytopenia) & DVT/PE. Avoid fetal exposure. Only available under a restricted distribution program called "RevAssist."

57 Highly concentrated. Check dose carefully.

58 Do not administer IV or by other parenteral routes. Deaths & serious, life-threatening adverse events have occurred when contents of capsules have been injected parenterally.

59 Renal impairment is the major toxicity. CI w/ nephrotoxic agents. Neutropenia reported. Carcinogenic, teratogenic & hyspospermic in animal studies.

60 Extreme caution w/ renal dysfunction. Monitor hematologic, renal & hepatic status.

61 Risk of fatal hepatotoxicity. CI w/ terfenadine, astemizole, cisapride, oral triazolam.

62 Increased risk of severe neurotoxic reactions w/ renal dysfunction. Avoid neurotoxic & nephrotoxic drugs.

63 Hematologic toxicity & opportunistic infections reported. Gradually increase dose to avoid infusion reactions.

64 Severe myelosuppression, hypersensitivity reactions & hepatotoxicity reported.

65 Fatal infusion reactions, tumor lysis syndrome, severe mucocutaneous reactions & progressive multifocal leukoencephalopathy reported.

66 NSAIDs may cause an increased risk of serious CV thrombotic events, MI, stroke & serious GI adverse events including bleeding, ulceration & perforation of the stomach or intestines.

67 CI for treatment of peri-operative pain in CABG surgery.

68 CI w/ PUD, GI bleeding/perforation, advanced renal impairment, risk of renal failure due to volume depletion, CV bleeding, hemorrhagic diathesis, incomplete hemostasis, high risk of bleeding, prophylactic analgesic before major surgery, intra-operatively when hemostasis is critical, intrathecal/epidural use, L&D, nursing & w/ ASA, NSAIDs, or probenecid.

69 Contains potent CII opioid agonist w/ high potential for abuse & risk of respiratory depression. HP formulation is highly concentrated; do not confuse w/ standard parenteral formulations.

70 Dermatologic toxicities & severe infusion reactions reported.

71 CI w/ myasthenia gravis.

72 Deaths, cardiac & respiratory, reported during initiation & conversion of pain patients to methadone treatment from treatment w/ other opioid agonists.

73 Life-threatening anaphylactic reactions, severe allergic reactions & immune mediated reactions observed. Appropriate medical support should be readily available. Risk of cardiorespiratory failure.

74 Not for use as prn analgesic. May cause fatal respiratory depression if not already tolerant to high doses of opioids. Swallow caps whole, sprinkle contents on applesauce, or dissolve in water & give thru 16 French G-tube. Do not crush, chew, or dissolve cap pellets.

75 (Aranesp, Epogen, Procrit) Chronic Kidney Disease: Greater risks for death, serious adverse CV reactions, and stroke when administered ESAs to target a hemoglobin level >11 g/dL. Cancer: ESAs shortened overall survival and/or increased the risk of tumor progression or recurrence in patients with breast, non-small cell lung, head and neck, lymphoid, and cervical cancers. Must enroll in and comply with the ESA APPRISE Oncology Program to prescribe and/or dispense. Use the lowest dose to reduce the need for RBC transfusions and d/c following completion of chemo. (Epogen, Procrit) Perisurgery: Due to increased risk of DVT, DVT prophylaxis is recommended.

77 Increases risk of meningococcal infections; vaccinate 2 wks prior to receiving 1st dose.

78 May cause fetal harm if taken during pregnancy. Exclude pregnancy before the start of treatment. Prevent pregnancy during treatment and for one month after stopping treatment by the use of two acceptable methods of contraception. Available through the LEAP program only.

79 Thiazolidinediones may cause or exacerbate CHF in some patients. Use not recommended in patients w/ symptomatic heart failure.

80 May lead to increased susceptibility to infection & possible development of lymphoma. Female users of childbearing potential must use contraception.

81 CI in combination w/ capecitabine if AST/ALT >2.5x ULN or bilirubin >1x ULN due to increased toxicity & neutropenia-related death.

82 Thiazolidinediones may cause or exacerbate CHF in some patients. Use not recommended w/ symptomatic heart failure. Studies have shown an increased risk of myocardial ischemic events.

83 Metronidazole has been shown to be carcinogenic in mice & rats. Unnecessary use should be avoided.

84 *C.difficile*-associated diarrhea reported.

85 Increases risk of progressive multifocal leukoencephalopathy (PML). Available only through special restricted distribution program called the TOUCH™ Prescribing Program.

86 Serious infections, including TB, bacterial sepsis & other opportunistic infections, reported. Evaluate for TB risk factors & test for latent TB infection prior to initiation.

87 Serious, sometimes fatal, dermatologic reactions, aplastic anemia & agranulocytosis reported.

88 Abnormal elevation of serum K^+ levels (≥5.5 mEq/L) can occur w/ all K^+-sparing agents, including triamterene; monitor serum K^+ at frequent intervals.

89 May cause QT interval prolongation, complete AV block, or APL differentiation syndrome. Monitor ECG, electrolytes & creatinine before & during therapy.

90 May increase susceptibility to infection & development of neoplasia. Neoral® & Sandimmune® are not bioequivalent. Increased skin malignancy risk w/ certain psoriasis therapies. May cause HTN & nephrotoxicity; monitor renal function.

91 Cardiomyopathy, infusion reactions & pulmonary toxicity reported.

92 Infections & progressive multifocal leukoencephalopathy may occur.

93 Myocardial damage, infusion-related reactions & myelosuppression may occur. Reduce dose w/ hepatic impairment. Avoid substitution w/ doxorubicin HCl.

94 May cause GI perforation, wound dehiscence & fatal pulmonary hemorrhage.

95 May cause negative inotropic effects. CI w/ cisapride, pimozide, quinidine, dofetilide, levacetylmethadol. Serious CV events reported w/ CYP3A4 inhibitors.

96 Life-threatening peripheral ischemia w/ concomitant potent CYP3A4 inhibitors.

97 Coadministration w/ certain nonsedating antihistamines, sedative hypnotics, antiarrhythmics, or ergot alkaloids may result in potentially serious/life-threatening adverse events.

98 Fluoroquinolones associated w/ increased risk of tendinitis & tendon rupture in all ages. Risk further increased if < 60 yo, taking corticosteroids, or w/ kidney, heart, or lung transplants. May exacerbate muscle weakness; avoid in patients with myasthenia gravis.

99 Abuse liability similar to other opioid analgesics. Not intended as prn analgesic. 100 mg & 200 mg tabs for use in opioid-tolerant patients only. Swallow whole.

100 May cause increased risk of serious cardiovascular thrombotic events, MI, stroke & serious GI adverse events.

101 Fatal hepatotoxicity reported (children <2 yo at higher risk); monitor closely & perform LFTs prior to therapy & then periodically. Teratogenic effects & life-threatening pancreatitis reported.

102 Give cautiously w/ history of drug dependence or alcoholism. Chronic abusive use may lead to marked tolerance & psychological dependence w/ varying degrees of abnormal behavior. Monitor closely during withdrawal from abusive use.

103 Acute phosphate nephropathy reported.

104 Virilization in children reported w/ secondary exposure to testosterone gel; cover & avoid contact w/ application site.

105 May cause significant, sometimes fatal, bleeding. Avoid w/ active pathological bleeding, history of TIA/stroke & prior to urgent CABG surgery. D/C at least 7 days prior to any surgery. Caution in elderly, hypotensive & recent surgical procedures, including coronary angiography, PCI & CABG.

106 May cause permanent vision loss. Risk increases w/ total dose & duration of use; may persist after stopping. Test vision before, during & after therapy. Only available through restricted distribution SHARE program.

107 Causes dose-dependent and treatment duration-dependent thyroid C-cell tumors at clinically relevant exposure in animal studies. Contraindicated with a personal or family history of MTC and with multiple endocrine neoplasia syndrome type 2.

108 Efficacy dependent on activation to its active metabolite via CYP2C19. Patients who are poor metabolizers (PM) of CYP2C19 will form less active metabolite. Tests are available to identify CYP2C19 PM prior to treatment; consider alternative treatment/strategies in those populations.

109 Rare reports of serious acute phosphate nephropathy. Patients at increased risk may include those with increased age, hypovolemia, increased bowel transit time (eg, bowel obstruction), active colitis, or baseline kidney disease, and those on medicines that affect renal perfusion or function (eg, diuretics, ACE inhibitors, ARBs, and possibly NSAIDs). Use the recommended dose and dosing regimen (pm/am split dose).

110 Profound myelosuppression reported. Give only under supervision of a physician experienced w/ allogenic hematopoietic stem cell transplantantation, antineoplastics & management of severe pancytopenia.

NAME	FORM/STRENGTH	DOSAGE	COMMENTS

ANALGESICS

Arthritis Therapy
SEE ALSO NSAIDs

NAME	FORM/STRENGTH	DOSAGE	COMMENTS
Abatacept (Orencia)	**Inj:** 250 mg; **Prefilled Syringe:** 125 mg/ml	**Adults: RA: IV Infusion: Initial: <60 kg:** 500 mg. **60-100 kg:** 750 mg. **>100 kg:** 1 gm. Infuse over 30 min. **Maint:** Give at 2 & 4 wks after initial infusion, then q4wks thereafter. **SC:** Following a single IV LD, give the 1st 125 mg SC w/in a d, followed by 125 mg SC once wkly. Refer to PI for remaining SC dosing parameters. **Peds: 6-17 yo: JIA: <75 kg: Initial:** 10 mg/kg. **Maint:** Give at 2 & 4 wks after initial infusion, then q4wks thereafter. **>75 kg:** Follow adult dosing. **Max:** 1000 mg.	⊞C ❀v
Adalimumab (Humira)	**Inj:** 20 mg/0.4 ml, 40 mg/0.8 ml	**Adults: RA/PsA/AS:** 40 mg SC qow. RA patients not taking MTX may derive additional benefit increasing to 40 mg qwk. **Peds: 4-17 yo: JIA: 15 kg-<30 kg:** 20 mg SC qow. **≥30 kg:** 40 mg SC qow.	⊞B ❀v W [86]
Anakinra (Kineret)	**Inj:** 100 mg/0.67 ml	**RA: Adults:** 100 mg SC qd.	⊞B ❀> R
Auranofin (Ridaura)	**Cap:** 3 mg	**RA: Adults: Usual:** 3 mg bid or 6 mg qd. May increase to 3 mg tid if response is inadequate after 6 mths; d/c if unresponsive after a 3 mth trial of 9 mg qd. **Max:** 9 mg/d.	⊞C ❀v May cause gold toxicity.

Azathioprine (Azasan)	Tab: 75 mg, 100 mg	RA: Adults: Initial: 1 mg/kg/d (50-100 mg) given qd-bid. Titrate: May increase by 0.5 mg/kg/d after 6-8 wks, then q4wks if no serious toxicities and initial response unsatisfactory. Max: 2.5 mg/kg/d. Maint: May decrease by 0.5 mg/kg/d or 25 mg/d q4wks until lowest effective dose. If no response after 12 wks, consider patient refractory.	⊕D ❄v Risk of neoplasia, mutagenesis & hematologic toxicities. R
Azathioprine (Imuran)	Tab: 50 mg	RA: Adults: Initial: 1 mg/kg/d (50-100 mg) given qd-bid. Titrate: May increase by 0.5 mg/kg/d after 6-8 wks, then q4wks. Max: 2.5 mg/kg/d. Maint: May decrease by 0.5 mg/kg/d or 25 mg/d q4wks to lowest effective dose. If no response by Week 12, consider patient refractory.	⊕D ❄v Risk of neoplasia, mutagenesis & hematologic toxicities. R
Celecoxib (Celebrex)	Cap: 50 mg, 100 mg, 200 mg, 400 mg	Adults: ≥18 yo: OA: 200 mg qd or 100 mg bid. RA: 100-200 mg bid. AS: Initial: 200 mg qd or 100 mg bid. Titrate: May increase to 400 mg/d after 6 wks. Peds: ≥2 yo: JRA: 10-25 kg: 50 mg bid. >25 kg: 100 mg bid. Poor Metabolizers of CYP2C9 Substrates: Half lowest recommended dose.	⊕C ⊕D (≥30 wks gestation) ❄v H W [66, 67]
Certolizumab Pegol (Cimzia)	Inj: 200 mg/ml	RA: Adults: Initial: 400 mg SC, and at Weeks 2 & 4, followed by 200 mg qow. Maint: 400 mg SC q4wks. Concomitant w/ MTX: 200 mg SC qow.	⊕B ❄v W [86]

NAME	FORM/STRENGTH	DOSAGE	COMMENTS
Etanercept (Enbrel)	Inj: 25 mg, 50 mg	**Adults: RA/PsA/AS:** 50 mg SC qwk. May continue MTX, glucocorticoids, salicylates, NSAIDs, or analgesics. **Max:** 50 mg/wk. **Peds: ≥2 yo: JIA: <63 kg:** 0.8 mg/kg SC qwk. **≥63 kg:** 50 mg SC qwk. May continue glucocorticoids, NSAIDs, or analgesics.	●B ❋v W [86]
Golimumab (Simponi)	Inj: 50 mg/0.5 ml	**Adults: RA:** 50 mg SC once a mth w/ MTX. **PsA/AS:** 50 mg SC once a mth.	●B ❋v W [86]
Hydroxychloroquine Sulfate (Plaquenil)	Tab: 200 mg	**RA: Adults: Initial:** 400-600 mg/d. Increase dose in 5-10d until optimum response. **Maint:** After 4-12 wks, 200-400 mg/d.	●N ❋>
Infliximab (Remicade)	Inj: 100 mg	**Adults: RA (Combo w/ MTX): Induction:** 3 mg/kg IV at 0, 2, 6 wks. **Maint:** 3 mg/kg q8wks. **Incomplete Response:** May increase to 10 mg/kg or give q4wks. **AS: Induction:** 5 mg/kg IV at 0, 2, & 6 wks. **Maint:** 5 mg/kg q6wks. **PsA: Induction:** 5 mg/kg IV at 0, 2, & 6 wks. **Maint:** 5 mg/kg q8wks.	●B ❋v Hepatosplenic T-cell lymphoma & other malignancies reported. W [86]
Leflunomide (Arava)	Tab: 10 mg, 20 mg, 100 mg	**RA: Adults: LD:** 100 mg qd x 3d. **Maint:** 20 mg qd. **Max:** 20 mg/d. If dose not tolerated, reduce dose to 10 mg qd.	●X ❋v Hepatotoxicity. CI in pregnancy. H
Meloxicam (Mobic)	Susp: 7.5 mg/5 ml; Tab: 7.5 mg, 15 mg	**Adults: OA/RA: Initial/Maint:** 7.5 mg qd. **Max:** 15 mg/d. **Peds: ≥2 yo: JRA:** 0.125 mg/kg qd. **Max:** 7.5 mg/d.	●C ❋v W [66, 67]

Methotrexate	Tab: 2.5 mg	**Adults: RA: Initial:** 7.5 mg once wkly or 2.5 mg q12h x 3 doses wkly. **Max:** 20 mg/wk. **Peds: 2-16 yo: JRA:** 10 mg/m^2 once wkly. Adjust dose to optimal response. **Max:** 30 mg/m^2/wk.	⊙X ❀v CI in pregnancy & nursing. **R W** [3, 19]
Rituximab (Rituxan)	Inj: 10 mg/ml, 500 mg/50 ml	**Adults: RA:** Give w/ MTX. Give two 1000-mg IV infusions separated by 2 wks. Give subsequent courses q16-24wks. Give methylprednisolone 100 mg IV (or equivalent) 30 min prior to each infusion to reduce infusion reactions.	⊙C ❀> **W** [65]
Tocilizumab (Actemra)	Inj: 20 mg/ml	**Adults: RA: Initial:** 4 mg/kg IV q4wks infused over 60 min. **Titrate:** Increase to 8 mg/kg based on clinical response. **Max:** 800 mg/infusion. **Peds: Systemic JIA: ≥2 yo: <30 kg:** 12 mg/kg IV q2wks infused over 60 min. **≥30 kg:** 8 mg/kg IV q2wks over 60 min.	⊙C ❀v **H W** [86]

Narcotics

| Buprenorphine HCl CIII
(Buprenex) | Inj: 0.3 mg/ml | **Adults & Peds: ≥13 yo:** 0.3mg IM/IV q6h prn. Repeat if needed, 30-60 min after initial dose & then prn. **High-Risk Patients/Concomitant CNS Depressants:** Reduce dose by approx. 50%. May use single doses ≤0.6 mg IM if not at high risk. **Peds: 2-12 yo:** 2-6 mcg/kg IM/IV q4-6h. | ⊙C
❀v Respiratory depression reported. |

NAME	FORM/STRENGTH	DOSAGE	COMMENTS
Buprenorphine CIII (Butrans)	**Patch:** 5 mcg/h, 10 mcg/h, 20 mcg/h	**Adults:** Individualize dose. **Conversion from Other Opioids:** Refer to PI. **Opioid-Naive: Initial:** 5 mcg/h. **Titrate:** Titrate dose based on response after a minimum interval of 72h to a level that provides adequate analgesia. **Max:** 20 mcg/h.	●C ❀v Potential for abuse. Do not exceed one 20 mcg/h system.
Codeine/Acetaminophen CIII (Tylenol w/ Codeine)	**Sol:** 12-120 mg/5 ml; **Tab:** (Tylenol w/ Codeine) (#3) 30-300 mg, (#4) 60-300 mg (Generic) 15-300 mg, 30-300 mg, 60-300 mg	**Tab: Adults:** 15-60 mg codeine/dose & 300 mg-1 gm APAP/dose up to q4h. **Max:** 360 mg codeine & 4 gm APAP/24h. **Sol: Adults:** 15 ml q4h prn. **Peds:** 0.5 mg/kg of codeine. **7-12 yo:** 10 ml tid-qid. **3-6 yo:** 5 ml tid-qid.	●C ❀v H R W [42]
Fentanyl CII (Duragesic)	**Patch:** 12.5 mcg/h, 25 mcg/h, 50 mcg/h, 75 mcg/h, 100 mcg/h	**Adults & Peds:** ≥2 yo: **Opioid-Tolerant:** Individualize dose. **Minimum Initial Dose:** 25 mcg/hr x 72h. **Titrate:** Initial dose may be increased after 3d; further increase should be made after higher dose is worn thru two applications. Dosage increments based on daily dose of supplementary opioids; use ratio of 45 mg/24h of PO morphine to a 12.5 mcg/h increase in dose.	●C ❀v Not for prn use. May cause fatal respiratory depression if not already tolerant to high doses of opioids. H R W [102]

Fentanyl Citrate CII (Actiq)	**Loz:** 200 mcg, 400 mcg, 600 mcg, 800 mcg, 1200 mcg, 1600 mcg	**Adults & Peds: ≥16 yo: Breakthrough Cancer Pain: Initial:** 200 mcg (consume over 15 min). **Titrate:** If breakthrough pain episode not relieved 15 min after completion of unit, take only 1 additional dose of same strength. **Maint:** 1 unit/pain episode. **Max:** 2 units/pain episode or 4 units/d.	◒C ✣v CI in acute or post-op pain, nonopioid-tolerant patients.
Fentanyl Citrate CII (Fentora)	**Tab, Buccal:** 100 mcg, 200 mcg, 400 mcg, 600 mcg, 800 mcg	**Adults: Breakthough Pain Associated w/ Cancer: Initial:** 100 mcg. Repeat once (30 min after starting dose) during a single episode. **Titration >100 mcg:** Use two 100-mcg tabs (1 on each side of buccal cavity); if not controlled, use two 100-mcg tabs on each side (total four 100-mcg tabs). **Titration >400 mcg:** Use 200-mcg tab increments. **Max:** Not >4 tabs simultaneously.	◒C ✣v CI in acute or post-op pain, nonopioid-tolerant patients.
Fentanyl CII (Lazanda)	**Spr:** 100 mcg/spr, 400 mcg/spr	**Adults: ≥18 yo: Initial** (including switching from another fentanyl product): One 100 mcg spr. **Maint:** If adequate analgesia w/in 30 min w/ 100 mcg, treat subsequent episodes w/ this dose. **Titrate:** Individualize. If adequate analgesia not achieved w/ 100 mcg dose, escalate dose in stepwise manner (200 mcg, then 400 mcg, then 800 mcg) over consecutive breakthrough episodes until adequate analgesia w/ tolerable side effects; allow ≥2h before treating another episode. **Max:** 800 mcg. Refer to PI for maintenance, titration, readjustment, and d/c.	◒C ✣v CI in acute or post-op pain, nonopioid-tolerant patients. Abuse potential.

NAME	FORM/STRENGTH	DOSAGE	COMMENTS
Fentanyl CII (Onsolis)	**Film, Buccal:** 200 mcg, 400 mcg, 600 mcg, 800 mcg, 1200 mcg	**Adults: Initial:** 200 mcg. **Titrate:** May use multiples of 200 mcg. Do not use >4 of 200-mcg films simultaneously. If inadequate pain relief after 800 mcg, & patient has tolerated the 800-mcg dose, may treat next episode w/ one 1200-mcg film. **Max:** 1200 mcg. Use single doses only once/episode; separate by ≥2h. If adequate pain relief is not achieved w/in 30 min, use rescue medication as directed. Limit to ≤4 doses/d. If >4 breakthrough pain episodes/d, may increase around-the-clock opioid medicine. **Switching from Another Oral Transmucosal Fentanyl: Initial:** ≤200 mcg. Do not switch on a mcg-per-mcg basis.	▣C ❂v CI in acute or post-op pain, nonopioid-tolerant patients.
Fentanyl CII (Subsys)	**Spr:** 100 mcg/spr, 200 mcg/spr, 400 mcg/spr, 600 mcg/spr, 800 mcg/spr	**Adults: ≥18 yo: Initial:** 100 mcg. **Titrate:** May take only 1 additional dose of the same strength if breakthrough pain episode is not relieved 30 min after completion of previous dose. Do not take >2 doses per breakthrough pain episode; wait at least 4h before treating another episode of breakthrough pain. Refer to PI for complete titration and maint dosing.	▣C ❂v CI in acute or post-op pain, nonopioid-tolerant patients. Abuse potential.
Hydrocodone Bitartrate/ Acetaminophen CIII (Hycet, Lortab)	**Sol:** (Hycet) 7.5-325 mg/ 15 ml, (Lortab) 7.5-500 mg/15 ml; **Tab:** (Lortab) 5-500 mg, 7.5-500 mg, 10-500 mg	**Adults: Tab:** (5-500 mg) 1-2 tabs q4-6h prn. **Max:** 8 tabs/d. (7.5-500 mg, 10-500 mg) 1 tab q4-6h prn. **Max:** 6 tabs/d. **Sol:** 15 ml q4-6h prn. **Max:** 90 ml/d. **Peds: ≥2 yo: Sol:** Give q4-6h prn. **12-15 kg:** 3.75 ml. **Max:** 22.5 ml/d. **16-22 kg:** 5 ml. **Max:** 30 ml/d. **23-31 kg:** 7.5 ml. **Max:** 45 ml/d. **32-45 kg:** 10 ml. **Max:** 60 ml/d. **≥46 kg:** 15 ml. **Max:** 90 ml/d.	▣C ❂v H R W [42]

Drug	Formulations	Dosing	
Hydrocodone Bitartrate/ Acetaminophen CIII (Vicodin, Vicodin ES, Vicodin HP)	**Tab:** (Vicodin) 5-500 mg; (Vicodin ES) 7.5-750 mg; (Vicodin HP) 10-660 mg	**Adults: Usual: Vicodin:** 1-2 tabs q4-6h prn. **Max:** 8 tabs/d. **Vicodin ES:** 1 tab q4-6h prn. **Max:** 5 tabs/d. **Vicodin HP:** 1 tab q4-6h prn. **Max:** 6 tabs/d.	⊕C ❄v H R W [42]
Hydrocodone Bitartrate/ Ibuprofen CIII (Reprexain, Vicoprofen)	**Tab:** (Reprexain) 2.5-200 mg, 5-200 mg, 7.5 mg-200 mg; (Vicoprofen) 7.5-200 mg	**Adults & Peds: ≥16 yo: Usual:** 1 tab q4-6h prn. **Max:** 5 tabs/d.	⊕C ❄v
Hydromorphone HCl CII (Dilaudid, Dilaudid-HP)	**Inj:** 1 mg/ml, 2 mg/ml, 4 mg/ml; (Dilaudid-HP) 10 mg/ml, 50 mg/5 ml, 500 mg/50 ml, 250 mg; **Sol:** 1 mg/ml; **Tab:** 2 mg, 4 mg, 8 mg	**Adults:** Individualize dose. **Inj (Opioid-Naive): SC/IM: Initial:** 1-2 mg q2-3h prn. **IV: Initial:** 0.2-1 mg q2-3h given slowly, over 2-3 min. **HP (Opioid-Tolerant):** If switching from regular Dilaudid to Dilaudid-HP, similar doses should be used. **Conversion from Different Opioid:** See PI. Adjust dose based on response. **Sol: Usual:** 2.5-10 mg PO q3-6h ud. **Tab: Initial:** 2-4 mg PO q4-6h. Adjust dose based on response. **Conversion from Different Opioid:** See PI.	⊕C ❄v H R W [69]
Meperidine HCl CII (Demerol Oral)	**Sol:** (Generic) 50 mg/ 5ml; **Tab:** (Demerol) 50 mg, 100 mg	**Adults: Usual:** 50-150 mg PO q3-4h prn. **Peds: Usual:** 1.1-1.8 mg/kg PO, up to adult dose, q3-4h prn. **Concomitant Phenothiazines/Other Tranquilizers:** Reduce dose by 25-50%.	⊕C ❄v CI w/ MAOI use w/in 14d.

NAME	FORM/STRENGTH	DOSAGE	COMMENTS
Morphine Sulfate CII (Avinza)	**Cap,ER:** 30 mg, 60 mg, 75 mg, 90 mg, 120 mg	**Adults: ≥18 yo: Conversion from PO Morphine:** Give total daily morphine dose as a single dose q24h. **Conversion from Parenteral Morphine: Initial:** Give about 3x previous daily parenteral morphine requirement. **Conversion from Other Parenteral or PO Non-Morphine Opioids: Initial:** Give 1/2 of estimated daily morphine requirement q24h. May supplement w/ IR morphine or short-acting analgesics. **Titrate:** Adjust as frequently as qod. **Nonopioid-Tolerant: Initial:** 30 mg q24h. **Titrate:** Increase by no more than 30 mg q4d. **Max:** 1600 mg/d. The 60, 90, & 120 mg caps are for opioid-tolerant patients.	▣C ❀v W [51]
Morphine Sulfate CII (Kadian)	**Cap,ER:** 10 mg, 20 mg, 30 mg, 50 mg, 60 mg, 80 mg, 100 mg, 200 mg	**Adults: Conversion from Other PO Morphine:** Give 50% of daily PO morphine dose q12h or 100% q24h. **Conversion from Parenteral Morphine:** PO dose of 3x the daily parenteral morphine requirement may be sufficient in chronic settings. **Conversion from Other Parenteral or PO Opioids: Initial:** Give 1/2 of estimated daily morphine requirement q24h or give 1/4 of estimated daily morphine requirement q12h. May supplement w/ IR morphine or short-acting analgesics. **Titrate:** Adjust as frequently as qod. **Nonopioid-Tolerant:** 20 mg q24h. **Titrate:** Increase by no more than 20 mg qod. **Max:** No ceiling dose.	▣C ❀v W [74]

Morphine Sulfate CII (MS Contin)	Tab,ER: 15 mg, 30 mg, 60 mg, 100 mg, 200 mg	**Adults: Conversion from Immediate-Release Oral Morphine:** Give 1/2 of patient's 24h requirement as MS Contin q12h or give 1/3 of daily requirement as MS Contin q8h. **Conversion from Parenteral Morphine: Initial:** If daily morphine dose ≤120 mg/d, give MS Contin 30 mg. **Titrate:** Switch to 60 mg or 100 mg MS Contin. Taper dose; do not d/c abruptly. Swallow whole.	⊙C ❄v W [99]
Oxycodone HCl CII (OxyContin)	Tab,ER: 10 mg, 15 mg, 20 mg, 30 mg, 40 mg, 60 mg, 80 mg	**Adults:** Individualize dose. **Initial: 1st Opioid Analgesic:** 10 mg q12h. **Conversion from other PO Oxycodone:** 1/2 of total daily dose q12h. **Conversion from Other Opioids:** 1/2 estimated daily requirement. **Conversion from Transdermal Fentanyl:** 10 mg q12h for each 25 mcg/ hr fentanyl patch 18h after removing patch. **Titrate:** May increase total daily dose by 25-50% of current dose q1-2d, or as indicated.	⊙B ❄v For continuous analgesia. Abuse potential. 60-mg and 80-mg tabs only for opioid-tolerant patients. Swallow whole. **H**
Oxycodone HCl/ Acetaminophen CII (Endocet, Percocet)	Tab: 5-325 mg, 7.5-325 mg, 7.5-500 mg, 10-325 mg, 10-650 mg (Percocet) 2.5-325 mg	**Adults:** (2.5-325 mg) 1-2 tabs q6h. **Max:** 12 tabs/d. (5-325 mg) 1 tab q6h prn. **Max:** 12 tabs/d. (7.5-325 mg) 1 tab q6h prn. **Max:** 8 tabs/d. (7.5-500 mg) 1 tab q6h prn. **Max:** 8 tabs/d. (10-325 mg) 1 tab q6h prn. **Max:** 6 tabs/d. (10-650 mg) 1 tab q6h prn. **Max:** 6 tabs/d. Do not exceed 4 gm APAP/d.	⊙C ❄v H R W [42]

NAME	FORM/STRENGTH	DOSAGE	COMMENTS
Oxycodone HCl/Aspirin CII (Endodan, Percodan)	**Tab:** 4.8355-325 mg	**Adults: Usual:** 1 tab q6h prn. **Max:** 12 tabs/d.	⊞B (Oxycodone) ⊞D (ASA) ❄v
Oxymorphone HCl CII (Opana, Opana ER)	**Tab:** (Opana) 5 mg, 10 mg; **Tab,ER:** (Opana ER) 5 mg, 7.5 mg, 10 mg, 15 mg, 20 mg, 30 mg, 40 mg	**Adults:** Individualize dose. **Opana: Opioid-Naive: Initial:** 10-20 mg q4-6h. Titrate based on response. **Max:** 20 mg/dose. **Conversion from Parenteral Oxymorphone:** Give 10x total daily parenteral oxymorphone dose in 4 or 6 equally divided doses. **Conversion from Other Oral Opioids:** Give half of calculated total daily dose in 4-6 equally divided doses, q4-6h. **Opana ER: Opioid-Naive: Initial:** 5 mg q12h. Titrate based on response. **Usual:** Increase dose by 5-10 mg q12h q3-7d. **Conversion from Opana:** Divide 24h Opana dose in half to obtain q12h dose. **Conversion from Parenteral Oxymorphone:** Give 10x total daily parenteral oxymorphone dose in 2 equally divided doses. **Conversion from Other Oral Opioids:** Divide calculated 24h opioid dose (refer to PI for conversion ratios) in half to obtain q12h dose.	⊞C ❄> Abuse potential. Do not crush, chew, or break ER tabs. H R
Tapentadol CII (Nucynta)	**Tab:** 50 mg, 75 mg, 100 mg	**Adults:** Individualize dose. **Usual:** 50 mg, 75 mg, or 100 mg q4-6h depending upon pain intensity. **Day 1:** May give 2nd dose 1h after 1st dose, if pain relief inadequate. **Max:** 700 mg on Day 1, then 600 mg/d thereafter.	⊞C ❄v H R

NSAIDs

Celecoxib (Celebrex)	**Cap:** 50 mg, 100 mg, 200 mg, 400 mg	**Adults: ≥18 yo: Acute Pain/Primary Dysmenorrhea: Day 1:** 400 mg, then 200 mg if needed. **Maint:** 200 mg bid prn. **OA:** 200 mg qd or 100 mg bid. **RA:** 100-200 mg bid. **AS:** 200 mg qd or 100 mg bid. **Titrate:** May increase to 400 mg/d after 6 wks. **Peds: ≥2 yo: JRA: 10-25 kg:** 50 mg bid. **>25 kg:** 100 mg bid. **Poor Metabolizers of CYP2C9 Substrates:** Half lowest recommended dose.	⊕C ⊕D (≥30 wks gestation) ✿v H W [66, 67]
Diclofenac Epolamine (Flector)	**Patch:** 180 mg (1.3%)	**Adults:** Apply 1 patch to most painful area bid.	⊕C ⊕D (≥30 wks gestation) ✿v H R W [66, 67]
Diclofenac Potassium (Zipsor)	**Cap:** 25 mg	**Adults: ≥18 yo:** 25 mg qid.	⊕C ⊕D (≥30 wks gestation) ✿v H R W [66, 67]
Diclofenac Sodium (Voltaren)	**Tab,ER:** 100 mg	**Adults: OA:** 100 mg qd. **RA:** 100 mg qd-bid.	⊕C ✿v W [66, 67]
Esomeprazole Magnesium/ Naproxen (Vimovo)	**Tab,Delay:** 20-375 mg, 20-500 mg	**Adults:** 20-375 mg or 20-500 mg bid ≥30 min ac. Use lowest effective dose.	⊕C ⊕ D (≥30 wks gestation) ✿v H R W [66, 67]

NAME	FORM/STRENGTH	DOSAGE	COMM
Ibuprofen (Caldolor)	Inj: 100 mg/ml	**Adults: Analgesia:** 400-800 mg IV q6h prn. Infusion time must be no less than 30 min. **Antipyretic:** 400 mg IV followed by 400 mg q4-6h or 100-200 mg q4h prn. Infusion time must be no less than 30 min.	⊕C ⊕D(≥ gestati ❄v R W [66, 67]
Ibuprofen (Motrin IB)	Tab: 200 mg	**Adults & Peds: ≥12 yo:** 200 mg q4-6h while symptoms persist, may increase to 400 mg if pain or fever does not respond. **Max:** 1200 mg/24h. Take w/ food/milk if stomach upset occurs.	⊕N ❄>
Meloxicam (Mobic)	Susp: 7.5 mg/5 ml; Tab: 7.5 mg, 15 mg	**Adults: OA/RA: Initial/Maint:** 7.5 mg qd. **Max:** 15 mg/d. **JRA: Peds: ≥2 yo:** 0.125 mg/kg qd. **Max:** 7.5 mg/d.	⊕C ❄v W [66, 67]
Naproxen (Anaprox, Anaprox DS, EC-Naprosyn, Naprosyn)	Susp: (Naprosyn) 125 mg/5 ml; Tab: (Naprosyn) 250 mg, 375 mg, 500 mg; (Anaprox) 275 mg, (Anaprox DS) 550 mg; Tab, Delay: (EC- Naprosyn) 375 mg, 500 mg	**Adults: RA/OA/AS:** Naprosyn: 250-500 mg bid. EC-Naprosyn: 375-500 mg bid. Anaprox: 275 mg bid. Anaprox DS: 550 mg bid. **Titrate:** Adjust dose/frequency up or down depending on clinical response; may increase to 1500 mg/d for ≤6 mths if patient can tolerate lower doses well. **Pain/Tendonitis/Bursitis: Initial:** Anaprox/Anaprox DS: 550 mg, then 550 mg q12h or 275 mg q6-8h prn. **Max:** 1375 mg/d initially, then 1100 mg/d thereafter. **Acute Gout: Initial:** Naprosyn: 750 mg, then 250 mg q8h until attack subsides. **Initial:** Anaprox: 825 mg, then 275 mg q8h until attack subsides. **Peds: ≥2 yo: JRA:** 5 mg/kg bid.	⊕C ❄v H R W [66, 67]

Miscellaneous

Acetaminophen (Ofirmev)	Inj: 10 mg/ml	**Pain/Fever: Adults & Peds: ≥13 yo: ≥50 kg:** 1000 mg q6h or 650 mg q4h. **Max:** 4000 mg/d or 1000 mg/dose. **<50 kg:** 15 mg/kg q6h or 12.5 mg/kg q4h. **Max:** 75 mg/kg/d or 15 mg/kg/dose. **2-12 yo:** 15 mg/kg q6h or 12.5 mg/kg q4h. **Max:** 75 mg/kg/d or 15 mg/kg/dose. Minimum dosing interval should be 4h.	⊙C ❀> H
Capsaicin (Qutenza)	Patch: 179 mg [8%]	**Postherpetic Neuralgia: Adults:** Single 60 min application of up to 4 patches. May repeat q3 mths or as warranted by the return of pain (not >q3 mths).	⊙B
Duloxetine HCl (Cymbalta)	Cap,Delay: 20 mg, 30 mg, 60 mg	**Adults: Chronic Musculoskeletal Pain: Initial:** 60 mg qd or 30 mg qd x 1 wk before increasing to 60 mg qd. **Maint:** 60 mg qd x up to 13 wks. **Diabetic Peripheral Neuropathic Pain: Initial:** 60 mg qd. May lower starting dose if tolerability is a concern. **Maint:** Individualize dose. Treat x up to 12 wks. **Max:** 60 mg qd. **Fibromyalgia: Initial:** 60 mg qd or 30 mg qd x 1 wk before increasing to 60 mg qd. **Maint:** Based on response. **Max:** 60 mg qd.	⊙C ❀v H R W [29]
Gabapentin (Gralise)	Tab: 300 mg, 600 mg	**Postherpetic Neuralgia: Adults:** Take w/ pm meal. **Initial: Day 1:** 300 mg qd. **Titrate: Day 2:** 600 mg qd. **Days 3-6:** 900 mg qd. **Days 7-10:** 1200 mg qd. **Days 11-14:** 1500 mg qd. **Day 15:** 1800 mg qd.	⊙C ❀> R

NAME	FORM/STRENGTH	DOSAGE	COMMENTS
Gabapentin (Neurontin)	**Cap:** 100 mg, 300 mg, 400 mg; **Sol:** 250 mg/5 ml; **Tab:** 600 mg, 800 mg	**Postherpetic Neuralgia: Adults: Titrate: Day 1:** 300 mg single dose. **Day 2:** 300 mg bid. **Day 3:** 300 mg tid. Increase further prn. **Max:** 1800 mg/d.	●C ❄️> R
Lidocaine (Lidoderm Patch)	**Patch:** 5%	**Postherpetic Neuralgia: Adults:** Apply up to 3 patches to intact skin qd for up to 12h w/in 24h period; cover most painful area.	●B ❄️>
Milnacipran HCl (Savella)	**Tab:** 12.5 mg, 25 mg, 50 mg, 100 mg	**Fibromyalgia: Adults: Usual:** 100 mg qd (50 mg bid). **Titrate: Day 1:** 12.5 mg once. **Days 2-3:** 25 mg/d (12.5 mg bid). **Days 4-7:** 50 mg/d (25 mg bid). **After Day 7:** 100 mg/d (50 mg bid). May increase to 200 mg/d (100 mg bid) based on individual response. **Max:** 200 mg/d. **Switching to or from MAOI:** See PI.	●C ❄️v H R W [29]
Pregabalin CV (Lyrica)	**Cap:** 25 mg, 50 mg, 75 mg, 100 mg, 150 mg, 200 mg, 225 mg, 300 mg; **Sol:** 20 mg/ml	**Adults: Neuropathic Pain: Initial:** 50 mg tid. **Titrate:** May increase to 300 mg/d w/in 1 wk based on efficacy & tolerability. **Max:** 100 mg tid (300 mg/d). **Postherpetic Neuralgia: Initial:** 150 mg/d divided bid or tid. **Titrate:** May increase to 300 mg/d w/in 1 wk based on efficacy & tolerability. May increase up to 600 mg/d given bid or tid if no relief following 2-4 wks of treatment w/ 300 mg/d. **Usual:** 150-300 mg/d. **Fibromyalgia: Initial:** 75 mg bid. **Titrate:** May increase to 150 mg bid (300 mg/d) w/in 1 wk based on efficacy & tolerability. May further increase to 225 mg bid (450 mg/d) if needed. **Usual:** 300-450 mg/d. **Max:** 450 mg/d. **D/C:** Taper over minimum of 1 wk.	●C ❄️v R

Tramadol HCl (Rybix ODT)	Tab, Dissolve: 50 mg	**Moderate to Moderately Severe Pain: Adults:** ≥17 yo: Individualize dose. **Titrate:** Increase by 50 mg q3d to reach 50 mg qid. **Maint:** 50-100 mg q4-6h prn. **Max:** 400 mg/d. **Rapid Onset Required:** May start at maint. **Elderly:** Start at lower end of dosing range.	⊕C ❀v H R
Tramadol HCl (Ryzolt)	Tab, ER: 100 mg, 200 mg, 300 mg	**Moderate to Moderately Severe Chronic Pain: Adults:** Individualize dose. **Initial:** 100 mg/d. **Titrate:** 100 mg q2-3d to achieve adequate pain control and tolerability. For patients requiring 300 mg/d, titration should take at least 4d. **Usual:** 200-300 mg/d. **Max:** 300 mg/d. **Patients Currently on Tramadol IR Products:** Calculate 24h IR dose and initiate on a total daily dose rounded down to next lowest 100-mg increment. **Max:** 300 mg/d. **Elderly:** Start at low end of dosing range. Swallow whole w/ liq.	⊕C ❀v H R
Tramadol HCl (Ultram, Ultram ER)	Tab: 50 mg; Tab, ER: 100 mg, 200 mg, 300 mg	**Moderate to Moderately Severe Pain: Adults:** ≥17 yo: **Tab: Initial:** 25 mg qam. **Titrate:** Increase by 25 mg/d q3d to 25 mg qid, then by 50 mg/d q3d to 50 mg qid. **Maint:** 50-100 mg q4-6h prn. **Max:** 400 mg/d. **Tab, ER: Adults:** ≥18 yo: **Initial:** 100 mg qd. **Titrate:** Increase by 100-mg increments q5d. **Max:** 300 mg/d. **Patients Currently on Tramadol IR Products:** Calculate 24h IR dose & initiate on a total daily dose rounded down to next lowest 100-mg increment. **Max:** 300 mg/d.	⊕C ❀v H R

NAME	FORM/STRENGTH	DOSAGE	COMMENTS

ANTI-INFECTIVES

AIDS Therapy

CCR5 CO-RECEPTOR ANTAGONIST

NAME	FORM/STRENGTH	DOSAGE	COMMENTS
Maraviroc (Selzentry)	**Tab:** 150 mg, 300 mg	**Adults: ≥16 yo:** Give in combo w/ other antiretroviral medications. **W/ Potent CYP3A Inhibitors (W/ or w/o Potent CYP3A Inducer):** 150 mg bid. **W/ Other Medications (Tipranavir/Ritonavir, Nevirapine, Raltegravir, NRTIs, Enfuvirtide):** 300 mg bid. **W/ Potent CYP3A Inducers (W/o a Potent CYP3A Inhibitor):** 600 mg bid.	⊞B ✣v Hepatotoxicity reported. R

FUSION INHIBITOR

NAME	FORM/STRENGTH	DOSAGE	COMMENTS
Enfuvirtide (Fuzeon)	**Inj:** 90 mg/ml	**Adults:** 90 mg SC bid. **Peds: 6-16 yo:** 2 mg/kg SC bid. **Max:** 90 mg bid. Inject into upper arm, anterior thigh, or abdomen.	⊞B ✣v

HIV INTEGRASE STRAND TRANSFER INHIBITOR

NAME	FORM/STRENGTH	DOSAGE	COMMENTS
Raltegravir Potassium (Isentress)	**Chewtab:** 25 mg, 100 mg; **Tab:** 400 mg	**Adults: Tab:** 400 mg bid. **Concomitant w/ Rifampin: Tab:** 800 mg bid. **Peds: ≥12 yo: Tab:** 400 mg bid. **6-<12 yo: ≥25 kg: Tab:** 400 mg bid. **2-<12 yo: Chewtab: 10-<14 kg:** 75 mg bid. **14-<20 kg:** 100 mg bid. **20-<28 kg:** 150 mg bid. **28-<40 kg:** 200 mg bid. **≥40 kg:** 300 mg bid. **Max:** 300 mg bid.	⊞C ✣v

NON-NUCLEOSIDE REVERSE TRANSCRIPTASE INHIBITORS & COMBINATIONS

Delavirdine Mesylate (Rescriptor)	**Tab:** 100 mg, 200 mg	**Adults & Peds:** ≥16 yo: 400 mg tid.	⊕C ❋v
Efavirenz/Emtricitabine/ Tenofovir Disoproxil (Atripla)	**Tab:** 600-200-300 mg	**Adults & Peds:** ≥12 yo: 1 tab qd on empty stomach. HS dosing may improve tolerability of nervous system symptoms.	⊕D ❋v R W [31, 32]
Efavirenz (Sustiva)	**Cap:** 50 mg, 200 mg; **Tab:** 600 mg	**Adults:** 600 mg qd. **Concomitant Voriconazole:** Reduce dose to 300 mg qd using cap formulation; increase voriconazole maint dose to 400 mg q12h. **Concomitant Rifampin in Patients ≥50 kg:** Increase dose to 800 mg qd. **Peds:** ≥3 yo: 10-<15 kg: 200 mg qd. 15-<20 kg: 250 mg qd. 20-<25 kg: 300 mg qd. 25-<32.5 kg: 350 mg qd. 32.5-<40 kg: 400 mg qd. ≥40 kg: 600 mg qd. Take on empty stomach, preferably hs.	⊕D ❋v H
Etravirine (Intelence)	**Tab:** 100 mg, 200 mg	**Adults:** 200 mg bid pc.	⊕B ❋v
Nevirapine (Viramune, Viramune XR)	**Susp:** 50 mg/5 ml; **Tab:** 200 mg; **Tab,ER:** (XR) 400 mg	**Adults:** 200 mg qd x 14d (lead-in period), then 200 mg bid or (XR) 400 mg qd. **Peds:** ≥15d: (IR) 150 mg/m² qd x 14d (lead-in period), then 150 mg/m² bid. **Max:** 400 mg/d. Do not increase dose or begin dosing w/ XR if rash develops during the 14d lead-in period until rash resolves. **Max Duration of Lead-in Period:** 28d. Dose Interruption (>7d): Restart w/ 14d lead-in dose. **Dialysis Patients/Switching From IR To XR:** See PI.	⊕B ❋v Severe hepatotoxicity & skin reactions reported. H

NAME	FORM/STRENGTH	DOSAGE	COMMENTS
Rilpivirine (Edurant)	**Tab:** 25 mg	**Adults:** 25 mg PO qd w/ meal.	◉B ❀v
Tenofovir Disoproxil Fumarate/Rilpivirine/ Emtricitabine (Complera)	**Tab:** 200-25-300 mg	**Adults:** ≥18 yo: 1 tab qd w/ meal.	◉R ❀v R W [31, 32]

NUCLEOSIDE REVERSE TRANSCRIPTASE INHIBITORS & COMBINATIONS

NAME	FORM/STRENGTH	DOSAGE	COMMENTS
Abacavir Sulfate/Lamivudine (Epzicom)	**Tab:** 600-300 mg	**Adults:** CrCl ≥50 ml/min: 1 tab qd.	◉C ❀v H R W [31, 32, 33]
Abacavir Sulfate/Lamivudine/ Zidovudine (Trizivir)	**Tab:** 300-150-300 mg	**Adults & Adolescents:** ≥40 kg & CrCl ≥50 ml/min: 1 tab bid.	◉C ❀v H R W [31, 32, 33, 34]
Abacavir Sulfate (Ziagen)	**Sol:** 20 mg/ml; **Tab:** 300 mg	**Adults:** 300 mg bid or 600 mg qd. **Peds:** ≥3 mths: Sol: 8 mg/kg bid. **Max:** 300 mg bid. Tab: 14-21 kg: 150 mg (1/2 tab) bid (am and pm). >21-<30 kg: 150 mg (1/2 tab) am, 300 mg (1 tab) pm. ≥30 kg: 300 mg (1 tab) bid (am and pm).	◉C ❀v H W [31, 33]
Didanosine (Videx, Videx EC)	**Cap,Delay:** (Videx EC) 125 mg, 200 mg, 250 mg, 400 mg; **Sol:** (Videx) 2 gm, 4 gm	**Adults & Peds:** 25-<60 kg: Cap: 250 mg qd. ≥60 kg: Cap: 400 mg qd. Sol: 200 mg bid or 400 mg qd. 20-<25 kg: Cap: 200 mg qd. <60 kg: Sol: 125 mg bid or 250 mg qd. **Peds:** >8 mths-18 yrs: Sol: 120 mg/m² bid. 2 wks-8 mths: Sol: 100 mg/m² bid. Take on empty stomach.	◉B ❀v R W [31, 35]

Emtricitabine (Emtriva)	Cap: 200 mg; Sol: 10 mg/ml	Adults: ≥18 yo: Cap: 200 mg qd. Sol: 240 mg (24 ml) qd. Peds: 3 mths-17 yo: Cap: >33 kg: 200 mg qd. Sol: 6 mg/kg qd. Max: 240 mg (24 ml). 0-3 mths: Sol: 3 mg/kg qd.	⊕B ✿v R W [31, 32]
Lamivudine/Zidovudine (Combivir)	Tab: 150-300 mg	Adults & Peds: ≥30 kg: CrCl ≥50 ml/min: 1 tab bid. Avoid if w/ dose-limiting adverse reactions.	⊕C ✿v H R W [31, 32, 34]
Lamivudine (Epivir)	Sol: 10 mg/ml; Tab: 150 mg, 300 mg	Adults/Peds >16 yo: 150 mg bid or 300 mg qd. Peds: 3 mths-16 yo: Sol: 4 mg/kg bid. Max: 150 mg bid. Tab: 14-21 kg: 1/2 tab (75 mg) in am & 1/2 tab (75 mg) in pm. >21-<30 kg: 1/2 tab (75 mg) in am & 1 tab (150 mg) in pm. ≥30 kg: 1 tab (150 mg) in am & 1 tab (150 mg) in pm.	⊕C ✿v R W [31, 32]
Tenofovir Disoproxil Fumarate/Emtricitabine (Truvada)	Tab: 300-200 mg	Adults & Peds: ≥12 yo: CrCl ≥50 ml/min: 1 tab qd. CrCl: 30-49 ml/min: 1 tab q48h.	⊕B ✿v R W [31, 32]
Zidovudine (Retrovir)	Cap: 100 mg; Inj: 10 mg/ml; Syr: 10 mg/ml; Tab: 300 mg	Adults: PO: 600 mg/d in divided doses. Inj: 1 mg/kg IV over 1h 5-6X/d. Peds: 4 wks-<18 yo: 480 mg/m² PO in divided doses (240 mg/m² bid or 160 mg/m² tid). 4-<9 kg: 12 mg/kg bid or 8 mg/kg tid. ≥9-<30 kg: 9 mg/kg bid or 6 mg/kg tid. ≥30 kg: 300 mg bid or 200 mg tid. Do not exceed the recommended adult dose. Prevention of Maternal-Fetal HIV Transmission: Adults: >14 wks Pregnancy: 100 mg PO 5X/d until start of labor. During Labor & Delivery: 2 mg/kg IV over 1h followed by	⊕C ✿v R W [31, 34]

Continued on Next Page

NAME	FORM/STRENGTH	DOSAGE	COMMENTS
Zidovudine (Retrovir) *Continued*		1 mg/kg/h IV infusion until clamping of umbilical cord. **Neonates:** 2 mg/kg PO q6h (or 1.5 mg/kg IV over 30 min q6h) starting w/in 12h after birth & continue through 6 wks of age.	

NUCLEOTIDE REVERSE TRANSCRIPTASE INHIBITOR

NAME	FORM/STRENGTH	DOSAGE	COMMENTS
Tenofovir Disoproxil Fumarate (Viread)	Pow: 40 mg/gm; Tab: 150 mg, 200 mg, 250 mg, 300 mg	**Adults:** 300-mg tab qd. If unable to swallow tabs, may use 7.5 scoops of PO powder. **Peds: ≥2 yo:** 8 mg/kg qd PO powder mixed in soft food not requiring chewing. **Max:** 300 mg/d. **≥17 kg & Able to Swallow Intact Tab:** 1 tab qd. Refer to PI for dosing based on body wt.	●B ❄v R W [31, 32]

PROTEASE INHIBITORS

NAME	FORM/STRENGTH	DOSAGE	COMMENTS
Atazanavir Sulfate (Reyataz)	Cap: 100 mg, 150 mg, 200 mg, 300 mg	**Adults: Therapy-Naïve:** 300 mg w/ ritonavir (RTV) 100 mg qd. If intolerant to RTV, give atazanavir (ATV) 400 mg qd. **Therapy-Experienced:** 300 mg w/ RTV 100 mg qd. **Concomitant Therapy/Use During Pregnancy and Postpartum Period:** Refer to PI for dose adjustments. **Peds: 6-<18 yo: 15-<20 kg:** 150 mg w/ RTV 100 mg qd. **20-<40 kg:** 200 mg w/ RTV 100 mg qd. **≥40 kg:** 300 mg w/ RTV 100 mg qd. **Therapy-Naïve: ≥13 yo & ≥40 kg:** If intolerant to RTV, give ATV 400 mg qd. **Concomitant Tenofovir/H2-Receptor Antagonists/Proton-Pump Inhibitors:** Do not administer w/o RTV. Do not exceed adult dose. Take w/ food.	●B ❄v H R

Fosamprenavir Calcium (Lexiva)	**Tab:** 700 mg; **Susp:** 50 mg/ml	**Adults: Therapy-Naive:** 1400 mg bid or 1400 mg qd + ritonavir (RTV) 200 mg qd or 1400 mg qd + RTV 100 mg qd or 700 mg bid + RTV 100 mg bid. **PI-Experienced:** 700 mg bid + RTV 100 mg bid. **Peds: 4 wks-18 yo: Susp:** See PI for Twice-Daily Dose Regimens by Wt for Therapy-Naive (≥4 wks) and Therapy-Experienced (≥6 mths) patients.	⊙C ✣v H
Indinavir Sulfate (Crixivan)	**Cap:** 100 mg, 200 mg, 400 mg	**Adults: Usual:** 800 mg q8h. Take w/o food but w/ water 1h before or 2h after meals. Maintain adequate hydration (1.5 L fluid/24h). **Mild-Moderate Hepatic Insufficiency/ Concomitant Delavirdine, Itraconazole, Ketoconazole:** 600 mg q8h. **Concomitant Didanosine:** Administer at least 1h apart. **Concomitant Rifabutin:** 1 gm q8h (reduce rifabutin dose by 1/2).	⊙C ✣v H
Lopinavir/Ritonavir (Kaletra)	**Tab:** 100-25 mg, 200-50 mg; **Sol:** 80-20 mg/ml	**Adults:** 400-100 mg bid or 800-200 mg qd in patients w/ <3 lopinavir resistance-associated substitutions. **Concomitant Efavirenz/Nevirapine/Amprenavir/Nelfinavir: (Tab)** 500-125 mg bid; **(Sol)** 533/133 mg (6.5 ml) bid. **Peds: 6 mths-18 yo: (Sol) <15 kg:** 12-3 mg/kg bid. **≥15-40 kg:** 10-2.5 mg/kg bid. **Max:** 400-100 mg bid. **(Tab) 15-25 kg:** 200-50 mg bid. **>25-35 kg:** 300-75 mg bid. **>35 kg:** 400-100 mg bid. **14d-6 mths: (Sol)** 16-4 mg/kg bid. **Concomitant Efavirenz/Nevirapine/Amprenavir/ Nelfinavir: Treatment-Naive and Treatment-Experienced:**	⊙C ✣v

Continued on Next Page

NAME	FORM/STRENGTH	DOSAGE	COMMENTS
Lopinavir/Ritonavir (Kaletra) *Continued*		**6 mths-18 yo: (Sol) <15 kg:** 13-3.25 mg/kg bid. **≥15-45 kg:** 11-2.75 mg/kg bid. **Max:** 533-133 mg bid. **(Tab) 15-20 kg:** 200-50 mg bid. **>20-30 kg:** 300-75 mg bid. **>30-45 kg:** 400-100 mg bid. **>45 kg:** 500-125 mg bid. Refer to PI for BSA-based dosing.	
Nelfinavir Mesylate (Viracept)	**Pow:** 50 mg/gm; **Tab:** 250 mg, 625 mg	**Adults:** 1250 mg bid or 750 mg tid. **Max:** 2500 mg/d. **Peds: 2-13 yo:** 45-55 mg/kg bid or 25-35 mg tid. Refer to PI for further dosing guidelines. Take w/ food.	⊞B ✿v H
Ritonavir (Norvir)	**Cap:** 100 mg; **Sol:** 80 mg/ml; **Tab:** 100 mg	**Adults: Initial:** 300 mg bid. **Titrate:** Increase by 100 mg bid q2-3d. **Maint/Max:** 600 mg bid. **Peds: >1 mth: Initial:** 250 mg/m² bid. **Titrate:** Increase by 50 mg/m² bid q2-3d. **Maint:** 350-400 mg/m² bid or highest tolerated dose. **Max:** 600 mg bid. Take w/ meals.	⊞B ✿v W [97]
Saquinavir Mesylate (Invirase)	**Cap:** 200 mg; **Tab:** 500 mg	**Adults & Peds: >16 yo:** 1000 mg bid w/ lopinavir/RTV 400-100 mg (w/ no additional RTV) or RTV 100 mg bid. Take w/in 2h after full meal.	⊞B ✿v
Tipranavir (Aptivus)	**Cap:** 250 mg; **Sol:** 100 mg/ml	**Adults:** 500 mg w/ ritonavir 200 mg bid. **Peds: 2-18 yo:** 14 mg/kg w/ ritonavir 6 mg/kg (or 375 mg/m² w/ ritonavir 150 mg/m²) bid. **Max:** 500 mg w/ ritonavir 200 mg bid. **Intolerance or Toxicity:** Decrease dose to 12 mg/kg w/ ritonavir 5 mg/kg (or 290 mg/m² w/ ritonavir 115 mg/m²) bid. W/ ritonavir tab, take w/ food.	⊞C ✿v H W [45]

Antiviral Agents
HEPATITIS

Adefovir Dipivoxil (Hepsera)	**Tab:** 10 mg	**HBV: Adults & Peds: ≥12 yo:** 10 mg qd.	⊕C ❀v R W [31, 32, 37, 38]
Boceprevir (Victrelis)	**Cap:** 200 mg	**HCV: Adults: W/ Peginterferon Alfa & Ribavirin:** 800 mg tid (q7-9h) w/ food. Give after 4 wks of treatment w/ peginterferon alfa & ribavirin regimen. **Patients w/o Cirrhosis & Previously Untreated or Previous Partial Responders/Relapsers to Interferon & Ribavirin Therapy:** Refer to PI for duration of therapy using Response-Guided Therapy Guidelines. **Patients w/ Cirrhosis:** Treat w/ boceprevir in combination w/ peginterferon alfa & ribavirin x 44 wks. Refer to PIs for dose modification or d/c therapy.	⊕B, Category X in combination w/ peginterferon alfa & ribavirin. ❀v
Entecavir (Baraclude)	**Sol:** 0.05 mg/ml; **Tab:** 0.5 mg, 1 mg	**HBV: Adults & Peds: ≥16 yo: Compensated Liver Disease: Nucleoside-Treatment-Naive:** 0.5 mg qd. **History of Hepatitis B Viremia while Receiving Lamivudine or Known Lamivudine/Telbivudine Resistance Mutations:** 1 mg qd. **Decompensated Liver Disease:** 1 mg qd. Take on empty stomach.	⊕C ❀v R W [31, 32]
Lamivudine (Epivir-HBV)	**Sol:** 5 mg/ml; **Tab:** 100 mg	**HBV: Adults:** 100 mg qd. **Peds: 2-17 yo:** 3 mg/kg qd. **Max:** 100 mg/d.	⊕C ❀v R W [31, 32]

NAME	FORM/STRENGTH	DOSAGE	COMMENTS
Peginterferon alfa-2a (Pegasys)	**Inj:** 180 mcg/0.5 ml, 135 mcg/0.5ml, 180 mcg/ml	**Adults: ≥18 yo: HCV & HCV/HIV: Monotherapy:** 180 mcg SC once wkly x 48 wks. **HCV: W/ Copegus:** 180 mcg SC once wkly x 48 wks (genotypes 1, 4); x 24 wks (genotypes 2, 3). **HCV/HIV: W/ Copegus:** 180 mcg once wkly x 48 wks regardless of genotype. **HBV: Monotherapy:** 180 mcg SC once wkly x 48 wks. **Peds: ≥5 yo: HCV: W/ Copegus:** 180 mcg/1.73 m² x BSA SC once wkly. **Max:** 180 mcg SC once wkly x 24 wks (genotype 2,3); 48 wks (other genotypes). Refer to PI for dose modification.	▣C (monotherapy) ▣X (w/ ribavirin) ❄v **H R W** [13]
Peginterferon alfa-2b (Peg-Intron)	**Inj:** 50 mcg/0.5 ml, 80 mcg/0.5 ml, 120 mcg/ 0.5 ml, 150 mcg/0.5 ml	**HCV: Adults: ≥18 yo: Monotherapy:** 1 mcg/kg/wk SC x 1 yr. **W/ Rebetol & NS3/4A Protease Inhibitor:** 1.5 mcg/kg/ wk SC w/ 800-1400 mg Rebetol PO based on wt; refer to PI of the specific HCV NS3/4A protease inhibitor for dosing regimen. **Interferon alfa-Naive Patients: Genotype 1:** Treat for 48 wks. **Genotype 2 & 3:** Treat for 24 wks. **Prior Treatment Failures:** Retreat for 48 wks, regardless of HCV genotype. **Pediatrics: 3-17 yo: W/ Ribavirin:** 60 mcg/ m²/wk SC w/ 15 mg/kg/d ribavirin PO in 2 divided doses. **Genotype 1:** Treat for 48 wks. **Genotype 2 & 3:** Treat for 24 wks. Refer to PI for dose modification and d/c.	▣C. Category X in combination w/ Rebetol. ❄v **R W** [13]
Ribavirin (Copegus)	**Tab:** 200 mg	**Adults: CHC Monoinfection:** Individualize dose. **Usual:** 800-1200 mg/d in 2 divided doses. Treat x 24-48 wks w/ Pegasys 180 mcg once wkly. **Genotypes 1 & 4: ≥75 kg:** 1200 mg/d x 48 wks. **<75 kg:** 1000 mg/d x 48 wks. **Genotypes 2 & 3:** 800 mg/d x 24 wks. **CHC w/ HIV**	▣X ❄v Hemolytic anemia reported. Avoid in significant

Coinfection: Usual: 800 mg/d. Treat x 48 wks w/ Pegasys 180 mcg SC once wkly. **Peds: ≥5 yo: CHC Monoinfection: ≥75 kg:** 600 mg qam and qpm. **60-74 kg:** 400 mg qam and 600 mg qpm. **47-59 kg:** 400 mg qam and qpm. **34-46 kg:** 200 mg qam and 400 mg qpm. **23-33 kg:** 200 mg qam and qpm. Treat x 24 wks in genotypes 2/3 or 48 wks in other genotypes w/ Pegasys 180 mcg/1.73m^2 x BSA SC once weekly. **Max Dose of Pegasys:** 180 mcg/wk. Remain on pediatric dosing if reached 18th birthday while receiving therapy. D/C if patient fails to demonstrate at least a 2 log$_{10}$ reduction from baseline in HCV RNA by 12 wks of therapy, or undetectable HCV RNA levels after 24 wks of therapy.

or unstable cardiac disease. **R**

Ribavirin (Rebetol)	**Cap:** 200 mg; **Sol:** 40 mg/ml	**HCV:** Take w/ food. **Adults: W/ Intron A: ≤75 kg:** 400 mg qam & 600 mg qpm. **>75 kg:** 600 mg qam & 600 mg qpm. **Interferon alfa-Naive:** Treat x 24-48 wks. **Retreatment:** Treat x 24 wks. **W/ PEG-Intron:** 800-1400 mg/d based on body wt; see PI. **Interferon alfa-Naive: Genotype 1:** Treat x 48 wks. **Genotype 2/3:** Treat x 24 wks. **Retreatment:** Treat x 48 wks. **Peds: ≥3 yo: W/ Intron A/PEG-Intron: <47 kg:** (Sol) 15 mg/kg/d given bid. **47-59 kg:** 400 mg qam & 400 mg qpm. **60-73 kg:** 400 mg qam & 600 mg qpm. **>73 kg:** 600 mg qam & 600 mg qpm. **Genotype 1:** Treat x 48 wks. **Genotype 2/3:** Treat x 24 wks. Refer to PI for dose modifications and d/c.	⊠X ✽v Hemolytic anemia reported. Avoid in significant or unstable cardiac disease. **R**

NAME	FORM/STRENGTH	DOSAGE	COMMENTS
Telaprevir (Incivek)	**Tab:** 375 mg	**HCV: Adults: W/Peginterferon Alfa/Ribavirin:** 750 mg tid (q7-9h) w/ food (not low fat) x 12 wks. Refer to PI for treatment duration, dose reduction & d/c.	⬤B, Category X in combination w/ peginterferon alfa & ribavirin. ❄v H
Telbivudine (Tyzeka)	**Tab:** 600 mg; **Sol:** 100 mg/5 ml	**HBV: Adults: ≥16 yo: Tab:** 600 mg qd. **Sol:** 30 ml qd.	⬤B ❄v R W [31, 32]
Tenofovir Disoproxil Fumarate (Viread)	**Pow:** 40 mg/gm; **Tab:** 150 mg, 200 mg, 250 mg, 300 mg	**HBV: Adults:** 300-mg tab qd. If unable to swallow tabs, may use 7.5 scoops of oral powder.	⬤B ❄v R W [31, 32]
HERPES INFECTION			
Acyclovir Sodium	**Inj:** 50 mg/ml	**Mucosal/Cutaneous Herpes Simplex: Adults & Peds: ≥12 yo:** 5 mg/kg IV q8h x 7d. **<12 yo:** 10 mg/kg IV q8h x 7d. **Neonatal Herpes Simplex: Birth-3 mths:** 10 mg/kg q8h IV x 10d. **Genital Herpes: Adults & Peds: ≥12 yo:** 5 mg/kg IV q8h x 5d. **Herpes Simplex Encephalitis: Adults & Peds: ≥12 yo:** 10 mg/kg IV q8h x 10d. **3 mths-<12 yo:** 20 mg/kg IV q8h x 10d. **Zoster: Adults & Peds: ≥12 yo:** 10 mg/kg IV q8h x 7d. **<12 yo:** 20 mg/kg IV q8h x 7d.	⬤B ❄> R

Acyclovir (Zovirax Oral)	Cap: 200 mg; Susp: 200 mg/5 ml; Tab: 400 mg, 800 mg	Herpes Zoster: Adults: 800 mg q4h, 5x/d x 7-10d. Genital Herpes: Adults: Initial Therapy: 200 mg q4h, 5x/d x 10d. Chronic Therapy: 400 mg bid x 1 yr or 200 mg 3-5x/d x 1 yr. Intermittent Therapy: 200 mg q4h 5x/d x 5d; start at 1st sign/symptom of recurrence. Varicella: Adults & Peds: >40 kg: 800 mg qid x 5d. Peds: ≥2 yo: <40 kg: 20 mg/kg qid x 5d. Start at earliest sign/symptom.	⊞B ❄> R
Famciclovir (Famvir)	Tab: 125 mg, 250 mg, 500 mg	Adults: Immunocompetent: Recurrent Herpes Labialis: 1500 mg single dose. Genital Herpes: Recurrent Episodes: 1000 mg bid x 1d. Suppressive Therapy: 250 mg bid. Herpes Zoster: 500 mg q8h x 7d. HIV-Infected: Recurrent Orolabial or Genital Herpes: 500 mg bid x 7d.	⊞B ❄v R
Valacyclovir HCl (Valtrex)	Tab: 500 mg, 1 gm	Adults: Herpes Zoster: 1 gm tid x 7d. Start w/in 48h after onset of rash. Genital Herpes: Initial Episode: 1 gm bid x 10d. Start w/in 48h after onset of symptoms. Recurrent Episodes: 500 mg bid x 3d. Start at 1st sign/symptom of episode. Chronic Suppressive Therapy w/ Normal Immune Function: 1 gm qd. Alternative: History of ≤9 episodes/yr: 500 mg qd. Chronic Suppressive Therapy w/ HIV & CD4 ≥100 cells/mm³: 500 mg bid. Reduction of Transmission of Genital Herpes: History of ≤9 episodes/yr: 500 mg qd for source partner. Adults & Peds: ≥12 yo: Herpes Labialis: 2 gm q12h x 1d. Start at earliest	⊞B ❄> R

Continued on Next Page

NAME	FORM/STRENGTH	DOSAGE	COMMENTS
Valacyclovir HCl (Valtrex) *Continued*		symptom of cold sore. **Peds: 2-<18 yo: Chickenpox:** 20 mg/kg tid x 5d. **Max:** 1 gm tid. Start at earliest sign/ symptom of chickenpox.	

INFLUENZA

NAME	FORM/STRENGTH	DOSAGE	COMMENTS
Amantadine HCl	**Cap:** 100 mg; **Sol:** 50 mg/5 ml; **Tab:** 100 mg	**Influenza A Prophylaxis & Treatment: Adults:** 200 mg qd or 100 mg bid. **Elderly/Intolerant to 200 mg/d:** 100 mg qd. **Peds: 9-12 yo:** 100 mg bid. **1-9 yo:** 4.4-8.8 mg/kg/d. **Max:** 150 mg/d.	⊕C ❄v R
Oseltamivir Phosphate (Tamiflu)	**Cap:** 30 mg, 45 mg, 75 mg; **Susp:** 6 mg/ml	**Adults & Peds: Prophylaxis:** Begin w/in 2d of exposure, may continue up to 6 wks w/ community outbreak. **≥13 yo:** 75 mg qd x ≥10d. **≥1 yo: ≤15 kg:** 30 mg qd x 10d. **16-23 kg:** 45 mg qd x 10d. **24-40 kg:** 60 mg qd x 10d. **≥41 kg:** 75 mg qd x 10d. **Treatment: ≥13 yo:** 75 mg bid x 5d; begin w/in 2d of symptom onset. **≥1 yo: ≤15 kg:** 30 mg bid x 5d. **16-23 kg:** 45 mg bid x 5d. **24-40 kg:** 60 mg bid x 5d. **≥41 kg:** 75 mg bid x 5d.	⊕C ❄>R
Rimantadine HCl (Flumadine)	**Tab:** 100 mg	**Influenza A: Prophylaxis: Adults & Peds: ≥10 yo:** 100 mg bid. **1-9 yo:** 5 mg/kg qd. **Max:** 150 mg/d. **Treatment: Adults:** 100 mg bid; begin w/in 48h of symptom onset & treat x 7d from initial symptom onset.	⊕C ❄v H R

Bone and Joint Infection

AMINOGLYCOSIDES

Amikacin Sulfate	Inj: 50 mg/ml, 250 mg/ml	**IM/IV: Adults, Children & Older Infants:** 7.5 mg/kg q12h or 5 mg/kg q8h. **Max:** 1.5 gm/d. **Newborns: LD:** 10 mg/kg. **Maint:** 7.5 mg/kg q12h.	⊙D ❁v R W [1]
Gentamicin Sulfate	Inj: 40 mg/ml	**IM/IV: Adults:** 3 mg/kg/d given q8h. **Max:** 5 mg/kg/d in 3-4 doses. Reduce to 3 mg/kg/d as soon as clinically indicated. **Peds:** 2-2.5 mg/kg q8h. **Infants/Neonates:** 2.5 mg/kg q8h. ≤**1 wk:** 2.5 mg/kg q12h.	⊙N ❁>R W [1]
Tobramycin Sulfate (Tobramycin)	Inj: 10 mg/ml, 40 mg/ml	**IM/IV: Adults:** 3 mg/kg/d given q8h. **Max:** 5 mg/kg/d in 3-4 equal doses. Reduce to 3 mg/kg/d as soon as clinically indicated. **W/ Severe Cystic Fibrosis: Initial (as a guide only):** 10 mg/kg/d in 4 equal doses. **Peds: >1 wk:** 2-2.5 mg/kg q8h or 1.5-1.89 mg/kg q6h. ≤**1 wk:** Up to 2 mg/kg q12h.	⊙D ❁> R W [1]

CARBAPENEM

Cilastatin Sodium/Imipenem (Primaxin I.V.)	Inj: 250-250 mg, 500-500 mg	**IV: Adults: ≥70 kg: Mild:** 250-500 mg q6h. **Moderate:** 500 mg q6-8h or 1 gm q8h. **Severe:** 500 mg q6h or 1 gm q6-8h. **Max:** 50 mg/kg/d or 4 gm/d, whichever is lower. **Peds: ≥3 mths:** 15-25 mg/kg q6h. **Max:** 4 gm/d. **4 wks-3 mths & ≥1500 gm:** 25 mg/kg q6h. **1-4 wks & ≥1500 gm:** 25 mg/kg q8h. **<1 wk & ≥1500 gm:** 25 mg/kg q12h.	⊙C ❁> R

NAME	FORM/STRENGTH	DOSAGE	COMMENTS
CEPHALOSPORINS			
Cefazolin	Inj: 500 mg, 1 gm, 10 gm, 20 gm	**IM/IV: Adults: Usual:** 500 mg-1 gm q6-8h. **Peds: Usual:** 25-50 mg/kg/d given as tid-qid. **Max:** 100 mg/kg/d.	●B ❄> Safety in premies & neonates unknown. R
Cefotaxime Sodium (Claforan)	Inj: 500 mg, 1 gm, 2 gm, 10 gm	**Adults & Peds: ≥ 50 kg:** 1-2 gm IM/IV q8h. **Max:** 12 gm/d. **1 mth-12 yo: <50 kg:** 50-180 mg/kg/d IM/IV divided into 4-6 doses. **1-4 wks:** 50 mg/kg IV q8h. **0-1 wk:** 50 mg/kg IV q12h.	●B ❄> R
Cefoxitin	Inj: 1 gm, 1 gm/50 ml, 2 gm, 2 gm/50 ml, 10 gm	**IV: Adults:** 1 gm q4h or 2 gm q6-8h. **Peds: ≥3 mths:** 80-160 mg/kg/d given as q4-6h. **Max:** 12 gm/d.	●B ❄> R
Ceftazidime (Fortaz)	Inj: 500 mg, 1 gm, 2 gm, 6 gm	**Adults:** 2 gm IV q12h. **Peds: 1 mth-12 yo:** 30-50 mg/kg IV q8h, up to 6 gm/d. **Neonates: 0-4 wks:** 30 mg/kg IV q12h.	●B ❄> R
Ceftazidime (Tazicef)	Inj: 1 gm, 2 gm, 6 gm	**Adults:** 2 gm IV q12h. **Peds: 1 mth-12 yo:** 30-50 mg/kg IV q8h, up to 6 gm/d. **Neonates: 0-4 wks:** 30 mg/kg IV q12h.	●B ❄> R
Ceftriaxone Sodium (Rocephin)	Inj: (Rocephin) 500 mg, 1 gm; (Generic) 250 mg, 500 mg, 1 gm, 2 gm, 10 gm	**Adults: IM/IV: Usual:** 1-2 gm qd (or in equally divided doses bid). **Max:** 4 gm/d.	●B ❄>
Cefuroxime (Zinacef)	Inj: 750 mg, 1.5 gm, 7.5 gm	**IM/IV: Adults:** 1.5 gm q8h. **Peds: >3 mths:** 50 mg/kg q8h. **Max:** 4.5 gm/d.	●B ❄> R

| Cephalexin (Keflex) | (Keflex) Cap: 250 mg, 500 mg, 750 mg; (Generic) Cap: 250 mg, 500 mg; Susp: 125 mg/5 ml, 250 mg/5 ml | Adults: Usual: 250 mg q6h. Max: 4 gm/d. Peds: Usual: 25-50 mg/kg/d in divided doses. | ⊕B ❄> |

PENICILLINS

| Ticarcillin Disodium/ Clavulanate Potassium (Timentin) | Inj: 3 gm-100 mg | Adults: ≥60 kg: 3.1 gm (3 gm-100 mg) q4-6h. <60 kg: 200-300 mg/kg/d ticarcillin divided q4-6h. Peds: ≥3 mths & <60 kg: Mild-Moderate: 200 mg/kg/d ticarcillin divided q6h. Severe: 300 mg/kg/d ticarcillin divided q4h. ≥3 mths & ≥60 kg: Mild-Moderate: 3.1 gm q6h. Severe: 3.1 gm q4h. | ⊕B ❄> R |

QUINOLONES

| Ciprofloxacin HCl (Cipro Oral) | Susp: 250 mg/5 ml, 500 mg/5 ml; Tab: 250 mg, 500 mg | Adults: Mild-Moderate: 500 mg PO q12h x ≥4-6 wks. Severe-Complicated: 750 mg PO q12h x ≥4-6 wks. | ⊕C ❄v R W [98] |
| Ciprofloxacin (Cipro IV) | Inj: 400 mg/200 ml | Adults: Mild-Moderate: 400 mg IV q12h x ≥4-6 wks. Severe-Complicated: 400 mg IV q8h x ≥4-6 wks. | ⊕C ❄v R W [98] |

NAME	FORM/STRENGTH	DOSAGE	COMMENTS
MISCELLANEOUS			
Clindamycin (Cleocin)	**Inj:** 150 mg/ml, 300 mg/ 50 ml, 600 mg/50 ml, 900 mg/50 ml	**IM/IV: Adults:** 600-2700 mg/d in 2-4 doses. **Max:** 600 mg IM single dose. **Peds: 1 mth-16 yo:** 20-40 mg/kg/d in 3-4 doses. **<1 mth:** 15-20 mg/kg/d in 3-4 doses.	⬛B ❄v W [84]
Metronidazole (Flagyl)	**Cap:** 375 mg; **Tab:** 250 mg, 500 mg	**Adults: PO:** 7.5 mg/kg q6h x ≥7-10d. **Max:** 4 gm/d.	⬛B ❄v CI in 1st trimester in trichomoniasis. H W [83]
Metronidazole (Flagyl IV)	**Inj:** 5 mg/ml	**Adults: IV: LD:** 15 mg/kg over 1h. **Maint:** After 6h, 7.5 mg/kg q6h. **Max:** 4 gm/d.	⬛B ❄v H W [83]

Fungal Infection

Amphotericin B Lipid Complex (Abelcet)	**Inj:** 5 mg/ml	**Invasive Fungal Infections: Adults & Peds:** 5 mg/kg as a single IV infusion at 2.5 mg/kg/h.	⬛B ❄v
Amphotericin B Liposome (Ambisome)	**Inj:** 50 mg	**Adults & Peds:** Give over 120 min & reduce to 60 min if well tolerated. **Empiric Therapy in Febrile, Neutropenic Patients:** 3 mg/kg/d IV. *Aspergillus/Candida/Cryptococcus:* 3-5 mg/kg/d IV. **Cryptococcal Meningitis in HIV Patients:** 6 mg/kg/d IV. **Visceral Leishmaniasis:** (Immunocompetent) 3 mg/kg/d IV for Days 1-5, 14, 21. (Immunocompromised) 4 mg/kg/d IV for Days 1-5, 10, 17, 24, 31, 38.	⬛B ❄v

Anidulafungin (Eraxis)	**Inj:** 50 mg, 100 mg	**Adults:** Duration of treatment based on patient's clinical response. **Candidemia/Candida Infections (Intra-Abdominal Abscess & Peritonitis): LD:** 200 mg IV on Day 1. Follow w/ 100 mg IV qd thereafter. Continue therapy for at least 14d after last positive culture. **Esophageal Candidiasis: LD:** 100 mg IV on Day 1. Follow w/ 50 mg IV qd thereafter. Treat for minimum of 14d & for at least 7d after symptoms resolve.	⊜C ❄>
Fluconazole (Diflucan)	**Inj:** 200 mg/100 ml, 400 mg/200 ml; **Susp:** 50 mg/5 ml, 200 mg/5 ml; **Tab:** 50 mg, 100 mg, 150 mg, 200 mg	**Adults: PO: Vaginal Candidiasis:** 150 mg single dose. **IV/ PO: Oropharyngeal Candidiasis:** 200 mg on Day 1, then 100 mg qd x min 2 wks. **Esophageal Candidiasis:** 200 mg on Day 1, then 100 mg qd x min 3 wks & 2 wks after symptoms resolve. **Max:** 400 mg/d. **Systemic Candida Infections:** 400 mg/d. **UTI & Peritonitis:** 50-200 mg/d. **Cryptococcal Meningitis:** 400 mg on Day 1, then 200 mg qd x 10-12 wks after negative CSF culture. **Relapse Suppression in AIDS:** 200 mg qd. **Prophylaxis in BMT:** 400 mg qd. **Peds: IV/PO: Oropharyngeal Candidiasis:** 6 mg/kg on Day 1, then 3 mg/kg/d x min 2 wks. **Esophageal Candidiasis:** 6 mg/kg on Day 1, then 3 mg/kg/d x min 3 wks & 2 wks after symptoms resolve. **Max:** 12 mg/kg/d. **Systemic Candida Infections:** 6-12 mg/kg/d. **Cryptococcal Meningitis:** 12 mg/kg on	⊜C ❄v R

Continued on Next Page

NAME	FORM/STRENGTH	DOSAGE	COMMENTS
Fluconazole (Diflucan) *Continued*		Day 1, then 6 mg/kg/d x 10-12 wks after negative CSF culture. **Relapse Suppression in AIDS:** 6 mg/kg/d.	
Micafungin Sodium (Mycamine)	**Inj:** 50 mg, 100 mg	**Adults: Esophageal Candidiasis:** 150 mg/d IV. **Candidemia/Acute Disseminated Candidiasis/Candida Peritonitis & Abscesses:** 100 mg/d IV. **Candida Infection Prophylaxis in Hematopoietic Stem Cell Transplantation:** 50 mg/d IV.	●C ❀>
Miconazole (Oravig)	**Tab,Buccal:** 50 mg	**Oropharyngeal Candidiasis: Adults & Peds: ≥16 yo:** 50-mg tab to upper gum region (canine fossa) qd x 14d.	●C ❀> H
Posaconazole (Noxafil)	**Susp:** 40 mg/ml	**Adults & Peds: ≥13 yo: Prophylaxis of Invasive Fungal Infections:** 200 mg (5 ml) tid. Base duration of therapy on recovery from neutropenia or immunosuppression. **Oropharyngeal Candidiasis: LD:** 100 mg (2.5 ml) bid on Day 1, then 100 mg qd x 13d. **Oropharyngeal Candidiasis Refractory to Itraconazole and/or Fluconazole:** 400 mg (10 ml) bid. Base duration of therapy on severity of underlying disease & clinical response. Give each dose w/ full meal or nutritional supplement.	●C ❀v
Terbinafine HCl (Lamisil)	**Granules:** 125 mg/pkt, 187.5 mg/pkt; **Tab:** 250 mg	**Adults: Onychomycosis: Tab: Fingernail:** 250 mg qd x 6 wks. **Toenail:** 250 mg qd x 12 wks. **Adults & Peds: ≥4 yo: Tinea Capitis: Granules:** Take qd w/ food x 6 wks. **<25 kg:** 125 mg/d. **25-35 kg:** 187.5 mg/d. **>35 kg:** 250 mg/d.	●B ❀v H

| Voriconazole (Vfend) | Inj: 200 mg; Susp: 40 mg/ml; Tab: 50 mg, 200 mg | Adults: Invasive Aspergillosis/Scedosporiosis/Fusariosis: LD: 6 mg/kg IV q12h x 1st 24h. Maint: IV: 4 mg/kg q12h; continue for ≥7d. Switch to PO form when appropriate. PO: <40 kg: 100 mg q12h; increase to 150 mg q12h if inadequate response. ≥40 kg: 200 mg q12h; increase to 300 mg q12h if inadequate response. Candidemia (Non-Neutropenic Patients) and other Deep Tissue Candida Infections: LD: 6 mg/kg IV q12h x 1st 24h. Maint: IV: 3-4 mg/kg q12h. PO: Follow maint dose for aspergillosis. Treat for ≥14d after resolution of symptoms or last positive culture, whichever is longer. Esophageal Candidiasis: Maint: PO: Follow maint dose for aspergillosis. Treat for ≥14d & for ≥7d after resolution of symptoms. Intolerant to Dose Increase: IV: Reduce 4 mg/kg q12h to 3 mg/kg q12h. PO: Reduce by 50 mg steps to minimum of 200 mg q12h for ≥40 kg or 100 mg q12h for <40 kg. W/ Phenytoin: Maint: IV: 5 mg/kg q12h. PO: <40 kg: 200 mg q12h. ≥40 kg: 400 mg q12h. W/ Efavirenz: Maint: PO: 400 mg q12h and decrease efavirenz to 300 mg q24h. | ⊛D ✷v H R |

NAME	FORM/STRENGTH	DOSAGE	COMMENTS

Lower Respiratory Tract Infection
AMINOGLYCOSIDES

NAME	FORM/STRENGTH	DOSAGE	COMMENTS
Amikacin Sulfate	**Inj:** 50 mg/ml, 250 mg/ml	**IM/IV: Adults, Children & Older Infants:** 7.5 mg/ky q12h or 5 mg/kg q8h. **Max:** 1.5 gm/d. **Newborns: LD:** 10 mg/kg. **Maint:** 7.5 mg/kg q12h.	⊕D ❄v R W [1]
Gentamicin Sulfate	**Inj:** 40 mg/ml	**IV: Adults:** 3 mg/kg/d given q8h. **Max:** 5 mg/kg/d in 3-4 doses. Reduce to 3 mg/kg/d as soon as clinically indicated. **Peds:** 2-2.5 mg/kg q8h. **Infants/Neonates:** 2.5 mg/kg q8h. ≤1 wk: 2.5 mg/kg q12h.	⊕N ❄>R W [1]
Tobramycin Sulfate (Tobramycin)	**Inj:** 10 mg/ml, 40 mg/ml	**IM/IV: Adults:** 3 mg/kg/d given q8h. **Max:** 5 mg/kg/d in 3-4 equal doses. Reduce to 3 mg/kg/d as soon as clinically indicated. **W/ Severe Cystic Fibrosis: Initial (as a guide only):** 10 mg/kg/d in 4 equal doses. **Peds: >1 wk:** 2-2.5 mg/kg q8h or 1.5-1.89 mg/kg q6h. **≤1 wk:** Up to 2 mg/kg q12h.	⊕D ❄> R W [1]

CARBAPENEM

NAME	FORM/STRENGTH	DOSAGE	COMMENTS
Ertapenem (Invanz)	**Inj:** 1 gm	**CAP: Adults & Peds: ≥13 yo:** 1 gm IM/IV qd. **3 mths-12 yo:** 15 mg/kg IM/IV bid. **Max:** 1 gm/d. **Duration:** 10-14d. May give IV up to 14d; IM up to 7d.	⊕B ❄> R

CEPHALOSPORINS

Cefaclor	**Cap:** 250 mg, 500 mg; **Susp:** 125 mg/5 ml, 187 mg/5 ml, 250 mg/5 ml, 375 mg/5 ml	**Adults: Cap/Susp:** Usual: 250 mg q8h. **Severe Infections/Pneumonia:** 500 mg q8h. **Peds:** ≥1 mth: **Cap/Susp:** 20 mg/kg/d given q8h. **Serious Infections:** 40 mg/kg/d. **Max:** 1 gm/d.	⊕B ❄>
Cefdinir (Omnicef)	**Cap:** 300 mg; **Susp:** 125 mg/5 ml, 250 mg/5 ml	**Adults & Peds:** ≥13 yo: CAP: 300 mg q12h x 10d. **ABECB:** 300 mg q12h x 5-10d or 600 mg q24h 10d.	⊕B ❄> R
Cefepime HCl	**Inj:** 500 mg, 1 gm, 2 gm, 1 gm/50 ml, 2 gm/100 ml	**Adults:** Moderate-Severe: 1-2 gm IV q12h x 10d. **Peds: 2 mths-16 yo:** ≤40 kg: 50 mg/kg IV q12h. **Max:** Do not exceed adult dose.	⊕B ❄> R
Cefixime (Suprax)	**Susp:** 100 mg/5 ml; **Tab:** 400 mg	**Acute Bronchitis/ABECB: Adults & Peds:** >12 yo or >50 kg: **Tab/Susp:** 400 mg qd or 200 mg bid. ≤50 kg or ≥6 mths: **Susp:** 8 mg/kg qd or 4 mg/kg bid.	⊕B ❄v R
Cefpodoxime Proxetil (Vantin)	**Susp:** 50 mg/5 ml, 100 mg/5 ml; **Tab:** 100 mg, 200 mg	**Adults & Peds:** ≥12 yo: 200 mg q12h x 10-14d.	⊕B ❄v R
Cefprozil (Cefzil)	**Susp:** 125 mg/5 ml, 250 mg/5 ml; **Tab:** 250 mg, 500 mg	**Acute Bronchitis/ABECB: Adults & Peds:** ≥13 yo: 500 mg q12h x 10d.	⊕B ❄> R
Ceftaroline Fosamil (Teflaro)	**Inj:** 400 mg, 600 mg	**Adults:** ≥18 yo: CABP: 600 mg q12h IV over 1h x 5-7d.	⊕B ❄> R

NAME	FORM/STRENGTH	DOSAGE	COMMENTS
Ceftazidime (Fortaz)	**Inj:** 500 mg, 1 gm, 2 gm, 6 gm	**Uncomplicated Pneumonia: Adults:** 500-1000 mg IM/IV q8h. **Peds: 1 mth-12 yo:** 30-50 mg/kg IV q8h, up to 6 gm/d. **Neonates: 0-4 wks:** 30 mg/kg IV q12h.	◉B ✳> R
Ceftazidime (Tazicef)	**Inj:** 1 gm, 2 gm, 6 gm	**Uncomplicated Pneumonia: Adults:** 500-1000 mg IM/IV q8h. **Peds: 1 mth-12 yo:** 30-50 mg/kg IV q8h, up to 6 gm/d. **Neonates: 0-4 wks:** 30 mg/kg IV q12h.	◉B ✳> R
Ceftriaxone Sodium (Rocephin)	**Inj:** (Rocephin) 500 mg, 1 gm; (Generic) 250 mg, 500 mg, 1 gm, 2 gm, 10 gm	**Adults: IM/IV: Usual:** 1-2 gm qd (or in equally divided doses bid). **Max:** 4 gm/d.	◉B ✳>
Cefuroxime Axetil (Ceftin)	**Tab:** 250 mg, 500 mg	**Adults & Peds: ≥13 yo:** 250-500 mg bid x 5-10d.	◉B ✳v R
Cephalexin (Keflex)	(Keflex) **Cap:** 250 mg, 500 mg, 750 mg; (Generic) **Cap:** 250 mg, 500 mg; **Susp:** 125 mg/5 ml, 250 mg/5 ml	**Adults: Usual:** 250 mg q6h. **Max:** 4 gm/d. **Peds: Usual:** 25-50 mg/kg/d in divided doses.	◉B ✳>

KETOLIDE

NAME	FORM/STRENGTH	DOSAGE	COMMENTS
Telithromycin (Ketek)	**Tab:** 300 mg, 400 mg	**Mild-to-Moderate CAP: Adults:** 800 mg qd x 7-10d.	◉C ✳> H R W [71]

MACROLIDES

Azithromycin (Zithromax)	**Inj:** 500 mg; **Susp:** 100 mg/5 ml, 200 mg/5 ml; **Tab:** 250 mg, 500 mg	**CAP: Adults: ≥16 yo: PO:** 500 mg on Day 1, then 250 mg qd on Days 2-5. **IV:** 500 mg qd x ≥2d, then 500 mg PO qd to complete 7-10d course. **Peds: ≥6 mths: Susp:** 10 mg/kg on Day 1, then 5 mg/kg on Days 2-5. **COPD: Adults: PO:** 500 mg qd x 3d or 500 mg on Day 1, then 250 mg qd on Days 2-5.	⊕B ✤>
Azithromycin (Zmax)	**Susp,ER:** 2 gm	**CAP: Adults:** 2 gm single dose. **Peds: ≥6 mths:** 60 mg/kg single dose. Patients weighing ≥34 kg should receive adult dose. See PI for specific pediatric dosage info. Take on empty stomach (at least 1h ac or 2h pc).	⊕B ✤>
Clarithromycin (Biaxin)	**Susp:** 125 mg/5 ml, 250 mg/5 ml; **Tab:** 250 mg, 500 mg	**Adults: ABECB:** 250-500 mg q12h x 7-14d. **CAP:** 250 mg q12h x 7-14d. **Peds: ≥6 mths: Usual:** 7.5 mg/kg q12h x 10d.	⊕C ✤> R
Erythromycin Ethylsuccinate (E.E.S.)	**Susp:** 200 mg/5 ml, 400 mg/5 ml; **Tab:** 400 mg	**Adults: Usual:** 1600 mg/d in divided doses given q6h, q8h, or q12h. **Max:** 4 gm/d. **Peds: Usual:** 30-50 mg/kg/d in divided doses given q6h, q8h, or q12h. May double dose for more severe infections.	⊕B ✤>
Erythromycin Ethylsuccinate (EryPed)	**Susp:** 200 mg/5 ml, 400 mg/5 ml	**Adults: Usual:** 1600 mg/d in divided doses given q6h, q8h, or q12h. **Max:** 4 gm/d. **Peds: Usual:** 30-50 mg/kg/d in divided doses given q6h, q8h, or q12h. May double dose for more severe infections.	⊕B ✤>
Erythromycin Stearate (Erythrocin)	**Tab:** 250 mg, 500 mg	**Adults: Usual:** 250 mg q6h or 500 mg q12h. **Peds: Usual:** 30-50 mg/kg/d in divided doses. **Max:** 4 gm/d.	⊕B ✤>

NAME	FORM/STRENGTH	DOSAGE	COMMENTS
Erythromycin (Ery-Tab)	Tab,Delay: 250 mg, 333 mg, 500 mg	Adults: Usual: 250 mg qid, 333 mg q8h, or 500 mg q12h. Peds: Usual: 30-50 mg/kg/d in divided doses. Max: 4 gm/d.	◉B ❄>
Erythromycin (PCE)	Tab: 333 mg, 500 mg	Adults: Usual: 333 mg q8h or 500 mg q12h. Peds: Usual: 30-50 mg/kg/d in divided doses. Max: 4 gm/d.	◉B ❄>
OXAZOLIDINONE			
Linezolid (Zyvox)	Inj: 2 mg/ml; Susp: 100 mg/5 ml; Tab: 600 mg	CAP/Nosocomial Pneumonia: Treat x 10-14d. Adults & Peds: ≥12 yo: 600 mg IV/PO q12h. Birth-11 yo: 10 mg/kg IV/PO q8h.	◉C ❄>
PENICILLINS			
Amoxicillin	Cap: 250 mg, 500 mg; Chewtab: 125 mg, 250 mg; Susp: 125 mg/5 ml, 200 mg/5 ml, 250 mg/5 ml, 400 mg/5 ml; Tab: 500 mg, 875 mg	Adults & Peds: ≥40 kg: 875 mg q12h or 500 mg q8h. >3 mths & <40 kg: 45 mg/kg/d divided q12h or 40 mg/kg/d divided q8h. ≤3 mths: Max: 30 mg/kg/d divided q12h.	◉B ❄> R
Amoxicillin/Clavulanate (Augmentin)	Chewtab: 125-31.25 mg, 200-28.5 mg, 250-62.5 mg, 400-57 mg; Susp: (per 5 ml) 125-31.25 mg,	Adults & Peds: Dose based on amoxicillin component. ≥40 kg: Tab: 875 mg q12h or 500 mg q8h. May use 125 mg/5 ml or 250 mg/5 ml susp in place of 500-mg tab & 200 mg/5 ml or 400 mg/5 ml susp in place of 875-mg tab. Chewtab/Susp: ≥12 wks: 45 mg/kg/d given q12h or	◉B ❄> (2) 250-mg tabs are not equivalent to (1) 500-mg tab.

	200-28.5 mg, 250-62.5 mg, 400-57 mg; **Tab:** 250-125 mg, 500-125 mg, 875-125 mg	40 mg/kg/d given q8h. **<12 wks:** 30 mg/kg/d given q12h (use 125 mg/5 ml susp).	Only use 250-mg tab if peds ≥40 kg. Chewtab & tab not interchangeable. **H R**
Ampicillin	**Cap:** 250 mg, 500 mg; **Susp:** 125 mg/5 ml, 250 mg/5 ml	**Adults & Peds: >20 kg:** 250 mg qid. **≤20 kg:** 50 mg/kg/d given tid-qid.	⊕B ✿v
Clavulanate Potassium/ Amoxicillin (Augmentin XR)	**Tab,ER:** 1000-62.5 mg	**CAP: Adults & Peds: ≥40 kg:** 2 tabs q12h x 7-10d.	⊕ B ✿> **H R**
Penicillin V Potassium (Penicillin VK)	**Susp:** 125 mg/5 ml, 250 mg/5 ml; **Tab:** 250 mg, 500 mg	**Pneumococcal: Adults & Peds: ≥12 yo:** 250-500 mg q6h until afebrile x 2d.	⊕N ✿>
Piperacillin Sodium/ Tazobactam Sodium (Zosyn)	**Inj:** 2-0.25 gm/50 ml, 3-0.375 gm/50 ml, 4-0.5 gm/100 ml, 2-0.25 gm, 3-0.375 gm, 4-0.5 gm	**Adults: Usual:** 3.375 gm IV q6h x 7-10d. **Nosocomial Pneumonia:** 4.5 gm IV q6h x 7-14d plus aminoglycoside. Infuse over 30 min.	⊕B ✿> **R**

NAME	FORM/STRENGTH	DOSAGE	COMMENTS
QUINOLONES			
Ciprofloxacin HCl (Cipro Oral)	**Susp:** 250 mg/5 ml, 500 mg/5 ml; **Tab:** 250 mg, 500 mg	**Adults: Mild-Moderate:** 500 mg PO q12h x 7-14d. **Severe-Complicated:** 750 mg PO q12h x 7-14d. **Inhalational Anthrax (Post-Exposure): Adults:** 500 mg PO q12h x 60d. **Peds:** 15 mg/kg PO q12h x 60d. **Max:** 500 mg PO per dose.	●C ❄v R W [98]
Ciprofloxacin (Cipro IV)	**Inj:** 400 mg/200 ml	**Adults: Mild-Moderate:** 400 mg IV q12h x 7-14d. **Severe-Complicated:** 400 mg IV q8h x 7-14d. **Nosocomial Pneumonia:** 400 mg IV q8h x 10-14d. **Inhalational Anthrax (Post-Exposure): Adults:** 400 mg IV q12h x 60d. **Peds:** 10 mg/kg IV q12h x 60d. **Max:** 400 mg IV per dose.	●C ❄v R W [98]
Gemifloxacin Mesylate (Factive)	**Tab:** 320 mg	**Adults: ≥18 yo: ABECB:** 320 mg qd x 5d. **CAP:** 320 mg qd x 5d (*S.pneumoniae, H.influenzae, M.pneumoniae, C.pneumoniae*) or 7d (multi-drug resistant *S.pneumoniae, K.pneumoniae,* or *M.catarrhalis*).	●C ❄v R W [98]
Levofloxacin (Levaquin)	**Inj:** 5 mg/ml, 25 mg/ml; **Sol:** 25 mg/ml; **Tab:** 250 mg, 500 mg, 750 mg	**Adults: ≥18 yo: CAP:** 500 mg IV/PO qd x 7-14d or 750 mg IV/PO qd x 5d. **Nosocomial Pneumonia:** 750 mg IV/PO qd x 7-14d. **ABECB:** 500 mg IV/PO x 7d. **Inhalational Anthrax (Post-Exposure):** 500 mg IV/PO qd x 60d. **Peds: ≥6 mths: Inhalation Anthrax (Post-Exposure): >50 kg:** 500 mg IV/PO q24h x 60d. **<50 kg:** 8 mg/kg PO/IV q12h x 60d. **Max:** 250 mg/dose.	●C ❄v R W [98]

| Moxifloxacin HCl (Avelox) | Inj: 400 mg/250 ml; Tab: 400 mg | **Adults:** ≥18 yo: **ABECB:** 400 mg IV/PO q24h x 5d. **CAP:** 400 mg IV/PO q24h x 7-14d. | ⊕C 🌼v W [98] |
| Ofloxacin | Tab: 200 mg, 300 mg, 400 mg | **ABECB/CAP: Adults:** ≥18 yo: 400 mg q12h x 10d. | ⊕C 🌼v H R W [98] |

TETRACYCLINES

Doxycycline Hyclate (Doryx)	Tab, Delay: 75 mg, 100 mg	**Adults:** 100 mg q12h on Day 1, then 100 mg qd or 50 mg q12h. **Severe:** 100 mg q12h. **Peds:** >8 yo & ≤100 lbs: 1 mg/lb bid on Day 1, then 1 mg/lb qd or 0.5 mg/lb bid. **Severe:** 2 mg/lb. >100 lbs: Adult dose. **Inhalation Anthrax (Post-Exposure): Adults:** 100 mg bid x 60d. **Peds:** >8 yo & <100 lbs: 1 mg/lb bid x 60d. ≥100 lbs: Adult dose.	⊕D 🌼v
Doxycycline Monohydrate (Monodox)	Cap: 50 mg, 75 mg, 100 mg	**Adults:** 100 mg q12h or 50 mg q6h on Day 1, then 100 mg qd or 50 mg q12h. **Severe:** 100 mg q12h. **Peds:** >8 yo & ≤100 lbs: 1 mg/lb bid on Day 1, then 1 mg/lb qd or 0.5 mg/lb bid. **Severe:** 2 mg/lb. >100 lbs: Adult dose. **Inhalation Anthrax (Post-Exposure): Adults:** 100 mg bid x 60d. **Peds:** >8 yo & <100 lbs: 1 mg/lb bid x 60d. ≥100 lbs: Adult dose.	⊕D 🌼v
Minocycline HCl (Dynacin)	Tab: 50 mg, 75 mg, 100 mg	**Adults:** 200 mg PO, then 100 mg q12h or 50 mg qid. **Peds:** >8 yo: 4 mg/kg PO, then 2 mg/kg q12h.	⊕D 🌼v R
Minocycline HCl (Minocin)	Cap: 50 mg, 100 mg; Inj: 100 mg	**Adults:** 200 mg PO/IV, then 100 mg q12h or 50 mg qid. **Peds:** >8 yo: 4 mg/kg PO/IV, then 2 mg/kg q12h.	⊕D 🌼v R

NAME	FORM/STRENGTH	DOSAGE	COMMENTS
Tetracycline HCl (Sumycin)	**Cap:** 250 mg, 500 mg; **Susp:** 125 mg/5 ml	**Adults:** 250 mg qid or 500 mg bid. **Peds: >8 yo:** 25-50 mg/kg divided bid-qid.	●D ❄v R

MISCELLANEOUS

NAME	FORM/STRENGTH	DOSAGE	COMMENTS
Clindamycin (Cleocin)	**Cap:** 75 mg, 150 mg, 300 mg; **Inj:** 150 mg/ml, 300 mg/50 ml, 600 mg/ 50 ml, 900 mg/50 ml; **Susp:** 75 mg/5 ml	**IM/IV: Adults:** 600-2700 mg/d in 2-4 doses. **Max:** 600 mg IM single dose. **Peds: 1 mth-16 yo:** 20-40 mg/kg/d in 3-4 doses. **<1 mth:** 15-20 mg/kg/d in 3-4 doses. **PO: Adults:** 150-450 mg q6h. **Peds: Cap:** 8-20 mg/kg/d in 3-4 doses. **Susp:** 8-25 mg/kg/d in 3-4 doses.	●B ❄v (IV) ❄> (PO) W [84]
Tigecycline (Tygacil)	**Inj:** 50 mg/5 ml, 50 mg/10 ml	**Adults: CAP: Initial:** 100 mg IV over 30-60 min. **Maint:** 50 mg IV q12h over 30-60 min x 7-14d.	●D ❄> H

Meningitis, Bacterial
AMINOGLYCOSIDES

NAME	FORM/STRENGTH	DOSAGE	COMMENTS
Amikacin Sulfate	**Inj:** 50 mg/ml, 250 mg/ml	**IM/IV: Adults, Children & Older Infants:** 7.5 mg/kg q12h or 5 mg/kg q8h. **Max:** 1.5 gm/d. **Newborns: LD:** 10 mg/kg. **Maint:** 7.5 mg/kg q12h.	●D ❄v R W [1]
Gentamicin Sulfate	**Inj:** 40 mg/ml	**IV: Adults:** 3 mg/kg/d given q8h. **Max:** 5 mg/kg/d in 3-4 doses. Reduce to 3 mg/kg/d as soon as clinically indicated. **Peds:** 2-2.5 mg/kg q8h. **Infants/Neonates:** 2.5 mg/kg q8h. **≤1 wk:** 2.5 mg/kg q12h.	●N ❄>R W [1]

Tobramycin Sulfate (Tobramycin)	**Inj:** 10 mg/ml, 40 mg/ml	**IM/IV: Adults:** 3 mg/kg/d given q8h. **Max:** 5 mg/kg/d in 3-4 equal doses. Reduce to 3 mg/kg/d as soon as clinically indicated. **W/ Severe Cystic Fibrosis: Initial (as a guide only):** 10 mg/kg/d in 4 equal doses. **Peds: >1 wk:** 2-2.5 mg/kg q8h or 1.5-1.89 mg/kg q6h. **≤1 wk:** Up to 2 mg/kg q12h.	⊕D ❄> R W [1]

CARBAPENEM

Meropenem (Merrem)	**Inj:** 500 mg, 1 gm	**IV: Peds: ≥3 mths: >50 kg:** 2 gm q8h. **≤50 kg:** 40 mg/kg q8h. **Max:** 2 gm q8h.	⊕B ❄> R

CEPHALOSPORINS

Cefotaxime Sodium (Claforan)	**Inj:** 500 mg, 1 gm, 2 gm, 10 gm	**Adults & Peds: ≥ 50 kg:** 2 gm IV q6-8h. **Max:** 12 gm/d. **1 mth-12 yo: <50 kg:** 50-180 mg/kg/d IM/IV divided into 4-6 doses. **1-4 wks:** 50 mg/kg IV q8h. **0-1 wk:** 50 mg/kg IV q12h.	⊕B ❄> R
Ceftazidime (Fortaz)	**Inj:** 500 mg, 1 gm, 2 gm, 6 gm	**Adults:** 2 gm IV q8h. **Peds: 1 mth-12 yo:** 30-50 mg/kg IV q8h, up to 6 gm/d. **Neonates: 0-4 wks:** 30 mg/kg IV q12h.	⊕B ❄> R
Ceftazidime (Tazicef)	**Inj:** 1 gm, 2 gm, 6 gm	**Adults:** 2 gm IV q8h. **Peds: 1 mth-12 yo:** 30-50 mg/kg IV q8h, up to 6 gm/d. **Neonates: 0-4 wks:** 30 mg/kg IV q12h.	⊕B ❄> R
Ceftriaxone Sodium (Rocephin)	**Inj:** (Rocephin) 500 mg, 1 gm; (Generic) 250 mg, 500 mg, 1 gm, 2 gm, 10 gm	**Adults: IV/IM: Usual:** 1-2 gm qd (or in equally divided doses bid). **Max:** 4 gm/d. **Peds: IV/IM: Initial:** 100 mg/kg then 100 mg/kg qd (or in equally divided doses q12h) x 7-14d. **Max:** 4 gm/d.	⊕B ❄>

NAME	FORM/STRENGTH	DOSAGE	COMMENTS
Cefuroxime (Zinacef)	**Inj:** 750 mg, 1.5 gm, 7.5 gm	**IV: Adults:** 1.5 gm q6h. **Max:** 3 gm q8h. **Peds:** >3 mths: 200-240 mg/kg/d divided q6-8h.	▣B ❄>R

PENICILLIN

| Ampicillin Sodium | **Inj:** 250 mg, 500 mg, 1 gm, 2 gm | **IV: Adults & Peds:** 150-200 mg/kg/d given q3-4h. | ▣B ❄> |

Mycobacterium Avium Complex

Azithromycin (Zithromax)	**Susp:** 1 gm/pkt; **Tab:** 600 mg	**Adults: Prevention:** 1200 mg qwk w/ or w/o rifabutin. **Treatment:** 600 mg qd w/ ethambutol 15 mg/kg/d.	▣B ❄>
Clarithromycin (Biaxin)	**Susp:** 125 mg/5 ml, 250 mg/5 ml; **Tab:** 250 mg, 500 mg	**Prevention & Treatment: Adults:** 500 mg bid. **Peds:** ≥**20 mths:** 7.5 mg/kg bid. **Max:** 500 mg bid.	▣C ❄>R
Rifabutin (Mycobutin)	**Cap:** 150 mg	**Adults:** 300 mg qd or 150 mg bid w/ food. Reduce dose w/ nelfinavir or indinavir.	▣B ❄vR

Otitis Media, Acute
CEPHALOSPORINS

| Cefaclor | **Cap:** 250 mg, 500 mg; **Susp:** 125 mg/5 ml, 187 mg/5 ml, 250 mg/5 ml, 375 mg/5 ml | **Peds:** ≥**1 mth:** 40 mg/kg/d given in divided doses. **Max:** 1 gm/d. | ▣B ❄> |

Cefdinir (Omnicef)	**Susp:** 125 mg/5 ml; 250 mg/5 ml	**Peds: 6 mths-12 yo:** 7 mg/kg q12h x 5-10d or 14 mg/kg q24h x 10d.	⊕B ❋> R
Cefixime (Suprax)	**Susp:** 100 mg/5 ml; **Tab:** 400 mg	**Adults & Peds: >12 yo or >50 kg: Tab/Susp:** 400 mg qd or 200 mg bid. **≤50 kg or >6 mths: Susp:** 8 mg/kg qd or 4 mg/kg bid.	⊕B ❋v R
Cefpodoxime Proxetil (Vantin)	**Susp:** 50 mg/5 ml, 100 mg/5 ml; **Tab:** 100 mg, 200 mg	**Peds: 2 mths-11 yo:** 5 mg/kg q12h x 5d.	⊕B ❋v R
Cefprozil (Cefzil)	**Susp:** 125 mg/5 ml, 250 mg/5 ml; **Tab:** 250 mg, 500 mg	**Peds: 6 mths-12 yo:** 15 mg/kg q12h x 10d.	⊕B ❋> R
Ceftriaxone Sodium (Rocephin)	**Inj:** (Rocephin) 500 mg, 1 gm; (Generic) 250 mg, 500 mg, 1 gm, 2 gm, 10 gm	**Peds: IM:** 50 mg/kg single dose. **Max:** 1 gm/dose.	⊕B ❋>
Cefuroxime Axetil (Ceftin)	**Susp:** 125 mg/5 ml, 250 mg/5 ml; **Tab:** 250 mg, 500 mg	**Peds: 3 mths-12 yo: Susp:** 15 mg/kg bid x 10d. **Max:** 1 gm/d. **Tab:** 250 mg bid x 10d.	⊕B ❋> Tabs & susp not bioequivalent. R

NAME	FORM/STRENGTH	DOSAGE	COMMENTS
Cephalexin (Keflex)	(Keflex) **Cap:** 250 mg, 500 mg, 750 mg; (Generic) **Cap:** 250 mg, 500 mg; **Susp:** 125 mg/5 ml, 250 mg/5 ml	**Peds:** 75-100 mg/kg/d in divided doses.	▣B ❄>

MACROLIDES

NAME	FORM/STRENGTH	DOSAGE	COMMENTS
Azithromycin (Zithromax)	**Susp:** 100 mg/5 ml, 200 mg/5 ml	**Peds:** ≥6 mths: 30 mg/kg x 1 dose; 10 mg/kg qd x 3d; or 10 mg/kg qd x 1d, then 5 mg/kg qd on Days 2-5.	▣B ❄>
Clarithromycin (Biaxin)	**Susp:** 125 mg/5 ml, 250 mg/5 ml; **Tab:** 250 mg, 500 mg	**Peds:** ≥6 mths: 7.5 mg/kg q12h x 10d.	▣C ❄> R

MACROLIDES AND COMBINATIONS

NAME	FORM/STRENGTH	DOSAGE	COMMENTS
Sulfisoxazole Acetyl/ Erythromycin Ethylsuccinate	**Susp:** 200-600 mg/5 ml	**Peds:** ≥2 mths: Dose based on 50 mg/kg/d erythromycin or 150 mg/kg/d sulfisoxazole given tid-qid x 10d. **Max:** 6 gm/d sulfisoxazole.	▣C ❄v

PENICILLINS

Amoxicillin	**Cap:** 250 mg, 500 mg; **Chewtab:** 125 mg, 250 mg; **Susp:** 125 mg/5 ml, 200 mg/5 ml, 250 mg/5 ml, 400 mg/5 ml; **Tab:** 500 mg, 875 mg	**Adults & Peds: ≥40 kg: Mild-Moderate:** 500 mg q12h or 250 mg q8h. **Severe:** 875 mg q12h or 500 mg q8h. **>3 mths & <40 kg: Mild-Moderate:** 25 mg/kg/d divided q12h or 20 mg/kg/d divided q8h. **Severe:** 45 mg/kg/d divided q12h or 40 mg/kg/d divided q8h. **≤3 mths: Max:** 30 mg/kg/d divided q12h.	⊕B ✿> R
Amoxicillin/Clavulanate (Augmentin ES-600)	**Susp:** 600-42.9 mg/5 ml	**Peds: ≥3 mths: <40 kg:** 90 mg/kg/d divided q12h x 10d. Based on amoxicillin component. Not interchangeable w/ other Augmentin susp.	⊕B ✿> H R
Amoxicillin/Clavulanate (Augmentin)	**Chewtab:** 125-31.25 mg, 200-28.5 mg, 250-62.5 mg, 400-57 mg; **Susp:** (per 5 ml) 125-31.25 mg, 200-28.5 mg, 250-62.5 mg, 400-57 mg; **Tab:** 250-125 mg, 500-125 mg, 875-125 mg	**Peds:** Dose based on amoxicillin component. **≥40 kg: Tab:** 500 mg q12h or 250 mg q8h. May use 125 mg/5 ml or 250 mg/5 ml susp in place of 500-mg tab & 200 mg/5 ml or 400 mg/5 ml susp in place of 875-mg tab. **≥12 wks: Susp/Chewtab:** 45 mg/kg/d given q12h or 40 mg/kg/d given q8h. **<12 wks: Susp:** 30 mg/kg/d given q12h (use 125 mg/5 ml susp).	⊕B ✿> (2) 250-mg tabs are not equivalent to (1) 500-mg tab. Only use 250-mg tab if peds ≥40 kg. Chewtab & tab not interchangeable. H R

NAME	FORM/STRENGTH	DOSAGE	COMMENTS
SULFONAMIDES AND COMBINATIONS			
Sulfamethoxazole/ Trimethoprim (Septra, Septra DS, Sulfatrim Pediatric)	**Susp:** 200-40 mg/5 ml; **Tab:** (SG) 400-00 mg, (DS) 800-160 mg	**Peds:** ≥2 mths: 4 mg/kg TMP & 20 mg/kg SMX q12h x 10d.	◐C ❄v Π Cl in pregnancy & nursing.

Pneumocystis Carinii Pneumonia

NAME	FORM/STRENGTH	DOSAGE	COMMENTS
Atovaquone (Mepron)	**Susp:** 750 mg/5 ml	**Adults & Peds:** ≥13 yo: Take w/ food. **Prevention:** 1500 mg qd. **Treatment:** 750 mg bid x 21d.	◐C ❄>
Sulfamethoxazole/ Trimethoprim (Septra, Septra DS, Sulfatrim Pediatric)	**Susp:** 200-40 mg/5 ml; **Tab:** (SS) 400-80 mg, (DS) 800-160 mg	**Treatment: Adults & Peds:** 75-100 mg/kg SMZ & 15-20 mg/kg TMP divided q6h x 14-21d. **Prophylaxis: Adults:** 1 DS tab qd. **Peds:** 750 mg/m^2/d SMZ & 150 mg/m^2/d TMP divided bid x 3 consecutive days/wk. **Max:** 1600 mg SMZ/320 mg TMP/d.	◐C ❄v Cl in pregnancy & nursing. **R**

Septicemia, Bacterial
AMINOGLYCOSIDES

NAME	FORM/STRENGTH	DOSAGE	COMMENTS
Amikacin Sulfate	**Inj:** 50 mg/ml, 250 mg/ml	**IM/IV: Adults, Children & Older Infants:** 7.5 mg/kg q12h or 5 mg/kg q8h. **Max:** 1.5 gm/d. **Newborns: LD:** 10 mg/kg. **Maint:** 7.5 mg/kg q12h.	◐D ❄v R W [1]

Gentamicin Sulfate	Inj: 10 mg/ml, 40 mg/ml	**Adults:** 3 mg/kg/d divided q8h. **Max:** 5 mg/kg/d. Reduce to 3 mg/kg/d as soon as clinically indicated. **Peds:** 2-2.5 mg/kg q8h. **Infants/Neonates:** 2.5 mg/kg q8h. ≤**1 wk:** 2.5 mg/kg q12h.	⊕D ❄v R W [1]
Tobramycin Sulfate (Tobramycin)	Inj: 10 mg/ml, 40 mg/ml	**IM/IV: Adults:** 3 mg/kg given q8h. **Max:** 5 mg/kg/d in 3-4 equal doses. Reduce to 3 mg/kg/d as soon as clinically indicated. **W/ Severe Cystic Fibrosis: Initial (as a guide only):** 10 mg/kg/d in 4 equal doses. **Peds: >1 wk:** 2-2.5 mg/kg q8h or 1.5-1.89 mg/kg q6h. ≤**1 wk:** Up to 2 mg/kg q12h.	⊕D ❄> R W [1]
CEPHALOSPORINS			
Cefazolin	Inj: 500 mg, 1 gm, 10 gm, 20 gm	**IV: Adults:** 1-1.5 gm q6h. **Peds:** 100 mg/kg/d given as tid-qid.	⊕B ❄> R Safety in prematures & neonates unknown.
Cefotaxime Sodium (Claforan)	Inj: 500 mg, 1 gm, 2 gm, 10 gm	**Adults & Peds:** ≥ 50 kg: 2 gm IV q6-8h. **Max:** 12 gm/d. **1 mth-12 yo:** <50 kg: 50-180 mg/kg/d IM/IV divided into 4-6 doses. **1-4 wks:** 50 mg/kg IV q8h. **0-1 wk:** 50 mg/kg IV q12h.	⊕B ❄> R
Cefoxitin	Inj: 1 gm, 1 gm/50 ml, 2 gm, 2 gm/50 ml, 10 gm	**IV: Adults:** 1 gm q4h or 2 gm q6-8h. **Peds:** ≥3 mths: 80-160 mg/kg/d given as q4-6h. **Max:** 12 gm/d.	⊕B ❄> R

NAME	FORM/STRENGTH	DOSAGE	COMMENTS
Ceftazidime (Fortaz)	Inj: 500 mg, 1 gm, 2 gm, 6 gm	**Adults:** 2 gm IV q8h. **Peds: 1 mth-12 yo:** 30-50 mg/kg IV q8h. **Max:** 6 gm/d. **Neonates: 0-4 wks:** 30 mg/kg IV q12h.	⊕B ✳> R
Ceftazidime (Tazicef)	Inj: 1 gm, 2 gm, 6 gm	**Adults:** 2 gm IV q8h. **Peds: 1 mth-12 yo:** 30-50 mg/kg IV q8h, up to 6 gm/d. **Neonates: 0-4 wks:** 30 mg/kg IV q12h.	⊕B ✳> R
Ceftriaxone Sodium (Rocephin)	Inj: (Rocephin) 500 mg, 1 gm; (Generic) 250 mg, 500 mg, 1 gm, 2 gm, 10 gm	**Adults: IV/IM: Usual:** 1-2 gm qd (or in equally divided doses bid). **Max:** 4 gm/d. **Peds: IV/IM:** 50-75 mg/kg in equally divided doses bid. **Max:** 2 gm/d.	⊕B ✳>
Cefuroxime (Zinacef)	Inj: 750 mg, 750 mg/ 50 ml, 1.5 gm, 1.5 gm/ 50 ml, 7.5 gm	**Adults:** 1.5 gm IV q6-8h. **Peds: >3 mths:** 100 mg/kg/d IV q6-8h. Not to exceed max adult dose.	⊕B ✳> R
MONOBACTAM			
Aztreonam (Azactam)	Inj: 1 gm, 2 gm, 1 gm/ 50 ml, 2 gm/50 ml	**Adults: Moderately Severe:** 1 or 2 gm q8 or 12h. **Max:** 8 gm/d. **Severe Systemic/Life-Threatening Infections/** *Pseudomonas aeruginosa:* 2 gm q6 or 8h. **Max:** 8 gm/d. **Peds: 9 mths-16 yo: Mild-Moderate Infections:** 30 mg/kg IV q8h. **Max:** 120 mg/kg/d. **Moderate-Severe:** 30 mg/kg IV q6 or 8h. **Max:** 120 mg/kg/d.	⊕B ✳v R

PENICILLIN

Ticarcillin Disodium/ Clavulanate Potassium (Timentin)	Inj: 3 gm-100mg	IV: Adults: ≥60 kg: 3.1 gm (3 gm-100 mg) q4-6h. <60 kg: 200-300 mg/kg/d ticarcillin divided q4-6h. Peds: ≥3 mths & <60 kg: Mild-Moderate: 200 mg/kg/d ticarcillin divided q6h. Severe: 300 mg/kg/d ticarcillin divided q4h. ≥3 mths & ≥60 kg: Mild-Moderate: 3.1 gm q6h. Severe: 3.1 gm q4h.	⊞B ❀> R

MISCELLANEOUS

Clindamycin (Cleocin)	Cap: 75 mg, 150 mg, 300 mg; Inj: 150 mg/ml, 300 mg/50 ml, 600 mg/ 50 ml, 900 mg/50 ml; Susp: 75 mg/5 ml	IM/IV: Adults: 600-2700 mg/d in 2-4 doses. Max: 600 mg IM single dose. Peds: 1 mth-16 yo: 20-40 mg/kg/d given tid-qid. <1 mth: 15-20 mg/kg/d in 3-4 doses. PO: Adults: 150-450 mg q6h. Peds: Cap: 8-20 mg/kg/d in 3-4 doses. Susp: 8-25 mg/kg/d in 3-4 doses.	❀> (PO) ⊞B ❀v (IV) W [84]
Vancomycin HCl	Inj: 500 mg, 1 gm, 5 gm, 10 gm	IV: Adults: 500 mg q6h or 1 gm q12h. Peds: 10 mg/kg q6h. Infants & Neonates: 15 mg/kg x 1 dose, then 10 mg/kg q12h for 1st wk of life & q8h up to 1 mth of age.	⊞C ❀v R

Skin/Skin Structure Infections
CARBAPENEMS

Ertapenem (Invanz)	Inj: 1 gm	Complicated: Adults & Peds: ≥13 yo: 1 gm IM/IV qd. 3 mths-12 yo: 15 mg/kg IM/IV bid. Max: 1 gm/d. Duration: 7-14d. May give IV up to 14d; IM up to 7d.	⊞B ❀> R

NAME	FORM/STRENGTH	DOSAGE	COMMENTS
Meropenem (Merrem)	**Inj:** 500 mg, 1 gm	**Complicated SSSI: IV: Adults:** 500 mg q8h. **Peds: ≥3 mths: >50 kg:** 500 mg q8h. **≤50 kg:** 10 mg/kg q8h. **Max:** 500 mg q8h.	●B ❄> R

CEPHALOSPORINS

NAME	FORM/STRENGTH	DOSAGE	COMMENTS
Cefaclor	**Cap:** 250 mg, 500 mg; **Susp:** 125 mg/5 ml, 187 mg/5 ml, 250 mg/5 ml, 375 mg/5 ml	**Adults: Cap/Susp: Usual:** 250 mg q8h. **Severe Infections:** 500 mg q8h. **Peds: ≥1 mth: Cap/Susp:** 20 mg/kg/d given q8h. **Serious Infections:** 40 mg/kg/d. **Max:** 1 gm/d.	●B ❄>
Cefadroxil	**Cap:** 500 mg; **Susp:** 250 mg/5 ml, 500 mg/5 ml; **Tab:** 1 gm	**Adults:** 1 gm qd or 500 mg bid. **Peds:** 15 mg/kg q12h (or 30 mg/kg qd for impetigo).	●B ❄> R
Cefdinir (Omnicef)	**Cap:** 300 mg; **Susp:** 125 mg/5 ml, 250 mg/5 ml	**Adults & Peds: ≥13 yo: Cap:** 300 mg q12h x 10d. **6 mths-12 yo: Susp:** 7 mg/kg q12h x 10d.	●B ❄> R
Cefepime HCl	**Inj:** 500 mg, 1 gm, 2 gm, 1 gm/50 ml, 2 gm/100 ml	**Adults: Moderate-Severe:** 2 gm IV q12h x 10d. **Peds: 2 mths-16 yo: ≤40 kg:** 50 mg/kg IV q12h. **Max:** Do not exceed adult dose.	●B ❄> R
Cefpodoxime Proxetil (Vantin)	**Susp:** 50 mg/5 ml, 100 mg/5 ml; **Tab:** 100 mg, 200 mg	**Adults & Peds: ≥12 yo:** 400 mg q12h x 7-14d.	●B ❄v R

Cefprozil (Cefzil)	**Susp:** 125 mg/5 ml, 250 mg/5 ml; **Tab:** 250 mg, 500 mg	**Uncomplicated: Adults & Peds: ≥13 yo:** 250-500 mg q12h or 500 mg q24h x 10d. **2-12 yo:** 20 mg/kg q24h x 10d.	⊕B ❀> R
Ceftaroline Fosamil (Teflaro)	**Inj:** 400 mg, 600 mg	**Adults: ≥18 yo: Acute:** 600 mg q12h IV over 1h x 5-14d.	⊕B ❀> R
Ceftazidime (Fortaz)	**Inj:** 500 mg, 1 gm, 2 gm, 6 gm	**Adults:** 500-1000 mg IM/IV q8h. **Peds: 1 mth-12 yo:** 30-50 mg/kg IV q8h. **Max:** 6 gm/d. **Neonates: 0-4 wks:** 30 mg/kg IV q12h.	⊕B ❀> R
Ceftazidime (Tazicef)	**Inj:** 1 gm, 2 gm, 6 gm	**Adults:** 500-1000 mg IM/IV q8h. **Peds: 1 mth-12 yo:** 30-50 mg/kg IV q8h, up to 6 gm/d. **Neonates: 0-4 wks:** 30 mg/kg IV q12h.	⊕B ❀> R
Ceftriaxone Sodium (Rocephin)	**Inj:** (Rocephin) 500 mg, 1 gm; (Generic) 250 mg, 500 mg, 1 gm, 2 gm, 10 gm	**Adults: IV/IM: Usual:** 1-2 gm qd (or in equally divided doses bid). **Max:** 4 gm/d. **Peds: IV/IM:** 50-75 mg/kg qd or in equally divided doses bid. **Max:** 2 gm/d.	⊕B ❀>
Cefuroxime Axetil (Ceftin)	**Susp:** 125 mg/5 ml, 250 mg/5 ml; **Tab:** 250 mg, 500 mg	**Adults & Peds: ≥13 yo: Tab:** 250-500 mg bid x 10d. **3 mths-12 yo: Susp:** 15 mg/kg/d bid x 10d for impetigo.	⊕B ❀v Tabs & susp not bioequivalent. R

NAME	FORM/STRENGTH	DOSAGE	COMMENTS
Cephalexin (Keflex)	(Keflex) **Cap:** 250 mg, 500 mg, 750 mg; (Generic) **Cap:** 250 mg, 500 mg; **Susp:** 125 mg/5 ml, 250 mg/5 ml	**Adults:** 500 mg q12h. **Max:** 4 gm/d. **Peds:** 25-50 mg/kg/d given q12h.	●B ❄>

MACROLIDES

NAME	FORM/STRENGTH	DOSAGE	COMMENTS
Azithromycin (Zithromax)	**Susp:** 100 mg/5 ml, 200 mg/5 ml; **Tab:** 250 mg, 500 mg	**Adults:** 500 mg qd x 1d, then 250 mg qd on Days 2-5.	●B ❄>
Clarithromycin (Biaxin)	**Susp:** 125 mg/5 ml, 250 mg/5 ml; **Tab:** 250 mg, 500 mg	**Adults:** 250 mg q12h x 7-14d. **Peds:** ≥6 mths: 7.5 mg/kg q12h x 10d.	●C ❄> R
Erythromycin (Erythromycin Base)	**Tab:** 250 mg, 500 mg	**Adults:** Usual: 250 mg q6h or 500 mg q12h. **Peds:** Usual: 30-50 mg/kg/d in divided doses. **Max:** 4 gm/d.	●B ❄>
Erythromycin Ethylsuccinate (E.E.S.)	**Susp:** 200 mg/5 ml, 400 mg/5 ml; **Tab:** 400 mg	**Adults:** Usual: 1600 mg/d in divided doses given q6h, q8h, or q12h. **Max:** 4 gm/d. **Peds:** Usual: 30-50 mg/kg/d in divided doses given q6h, q8h, or q12h. May double dose for more severe infections.	●B ❄>
Erythromycin Ethylsuccinate (EryPed)	**Susp:** 200 mg/5 ml, 400 mg/5 ml	**Adults:** Usual: 1600 mg/d in divided doses given q6h, q8h, or q12h. **Max:** 4 gm/d. **Peds:** Usual: 30-50 mg/kg/d in divided doses given q6h, q8h, or q12h. May double dose for more severe infections.	●B ❄>

Erythromycin Stearate (Erythrocin)	**Tab:** 250 mg, 500 mg	**Adults: Usual:** 250 mg q6h or 500 mg q12h. **Peds: Usual:** 30-50 mg/kg/d in divided doses. **Max:** 4 gm/d.	⊕B ❊>
Erythromycin (Ery-Tab)	**Tab,Delay:** 250 mg, 333 mg, 500 mg	**Adults: Usual:** 250 mg qid, 333 mg q8h, or 500 mg q12h. **Peds: Usual:** 30-50 mg/kg/d in divided doses. **Max:** 4 gm/d.	⊕B ❊>
Erythromycin (PCE)	**Tab:** 333 mg, 500 mg	**Adults: Usual:** 333 mg q8h or 500 mg q12h. **Peds: Usual:** 30-50 mg/kg/d in divided doses. **Max:** 4 gm/d.	⊕B ❊>
OXAZOLIDINONE			
Linezolid (Zyvox)	**Inj:** 2 mg/ml; **Susp:** 100 mg/5 ml; **Tab:** 600 mg	**Uncomplicated: Adults:** 400 mg PO q12h x 10-14d. **Peds:** **≥12 yo:** 600 mg PO q12h x 10-14d. **5-11 yo:** 10 mg/kg PO q12h x 10-14d. **<5 yo:** 10 mg/kg PO q8h x 10-14d. **Complicated: Adults & Peds:** **≥12 yo:** 600 mg IV/PO q12h x 10-14d. **Birth-11 yo:** 10 mg/kg IV/PO q8h x 10-14d.	⊕C ❊>
PENICILLINS			
Amoxicillin	**Cap:** 250 mg, 500 mg; **Chewtab:** 125 mg, 250 mg; **Susp:** 125 mg/ 5 ml, 200 mg/5 ml, 250 mg/5ml, 400 mg/ 5 ml; **Tab:** 500 mg, 875 mg	**Adults & Peds: ≥40 kg: Mild-Moderate:** 500 mg q12h or 250 mg q8h. **Severe:** 875 mg q12h or 500 mg q8h. **>3 mths & <40 kg: Mild-Moderate:** 25 mg/kg/d divided q12h or 20 mg/kg/d divided q8h. **Severe:** 45 mg/kg/d divided q12h or 40 mg/kg/d divided q8h. **≤3 mths: Max:** 30 mg/kg/d divided q12h.	⊕B ❊> R

NAME	FORM/STRENGTH	DOSAGE	COMMENTS
Amoxicillin/Clavulanate (Augmentin)	**Chewtab:** 125-31.25 mg, 200-28.5 mg, 250-62.5 mg, 400-57 mg **Tab:** 250-125-31.25 mg, 200-28.5 mg, 250-62.5 mg, 400-57 mg 875-125 mg **Susp:** (per 5 ml) 125 mg, 250-125 mg, 400-57 mg	**Adults & Peds:** Dose based on amoxicillin component. **>40 kg: Tab:** 500-875 mg q12h or 250-500 mg q8h, depending on severity. May use 125 mg/5 ml or 250 mg/5 ml susp in place of 500-mg tab & 200 mg/5 ml susp or 400 mg/5 ml susp in place of 875-mg tab. **>12 wks: Chewtab/Susp:** 25-45 mg/kg/d given q12h or 20-40 mg/kg/d given q8h, depending on severity. **<12 wks: Susp:** 30 mg/kg/d given q12h (use 125 mg/5 ml susp).	⊕B ❄> (2) 250-mg tabs are not equivalent to (1) 500-mg tab. Only use 250-mg tab if peds >40 kg. Chewtab & tab not interchangeable. H R
Ampicillin Sodium/Sulbactam Sodium (Unasyn)	**Inj:** 1-0.5 gm, 2-1 gm	**Adults & Peds: ≥40 kg:** 1.5-3 gm (ampicillin+sulbactam) IV/IM q6h. **Max:** 4 gm sulbactam/d. **Peds: ≥1 yo:** 300 mg/kg/d (ampicillin+sulbactam) IV in equally divided doses q6h. **Max:** 4 gm sulbactam/d. Therapy should not exceed 14d.	⊕B ❄> R
Penicillin V Potassium (Penicillin VK)	**Susp:** 125 mg/5 ml, 250 mg/5 ml. **Tab:** 250 mg, 500 mg	**Adults & Peds: ≥12 yo:** 250-500 mg q6-8h.	⊕X ❄>
Piperacillin Sodium/Tazobactam Sodium (Zosyn)	**Inj:** 2-0.25 gm/50 ml, 3-0.375 gm/50 ml, 4-0.5 gm/100 ml, 2-0.25 gm, 3-0.375 gm, 4-0.5 gm	**Adults:** 3.375 gm IV q6h, infuse over 30 min.	⊕B ❄> R

QUINOLONES

Ciprofloxacin HCl (Cipro Oral)	**Susp:** 250 mg/5 ml, 500 mg/5 ml; **Tab:** 250 mg, 500 mg	**Adults: Mild-Moderate:** 500 mg PO q12h x 7-14d. **Severe-Complicated:** 750 mg PO q12h x 7-14d.	⊞C ❀v R W [98]
Ciprofloxacin (Cipro IV)	**Inj:** 400 mg/200 ml	**Adults: Mild-Moderate:** 400 mg IV q12h x 7-14d. **Severe-Complicated:** 400 mg IV q8h x 7-14d.	⊞C ❀v R W [98]
Levofloxacin (Levaquin)	**Inj:** 5 mg/ml, 25 mg/ml; **Sol:** 25 mg/ml; **Tab:** 250 mg, 500 mg, 750 mg	**Adults: ≥18 yo: Uncomplicated:** 500 mg IV/PO qd x 7-10d. **Complicated:** 750 mg IV/PO qd x 7-14d.	⊞C ❀v R W [98]
Moxifloxacin HCl (Avelox)	**Inj:** 400 mg/250 ml; **Tab:** 400 mg	**Adults: ≥18 yo: Uncomplicated:** 400 mg IV/PO q24h x 7d. **Complicated:** 400 mg IV/PO q24h x 7-21d.	⊞C ❀v W [98]
Ofloxacin	**Tab:** 200 mg, 300 mg, 400 mg	**Adults: ≥18 yo:** 400 mg q12h x 10d.	⊞C ❀v H R W [98]

STREPTOGRAMIN AGENT

Dalfopristin/Quinupristin (Synercid)	**Inj:** 350-150 mg	**Adults & Peds: ≥12 yo: Complicated:** 7.5 mg/kg IV q12h x ≥7d.	⊞B ❀> H

NAME	FORM/STRENGTH	DOSAGE	COMMENTS
TETRACYCLINES			
Doxycycline Hyclate (Doryx)	**Cap, Delay:** 75 mg, 100 mg	**Adults:** 100 mg q12h on Day 1, then 100 mg qd or 50 mg q12h. **Severe:** 100 mg q12h. **Peds: >8 yo & ≤100 lbs:** 1 mg/lb bid on Day 1, then 1 mg/lb qd or 0.5 mg/lb bid. **Severe:** 2 mg/lb. **>100 lbs:** Adult dose.	◐D ❋v
Doxycycline Hyclate (Doxycycline IV)	**Inj:** 100 mg	**Adults:** 200 mg IV divided qd-bid on Day 1, then 100-200 mg/d IV depending on severity of infection, w/ 200 mg administered in 1 or 2 infusions. **Peds: >8 yo & ≤100 lbs:** 2 mg/lb IV divided qd-bid on Day 1, then 1-2 mg/lb/d IV divided qd-bid depending on severity of infection. **>100 lbs:** Adult dose.	◐N ❋>
Doxycycline Monohydrate (Monodox)	**Cap:** 50 mg, 75 mg, 100 mg	**Adults:** 100 mg q12h or 50 mg q6h on Day 1, then 100 mg qd or 50 mg q12h. **Severe:** 100 mg q12h. **Peds: >8 yo & ≤100 lbs:** 1 mg/lb bid on Day 1, then 1 mg/lb qd or 0.5 mg/lb bid. **Severe:** 2 mg/lb. **>100 lbs:** Adult dose.	◐D ❋v
Doxycycline Monohydrate (Vibramycin)	**Cap:** (Hyclate) 100 mg; **Susp:** (Monohydrate) 25 mg/5 ml; **Syr:** (Calcium) 50 mg/5 ml; (Vibra-Tabs) **Tab:** 100 mg	**Adults:** 100 mg q12h on Day 1, then 100 mg/d. **Severe:** 100 mg q12h. **Peds: >8 yo & ≤100 lbs:** 1 mg/lb bid on Day 1, then 1 mg/lb qd or 0.5 mg/lb bid. **Severe:** Up to 2 mg/lb. **>100 lbs:** Adult dose.	◐D ❋v
Minocycline HCl (Dynacin)	**Tab:** 50 mg, 75 mg, 100 mg	**Adults:** 200 mg PO, then 100 mg q12h or 50 mg qid. **Peds: >8 yo:** 4 mg/kg PO, then 2 mg/kg q12h.	◐D ❋v R

| Minocycline HCl (Minocin) | **Cap:** 50 mg, 100 mg; **Inj:** 100 mg | **Adults:** 200 mg PO/IV, then 100 mg q12h or 50 mg qid. **Peds: >8 yo:** 4 mg/kg PO/IV, then 2 mg/kg q12h. | ⊙D ❁v R |

MISCELLANEOUS

Clindamycin (Cleocin)	**Cap:** 75 mg, 150 mg, 300 mg; **Inj:** 150 mg/ml, 300 mg/50 ml, 600 mg/ 50 ml, 900 mg/50 ml; **Susp:** 75 mg/5 ml	**IM/IV: Adults:** 600-2700 mg/d in 2-4 doses. **Max:** 600 mg IM single dose. **Peds: 1 mth-16 yo:** 20-40 mg/kg/d in 3-4 doses. **<1 mth:** 15-20 mg/kg/d in 3-4 doses. **PO: Adults:** 150-450 mg q6h. **Peds: Cap:** 8-20 mg/kg/d given in 3-4 doses. **Susp:** 8-25 mg/kg/d given in 3-4 doses.	⊙B ❁v (IV) ❁> (PO) W [84]
Daptomycin (Cubicin)	**Inj:** 500 mg	**Complicated: Adults:** Administer as IV inj over 2 min or infusion over 30-min period. 4 mg/kg q24h x 7-14d. Do not dose more frequently than qd.	⊙B ❁> R
Telavancin (Vibativ)	**Inj:** 250 mg, 750 mg	**Adults: ≥18 yo:** 10 mg/kg IV infusion over 60 min q24h x 7-14d.	⊙C ❁> Avoid during pregnancy. R
Tigecycline (Tygacil)	**Inj:** 50 mg/5 ml, 50 mg/ 10 ml	**Adults: Initial:** 100 mg IV over 30-60 min. **Maint:** 50 mg IV q12h over 30-60 min x 5-14d.	⊙D ❁> H

NAME	FORM/STRENGTH	DOSAGE	COMMENTS

Upper Respiratory Tract Infection
CEPHALOSPORINS

NAME	FORM/STRENGTH	DOSAGE	COMMENTS
Cefaclor	Cap: 250 mg, 500 mg; Susp: 125 mg/5 ml, 187 mg/5 ml, 250 mg/ 5 ml, 375 mg/5 ml	**Pharyngitis/Tonsillitis: Adults:** Cap/Susp: 250 mg q8h. **Severe Infections:** 500 mg q8h. **Peds:** ≥1 mth: Cap/Susp: 20 mg/kg/d given q8h. **Serious Infections:** 40 mg/kg/d. **Max:** 1 gm/d.	●B ❄>
Cefadroxil	Cap: 500 mg; Susp: 250 mg/5 ml, 500 mg/ 5 ml; Tab: 1 gm	**Adults:** 1 gm qd or 500 mg bid x 10d. **Peds:** 15 mg/kg q12h or 30 mg/kg qd.	●B ❄> R
Cefdinir (Omnicef)	Cap: 300 mg; Susp: 125 mg/5 ml; 250 mg/ 5 ml	**Pharyngitis/Tonsillitis: Adults & Peds: ≥13 yo:** Cap: 300 mg q12h x 5-10d or 600 mg q24h x 10d. **6 mths-12 yo:** Susp: 7 mg/kg q12h x 5-10d or 14 mg/kg q24h x 10d. **Sinusitis: Adults & Peds: ≥13 yo:** Cap: 300 mg q12h or 600 mg q24h x 10d. **6 mths-12 yo:** Susp: 7 mg/kg q12h or 14 mg/kg q24h x 10d.	●B ❄> R
Cefixime (Suprax)	Susp: 100 mg/5 ml; Tab: 400 mg	**Pharyngitis/Tonsillitis: Adults & Peds: >12 yo or >50 kg:** Susp/Tab: 400 mg qd or 200 mg bid. **≤50 kg or >6 mths:** Susp: 8 mg/kg qd or 4 mg/kg bid.	●B ❄v R
Cefpodoxime Proxetil (Vantin)	Susp: 50 mg/5 ml, 100 mg/5 ml; Tab: 100 mg, 200 mg	**Pharyngitis/Tonsillitis: Adults & Peds: ≥12 yo:** 100 mg q12h x 5-10d. **2 mths-11 yo:** 5 mg/kg q12h x 5-10d. **Sinusitis: Adults & Peds: ≥12 yo:** 200 mg q12h x 10d. **2 mths-11 yo:** 5 mg/kg q12h x 10d.	●B ❄v R

Cefprozil (Cefzil)	**Susp:** 125 mg/5 ml, 250 mg/5 ml; **Tab:** 250 mg, 500 mg	**Pharyngitis/Tonsillitis: Adults & Peds: ≥13 yo:** 500 mg q24h x 10d. **2-12 yo:** 7.5 mg/kg q12h x 10d. **Max:** Adult dose. **Sinusitis: Adults & Peds: ≥13 yo:** 250-500 mg q12h x 10d. **6 mths-12 yo:** 7.5-15 mg/kg q12h x 10d. **Max:** Adult dose.	⊕B ✿> R
Cefuroxime Axetil (Ceftin)	**Susp:** 125 mg/5 ml, 250 mg/5 ml; **Tab:** 250 mg, 500 mg	**Pharyngitis/Tonsillitis/Sinusitis: Adults & Peds: ≥13 yo: Tab:** 250 mg bid x 10d. **3 mths-12 yo: Pharyngitis/Tonsillitis: Susp:** 10 mg/kg bid x 10d. **Tab:** 125 mg bid x 10d. **Max:** 500 mg/d. **Sinusitis: Susp:** 15 mg/kg bid x 10d. **Tab:** 250 mg bid x 10d. **Max:** 1 gm/d.	⊕B ✿v Tabs & susp not bioequivalent. R
Cephalexin (Keflex)	(Keflex) **Cap:** 250 mg, 500 mg, 750 mg; (Generic) **Cap:** 250 mg, 500 mg; **Susp:** 125 mg/5 ml, 250 mg/5 ml	**Adults: Usual:** 250 mg q6h. **Streptococcal Pharyngitis:** 500 mg q12h. **Max:** 4 gm/d. **Peds: >1 yo: Usual:** 25-50 mg/kg/d given q12h.	⊕B ✿>

MACROLIDES

| Azithromycin (Zithromax) | **Susp:** 100 mg/5 ml, 200 mg/5 ml; **Tab:** 250 mg, 500 mg | **Pharyngitis/Tonsillitis: Adults:** 500 mg on Day 1, then 250 mg qd on Days 2-5. **Peds: ≥2 yo:** 12 mg/kg/d x 5d. **Acute Bacterial Sinusitis: Adults:** 500 mg qd x 3d. **Peds: ≥6 mths:** 10 mg/kg/d x 3d. | ⊕B ✿> |
| Azithromycin (Zmax) | **Susp, ER:** 2 gm | **Adults: Acute Bacterial Sinusitis:** 2 gm single dose on an empty stomach (at least 1h ac or 2h pc). | ⊕B ✿> |

NAME	FORM/STRENGTH	DOSAGE	COMMENTS
Clarithromycin (Biaxin)	**Susp:** 125 mg/5 ml, 250 mg/5 ml; **Tab:** 250 mg, 500 mg	**Adults: Pharyngitis/Tonsillitis:** 250 mg q12h x 10d. **Sinusitis:** 500 mg q12h x 14d. **Peds: ≥6 mths:** Usual: 7.5 mg/kg q12h x 10d.	▣C ❄>R
Erythromycin (Erythromycin Base)	**Tab:** 250 mg, 500 mg	**Adults:** Usual: 250 mg q6h or 500 mg q12h. **Peds:** Usual: 30-50 mg/kg/d in divided doses. **Max:** 4 gm/d.	▣B ❄>
Erythromycin Ethylsuccinate (E.E.S.)	**Susp:** 200 mg/5 ml, 400 mg/5 ml; **Tab:** 400 mg	**Adults:** Usual: 1600 mg/d in divided doses given q6h, q8h, or q12h. **Max:** 4 gm/d. **Peds:** Usual: 30-50 mg/kg/d in divided doses given q6h, q8h, or q12h. May double dose for more severe infections.	▣B ❄>
Erythromycin Ethylsuccinate (EryPed)	**Susp:** 200 mg/5 ml, 400 mg/5 ml	**Adults:** Usual: 1600 mg/d in divided doses given q6h, q8h, or q12h. **Max:** 4 gm/d. **Peds:** Usual: 30-50 mg/kg/d in divided doses given q6h, q8h, or q12h. May double dose for more severe infections.	▣B ❄>
Erythromycin Stearate (Erythrocin)	**Tab:** 250 mg, 500 mg	**Adults:** Usual: 250 mg q6h or 500 mg q12h. **Peds:** Usual: 30-50 mg/kg/d in divided doses. **Max:** 4 gm/d.	▣B ❄>
Erythromycin (Ery-Tab)	**Tab, Delay:** 250 mg, 333 mg, 500 mg	**Adults:** Usual: 250 mg qid, 333 mg q8h, or 500 mg q12h. **Peds:** Usual: 30-50 mg/kg/d in divided doses. **Max:** 4 gm/d.	▣B ❄>
Erythromycin (PCE)	**Tab:** 333 mg, 500 mg	**Adults:** Usual: 333 mg q8h or 500 mg q12h. **Peds:** Usual: 30-50 mg/kg/d in divided doses. **Max:** 4 gm/d.	▣B ❄>

Amoxicillin	Cap: 250 mg, 500 mg; Chewtab: 125 mg, 250 mg; Susp: 125 mg/5 ml, 200 mg/5 ml, 250 mg/5 ml, 400 mg/5 ml; Tab: 500 mg, 875 mg	Adults & Peds: ≥40 kg: Mild-Moderate: 500 mg q12h or 250 mg q8h. Severe: 875 mg q12h or 500 mg q8h. >3 mths & <40 kg: Mild-Moderate: 25 mg/kg/d divided q12h or 20 mg/kg/d divided q8h. Severe: 45 mg/kg/d divided q12h or 40 mg/kg/d divided q8h. ≤3 mths: Max: 30 mg/kg/d divided q12h.	⊕B ✿> R
Amoxicillin/Clavulanate (Augmentin)	Chewtab: 125-31.25 mg, 200-28.5 mg, 250-62.5 mg, 400-57 mg; Susp: (per 5 ml) 125-31.25 mg, 200-28.5 mg, 250-62.5 mg, 400-57 mg; Tab: 250-125 mg, 500-125 mg, 875-125 mg	Adults & Peds: Dose based on amoxicillin component. ≥40 kg: Tab: 500-875 mg q12h or 250-500 mg q8h, depending on severity. May use 125 mg/5 ml or 250 mg/5 ml susp in place of 500-mg tab & 200 mg/5 ml susp or 400 mg/5 ml susp in place of 875-mg tab. ≥12 wks: Chewtab/Susp: 25-45 mg/kg/d given q12h or 20-40 mg/kg/d given q8h, depending on severity. <12 wks: Susp: 30 mg/kg/d given q12h (use 125 mg/5 ml susp).	⊕B ✿> (2) 250-mg tabs are not equivalent to (1) 500-mg tab. Only use 250-mg tab if peds ≥40 kg. Chewtab & tab not interchangeable. H R
Ampicillin Sodium	Inj: 250 mg, 500 mg, 1 gm, 2 gm, 10 gm	IM/IV: Adults & Peds: ≥40 kg: 250-500 mg q6h. <40 kg: 25-50 mg/kg/d given q6-8h.	⊕B ✿>
Ampicillin	Cap: 250 mg, 500 mg; Susp: 125 mg/5 ml, 250 mg/5 ml	Adults & Peds: >20 kg: 250 mg qid. ≤20 kg: 50 mg/kg/d given tid-qid.	⊕B ✿v

NAME	FORM/STRENGTH	DOSAGE	COMMENTS
Amoxicillin/ Clavulanate Potassium (Augmentin XR)	Tab,ER: 1000-62.5 mg	Sinusitis: Adults & Peds: ≥40 kg: 2 tabs q12h x10d.	B ▦ ✲< H R
Penicillin V Potassium (Penicillin VK)	Susp: 125 mg/5 ml, 250 mg/5 ml; Tab: 250 mg, 500 mg	Adults & Peds: ≥12 yo: Streptococcal: 125-250 mg q6-8h. Fusospirochetosis: (Oropharynx) 250-500 mg q6-8h x10d. Pneumococcal: 250-500 mg q6h until afebrile x2d.	ON ✲<
QUINOLONES			
Ciprofloxacin HCl (Cipro Oral)	Susp: 250 mg/5 ml, 500 mg/5 ml; Tab: 250 mg, 500 mg	Mild-Moderate Acute Sinusitis: Adults: 500 mg PO q12h x10d.	OC ✲∨ R W[98]
Ciprofloxacin (Cipro IV)	Inj: 400 mg/200 ml	Mild-Moderate Acute Sinusitis: Adults: 400 mg IV q12h x10d.	OC ✲∨ R W[98]
Levofloxacin (Levaquin)	Inj: 5 mg/ml, 25 mg/ml; Sol: 25 mg/ml; Tab: 250 mg, 500 mg, 750 mg	Adults: ≥18 yo: Acute Bacterial Sinusitis: 500 mg IV/PO qd x 10-14d or 750 mg IV/PO qd x 5d.	OC ✲∨ R W[98]
Moxifloxacin HCl (Avelox)	Tab: 400 mg; Inj: 400 mg/250 ml;	Sinusitis: Adults: ≥18 yo: 400 mg PO/IV q24h x10d.	OC ✲∨ W[98]
TETRACYCLINES			
Demeclocycline HCl	Tab: 150 mg, 300 mg	Adults: 150 mg qid or 300 mg bid. Peds: ≥8 yo: 7-13 mg/kg/d given bid-qid.	DD ✲∨

Doxycycline Hyclate (Doryx)	**Cap,Delay:** 75 mg, 100 mg	**Adults:** 100 mg q12h on Day 1, then 100 mg qd or 50 mg q12h. **Severe:** 100 mg q12h. **Peds: >8 yo & ≤100 lbs:** 1 mg/lb bid on Day 1, then 1 mg/lb qd or 0.5 mg/lb bid. **Severe:** 2 mg/lb. **>100 lbs:** Adult dose.	⊕D ❋v
Doxycycline Hyclate (Doxycycline IV)	**Inj:** 100 mg	**Adults:** 200 mg IV divided qd-bid on Day 1, then 100-200 mg/d IV depending on severity of infection, w/ 200 mg administered in 1 or 2 infusions. **Peds: >8 yo & ≤100 lbs:** 2 mg/lb IV divided qd-bid on Day 1, then 1-2 mg/lb/day IV divided qd-bid depending on severity of infection. **>100 lbs:** Adult dose.	⊕N ❋>
Doxycycline Monohydrate (Monodox)	**Cap:** 50 mg, 75 mg, 100 mg	**Adults:** 100 mg q12h or 50 mg q6h on Day 1, then 100 mg qd or 50 mg q12h. **Severe:** 100 mg q12h. **Peds: >8 yo & ≤100 lbs:** 1 mg/lb bid on Day 1, then 1 mg/lb qd or 0.5 mg/lb bid. **Severe:** 2 mg/lb. **>100 lbs:** Adult dose.	⊕D ❋v
Doxycycline Monohydrate (Vibramycin)	**Cap:** (Hyclate) 100 mg; **Susp:** (Monohydrate) 25 mg/5 ml; **Syr:** (Calcium) 50 mg/5 ml; (Vibra-Tabs) **Tab:** 100 mg	**Adults:** 100 mg q12h on Day 1, then 100 mg/d. **Severe:** 100 mg q12h. **Peds: >8 yo & ≤100 lbs:** 1 mg/lb bid on Day 1, then 1 mg/lb qd or 0.5 mg/lb bid. **Severe:** Up to 2 mg/lb. **>100 lbs:** Adult dose.	⊕D ❋v
Minocycline HCI (Dynacin)	**Tab:** 50 mg, 75 mg, 100 mg	**Adults:** 200 mg PO, then 100 mg q12h or 50 mg qid. **Peds: >8 yo:** 4 mg/kg PO, then 2 mg/kg q12h.	⊕D ❋v R
Minocycline HCI (Minocin)	**Cap:** 50 mg, 100 mg; **Inj:** 100 mg	**Adults:** 200 mg PO/IV, then 100 mg q12h or 50 mg qid. **Peds: >8 yo:** 4 mg/kg PO/IV, then 2 mg/kg q12h.	⊕D ❋v R

NAME	FORM/STRENGTH	DOSAGE	COMMENTS
Tetracycline HCl (Sumycin)	**Cap:** 250 mg, 500 mg; **Susp:** 125 mg/5 ml	**Adults:** 250 mg qid or 500 mg bid. **Peds: >8 yo:** 25-50 mg/kg divided bid-qid.	⊕D ❄v R

Urinary Tract Infection

CARBAPENEMS

NAME	FORM/STRENGTH	DOSAGE	COMMENTS
Doripenem (Doribax)	**Inj:** 250 mg, 500 mg	**Complicated UTI/Pyelonephritis: Adults: ≥18 yo:** 500 mg IV q8h x 10d. Infuse over 1h.	⊕B ❄> R
Ertapenem (Invanz)	**Inj:** 1 gm	**Complicated UTI/Acute Pelvic Infections: Adults & Peds:** **≥13 yo:** 1 gm IM/IV qd. **3 mths-12 yo:** 15 mg/kg IM/IV bid. **Max:** 1 gm/d. **Duration: Complicated UTI:** 10-14d. **Acute Pelvic Infections:** 3-10d. May give IV up to 14d; IM up to 7d.	⊕B ❄> R

CEPHALOSPORINS

NAME	FORM/STRENGTH	DOSAGE	COMMENTS
Cefaclor	**Cap:** 250 mg, 500 mg; **Susp:** 125 mg/5 ml, 187 mg/5 ml, 250 mg/ 5 ml, 375 mg/5 ml	**Adults:** 250 mg q8h. **Severe Infections:** 500 mg q8h. **Peds: ≥1 mth:** 20 mg/kg/d q8h. **Serious Infections:** 40 mg/kg/d. **Max:** 1 gm/d.	⊕B ❄>
Cefadroxil	**Cap:** 500 mg; **Susp:** 250 mg/5 ml, 500 mg/ 5 ml; **Tab:** 1 gm	**Adults: Uncomplicated Lower UTI:** 1-2 gm/d given qd-bid. **Other UTIs:** 1 gm bid. **Peds:** 15 mg/kg q12h.	⊕B ❄> R

Cefepime HCl	Inj: 500 mg, 1 gm, 2 gm, 1 gm/50 ml, 2 gm/100 ml	Adults: Mild-Moderate: 0.5-1 gm IM/IV q12h x 7-10d. Severe: 2 gm IV q12h x 10d. Peds: 2 mths-16 yo: ≤40 kg: 50 mg/kg IV q12h. Max: Do not exceed adult dose.	⊕B ✿> R
Cefixime (Suprax)	Susp: 100 mg/5 ml; Tab: 400 mg	Adults & Peds: >12 yo or >50 kg: Susp/Tab: 400 mg qd or 200 mg bid. ≤50 kg or >6 mths: Susp: 8 mg/kg qd or 4 mg/kg bid.	⊕B ✿v R
Cefpodoxime Proxetil (Vantin)	Susp: 50 mg/5 ml, 100 mg/5 ml; Tab: 100 mg, 200 mg	Uncomplicated UTI: Adults & Peds: ≥12 yo: 100 mg q12h x 7d.	⊕B ✿v R
Ceftazidime (Fortaz)	Inj: 500 mg, 1 gm, 2 gm, 6 gm	Adults: Uncomplicated UTI: 250 mg IM/IV q12h. Complicated UTI: 500 mg IM/IV q8-12h. Peds: 1 mth-12 yo: 30-50 mg/kg IV q8h, up to 6 gm/d. Neonates: 0-4 wks: 30 mg/kg IV q12h.	⊕B ✿> R
Ceftazidime (Tazicef)	Inj: 1 gm, 2 gm, 6 gm	Adults: Uncomplicated UTI: 250 mg IM/IV q12h. Complicated UTI: 500 mg IM/IV q8-12h. Peds: 1 mth-12 yo: 30-50 mg/kg IV q8h, up to 6 gm/d. Neonates: 0-4 wks: 30 mg/kg IV q12h.	⊕B ✿> R
Ceftriaxone Sodium (Rocephin)	Inj: (Rocephin) 500 mg, 1 gm; (Generic) 250 mg, 500 mg, 1 gm, 2 gm, 10 gm	Adults: IM/IV: Usual: 1-2 gm qd (or in equally divided doses bid). Max: 4 gm/d.	⊕B ✿>
Cefuroxime (Zinacef)	Inj: 750 mg, 1.5 gm, 7.5 gm	IM/IV: Adults: Uncomplicated UTI: 750 mg q8h x 5-10d. Severe-Complicated UTI: 1.5 gm q8h x 5-10d. Peds: >3 mths: 50-100 mg/kg/d given q6-8h. Max: 4.5 gm/d.	⊕B ✿> R

NAME	FORM/STRENGTH	DOSAGE	COMMENTS
Cefuroxime Axetil (Ceftin)	**Tab:** 250 mg, 500 mg	**Adults & Peds:** ≥13 yo: 125-250 mg bid x 7-10d.	▣B ❀v R
Cephalexin (Keflex)	(Keflex) **Cap:** 250 mg, 500 mg, 750 mg; (Generic) **Cap:** 250 mg, 500 mg; **Susp:** 125 mg/5 ml, 250 mg/5 ml	**Adults:** Usual: 250 mg q6h. **Uncomplicated Cystitis:** 500 mg q12h x 7-14d. **Max:** 4 gm/d. **Peds:** Usual: 25-50 mg/kg/d in divided doses.	▣B ❀>

MACROLIDE

NAME	FORM/STRENGTH	DOSAGE	COMMENTS
Azithromycin (Zithromax)	**Inj:** 500 mg; **Susp:** 100 mg/5 ml, 200 mg/5 ml, 1 gm/pkt; **Tab:** 250 mg, 500 mg, 600 mg	**Adults: Genital Ulcer Disease/Nongonococcal Urethritis & Cervicitis:** Single 1 gm dose. **Gonococcal Urethritis & Cervicitis:** Single 2 gm dose. **PID:** 500 mg IV qd x 1-2d followed by 250 mg PO qd to complete 7d course of therapy.	▣B ❀>

PENICILLINS

NAME	FORM/STRENGTH	DOSAGE	COMMENTS
Amoxicillin	**Cap:** 250 mg, 500 mg; **Chewtab:** 125 mg, 250 mg; **Susp:** 125 mg/5 ml, 200 mg/5 ml, 250 mg/5 ml, 400 mg/5 ml; **Tab:** 500 mg, 875 mg	**Adults & Peds: ≥40 kg: Mild-Moderate:** 500 mg q12h or 250 mg q8h. **Severe:** 875 mg q12h or 500 mg q8h. **>3 mths & <40 kg: Mild-Moderate:** 25 mg/kg/d divided q12h or 20 mg/kg/d divided q8h. **Severe:** 45 mg/kg/d divided q12h or 40 mg/kg/d divided q8h. **≤3 mths: Max:** 30 mg/kg/d divided q12h.	▣B ❀> R

Amoxicillin/Clavulanate (Augmentin)	Chewtab: 125-31.25 mg, 200-28.5 mg, 250-62.5 mg, 400-57 mg; Susp: (per 5 ml) 125-31.25 mg, 200-28.5 mg, 250-62.5 mg, 400-57 mg; Tab: 250-125 mg, 500-125 mg, 875-125 mg	Adults & Peds: Dose based on amoxicillin component. ≥40 kg: Tab: 500 mg q12h or 250 mg q8h. May use 125 mg/5 ml or 250 mg/5 ml susp in place of 500-mg tab & 200 mg/5 ml or 400 mg/5 ml susp in place of 875-mg tab. ≥12 wks: Chewtab/Susp: 25 mg/kg/d given q12h or 20 mg/kg/d given q8h. <12 wks: Susp: 30 mg/kg/d q12h (use 125 mg/5 ml susp).	⊕B ✿> (2) 250-mg tabs are not equivalent to (1) 500-mg tab. Only use 250-mg tab if peds ≥40 kg. Chewtab & tab not interchangeable. H R
Ampicillin	Cap: 250 mg, 500 mg; Susp: 125 mg/5 ml, 250 mg/5 ml	GU Tract: Adults & Peds: >20 kg: 500 mg qid. ≤20 kg: 100 mg/kg/d given qid.	⊕B ✿v
QUINOLONES			
Ciprofloxacin HCl (Cipro Oral)	Susp: 250 mg/5 ml, 500 mg/5 ml; Tab: 250 mg, 500 mg	Adults: Acute Uncomplicated UTI: 250 mg PO q12h x 3d. Mild-Moderate UTI: 250 mg PO q12h x 7-14d. Severe-Complicated UTI: 500 mg PO q12h x 7-14d. Mild-Moderate Chronic Bacterial Prostatitis: 500 mg PO q12h x 28d. Uncomplicated Urethral & Cervical Gonococcal Infections: 250 mg PO as single dose. Peds: 1-17 yo: Complicated UTI/Pyelonephritis: 10-20 mg/kg PO q12h x 10-21d. Max: 750 mg PO per dose.	⊕C ✿v R W [98]

NAME	FORM/STRENGTH	DOSAGE	COMMENTS
Ciprofloxacin HCl (Proquin XR)	**Tab,ER:** 500 mg	**Adults:** 500 mg qd x 3d.	⊕C ❄v W [98]
Ciprofloxacin (Cipro IV)	**Inj:** 400 mg/200 ml	**Adults: Mild-Moderate UTI:** 200 mg IV q12h x 7 14d. **Severe-Complicated UTI:** 400 mg IV q12h x 7-14d. **Chronic Bacterial Prostatitis:** 400 mg IV q12h x 28d. **Peds: 1-17 yo: Complicated UTI/Pyelonephritis:** 6-10 mg/kg IV q8h x 10-21d. **Max:** 400 mg IV per dose.	⊕C ❄v R W [98]
Ciprofloxacin (Cipro XR)	**Tab,ER:** 500 mg, 1000 mg	**Adults: Uncomplicated UTI (Acute Cystitis):** 500 mg q24h x 3d. **Complicated UTI/Acute Uncomplicated Pyelonephritis:** 1000 mg q24h x 7-14d.	⊕C ❄v R W [98]
Levofloxacin (Levaquin)	**Inj:** 5 mg/ml, 25 mg/ml; **Sol:** 25 mg/ml; **Tab:** 250 mg, 500 mg, 750 mg	**Adults: ≥18 yo: Complicated UTI/Acute Pyelonephritis:** 250 mg IV/PO qd x 10d or 750 mg IV/PO qd x 5d. **Uncomplicated UTI:** 250 mg IV/PO qd x 3d. **Chronic Bacterial Prostatitis:** 500 mg IV/PO qd x 28d.	⊕C ❄v R W [98]
Norfloxacin (Noroxin)	**Tab:** 400 mg	**Adults: Uncomplicated UTI:** 400 mg q12h x 3d (*K. pneumoniae, E. coli,* or *P. mirabilis*), or x 7-10d (other organisms). **Complicated UTI:** 400 mg q12h x 10-21d. **Acute/Chronic Prostatitis:** 400 mg q12h x 28d.	⊕C ❄v R W [98]
Ofloxacin	**Tab:** 200 mg, 300 mg, 400 mg	**Adults: ≥18 yo: Nongonococcal Cervicitis/Urethritis (C. trachomatis) or Mixed Infection of Urethra & Cervix (C. trachomatis & N.gonorrhoeae):** 300 mg q12h x 7d. **Acute PID:** 400 mg q12h x 10-14d. **Uncomplicated Cystitis:** 200 mg q12h x 3d (*E. coli* or *K. pneumoniae*) or 7d (other	⊕C ❄v H R W [98]

pathogens). **Complicated UTI:** 200 mg q12h x 10d.
Prostatitis (*E. coli*): 300 mg q12h x 6 wks.

SULFONAMIDES AND COMBINATIONS

Sulfamethoxazole/ Trimethoprim (Septra, Septra DS, Sulfatrim Pediatric)	**Susp:** 200-40 mg/5 ml; **Tab:** (SS) 400-80 mg, (DS) 800-160 mg	**PO: Adults:** 800 mg SMX & 160 mg TMP (1 DS tab, 2 SS tabs, or 20 ml) q12h x 10-14d. **Peds: ≥2 mths:** 4 mg/kg TMP & 20 mg/kg SMX q12h x 10d. **Severe: Adults & Peds: IV:** 8-10 mg/kg/d (based on TMP) given q6-12h up to 14d.	⊙C ❄v **R** Cl in pregnancy & nursing.

TETRACYCLINES

Doxycycline Hyclate (Doryx)	**Cap,Delay:** 75 mg, 100 mg	**Adults:** 100 mg q12h on Day 1, then 100 mg qd or 50 mg q12h. **Peds: >8 yo & ≤100 lbs:** 1 mg/lb bid on Day 1, then 1 mg/lb qd or 0.5 mg/lb bid. **>100 lbs:** Adult dose.	⊙D ❄v
Doxycycline Hyclate (Doxycycline IV)	**Inj:** 100 mg	**Adults:** 200 mg IV divided qd-bid on Day 1, then 100-200 mg/d IV depending on severity of infection, w/ 200 mg administered in 1 or 2 infusions. **Peds: >8 yo & ≤100 lbs:** 2 mg/lb IV divided qd-bid on Day 1, then 1-2 mg/lb/d IV divided qd-bid depending on severity of infection. **>100 lbs:** Adult dose.	⊙N ❄>
Doxycycline Monohydrate (Monodox)	**Cap:** 50 mg, 75 mg, 100 mg	**Adults:** 100 mg q12h or 50 mg q6h on Day 1, then 100 mg qd or 50 mg q12h. **Severe:** 100 mg q12h. **Peds: >8 yo & ≤100 lbs:** 1 mg/lb bid on Day 1, then 1 mg/lb qd or 0.5 mg/lb bid. **Severe:** 2 mg/lb. **>100 lbs:** Adult dose.	⊙D ❄v

NAME	FORM/STRENGTH	DOSAGE	COMMENTS
Doxycycline Monohydrate (Vibramycin)	**Cap:** (Hyclate) 100 mg; **Susp:** (Monohydrate) 25 mg/5 ml; **Syr:** (Calcium) 50 mg/5 ml; (Vibra-Tabs) **Tab:** 100 mg	**Adults:** 100 mg q12h on Day 1, then 100 mg/d. **Severe:** 100 mg q12h. **Peds: >8 yo & ≤100 lbs:** 1 mg/lb bid on Day 1, then 1 mg/lb qd or 0.5 mg/lb bid. **Severe:** Up to 2 mg/lb. **>100 lbs:** Adult dose.	✚D ❋v
Minocycline HCl (Dynacin)	**Tab:** 50 mg, 75 mg, 100 mg	**Adults:** 200 mg PO, then 100 mg q12h or 50 mg qid. **Peds: >8 yo:** 4 mg/kg PO, then 2 mg/kg q12h.	✚D ❋v R
Minocycline HCl (Minocin)	**Cap:** 50 mg, 100 mg; **Inj:** 100 mg	**Adults:** 200 mg PO/IV, then 100 mg q12h or 50 mg qid. **Peds: >8 yo:** 4 mg/kg PO/IV, then 2 mg/kg q12h.	✚D ❋v R
Tetracycline HCl (Sumycin)	**Cap:** 250 mg, 500 mg; **Susp:** 125 mg/5 ml	**Adults:** 250 mg qid or 500 mg bid. **Peds: >8 yo:** 25-50 mg/kg divided bid-qid.	✚D ❋v R

MISCELLANEOUS

NAME	FORM/STRENGTH	DOSAGE	COMMENTS
Nitrofurantoin Macrocrystals/ Nitrofurantoin Monohydrate (Macrobid)	**Cap:** 100 mg	**Adults & Peds: >12 yo:** 100 mg q12h x 7d.	✚B ❋v R
Nitrofurantoin, Macrocrystals (Macrodantin)	**Cap:** 25 mg, 50 mg, 100 mg	**Adults:** 50-100 mg qid for 1 wk or at least 3 days after sterility of the urine obtained. **Long-Term Suppressive Use:** 50-100mg q hs. **Peds: ≥1 mth:** 5-7 mg/kg/d given in 4 divided doses for 1 wk or at least 3 days after sterility of the urine obtained. **Long-Term Suppressive Use:** 1 mg/kg/d given in single dose or in 2 divided doses.	✚B ❋v R

Nitrofurantoin (Furadantin)	**Susp:** 25 mg/5 ml	**Adults:** 50-100 mg qid x 7d. **Peds:** >1 mth: 5-7 mg/kg/d divided qid x 7d.	⊕B ❖v R

Miscellaneous Anti-Infectives

Ciprofloxacin HCl (Cipro Oral)	**Susp:** 250 mg/5 ml, 500 mg/5 ml; **Tab:** 250 mg, 500 mg	**Adults: Complicated Intra-Abdominal (w/ Metronidazole):** 500 mg q12h x 7-14d. **Infectious Diarrhea:** 500 mg q12h x 5-7d.	⊕C ❖v R W [98]
Daptomycin (Cubicin)	**Inj:** 500 mg	***S. aureus* Bacteremia: Adults:** Administer as IV inj over 2 min or infusion over 30 min period. 6 mg/kg q24h x 2-6 wks. Limited safety data for use >28d. Do not dose more frequently than qd.	⊕B ❖> R
Doripenem (Doribax)	**Inj:** 250 mg, 500 mg	**Complicated Intra-Abdominal Infection: Adults:** ≥18 yo: 500 mg q8h IV over 1h x 5-14d.	⊕B ❖> R
Fidaxomicin (Dificid)	**Tab:** 200 mg	***Clostridium difficile*-Associated Diarrhea: Adults:** ≥18 yo: **Usual:** 200 mg bid x 10d w/or w/o food.	⊕B ❖>
Tinidazole (Tindamax)	**Tab:** 250 mg, 500 mg	**Giardiasis: Adults:** 2 gm single dose. **Peds:** >3 yo: 50 mg/kg single dose. **Max:** 2 gm/d. **Amebiasis: Intestinal: Adults:** 2 gm qd x 3d. **Peds:** >3 yo: 50 mg/kg qd x 3d. **Max:** 2 gm/d. **Amebic Liver Abscess: Adults:** 2 gm qd x 3-5d. **Peds:** >3 yo: 50 mg/kg qd x 3-5d. **Max:** 2 gm/d. Take w/ food.	⊕C ❖v CI in 1st trimester. W [83]

NAME	FORM/STRENGTH	DOSAGE	COMMENTS

ANTINEOPLASTICS

Antineoplastics

NAME	FORM/STRENGTH	DOSAGE	COMMENTS
Anastrozole (Arimidex)	Tab: 1 mg	**Adults: Postmenopausal Women: Adjuvant in Breast Cancer /1st-line Treatment of Advanced or Metastatic Breast Cancer/Treatment of Advanced Breast Cancer Following Tamoxifen:** 1 mg qd.	⊕X ❀v
Bicalutamide (Casodex)	Tab: 50 mg	**Stage D2 Metastatic Carcinoma of the Prostate: Adults:** 50 mg qd. Initiate w/ LHRH analog therapy.	⊕X ❀v **W** [3]
Cabazitaxel (Jevtana)	Inj: 60 mg/1.5 mL	**Hormone-Refractory Metastatic Prostate Cancer: Adults:** 25 mg/m² over 1h IV infusion q3wks in combination w/ PO prednisone 10 mg qd. Refer to PI for dosing modifications if experience adverse reactions.	⊕D ❀v Neutropenic deaths reported. Severe hypersensitivity can occur. **H**
Cetuximab (Erbitux)	Inj: 2 mg/ml	**Adults:** Premedication w/ H₁-antagonist (eg, diphenhydramine 50 mg IV) recommended; see PI. **Squamous Cell Carcinoma of Head & Neck (SCCHN): Combination Therapy: Initial:** 400 mg/m² IV over 120 min 1 wk prior to initiation of a course of radiation treatment or on the day of initiation of platinum-based therapy w/ 5-FU. Complete administration 1h prior to platinum-based therapy w/ 5-FU. **Maint:** 250 mg/m² IV over 60 min qwk for duration of radiation therapy (6-7 wks) or until disease	⊕C ❀v Infusion reactions and cardiopulmonary arrest.

		progression or unacceptable toxicity w/ platinum-based therapy w/ 5-FU. Complete administration 1h prior to radiation or platinum-based therapy w/ 5-FU. **SCCHN (Monotherapy)/Metastatic Colorectal Cancer (Monotherapy/In Combination w/ Irinotecan): Initial:** 400 mg/m^2 IV over 120 min. **Maint:** 250 mg/m^2 IV over 60 min qwk until disease progression or unacceptable toxicity. Adjust dose based on infusion reactions/dermatologic toxicity; see PI. **Max Infusion Rate:** 10 mg/min.	
Cisplatin	**Inj:** 50 mg, 100 mg	**Adults: Metastatic Testicular Tumors:** 20 mg/m^2 IV qd x 5d/cycle in combination w/ other approved chemo agents. **Metastatic Ovarian Tumors (w/ cyclophosphamide):** 75-100 mg/m^2 IV/cycle once q4wks. **Monotherapy:** 100 mg/m^2 IV/cycle once q4wks. **Advanced Bladder Cancer:** 50-70 mg/m^2 IV/cycle once q3-4wks. **Heavily Pretreated Patients: Initial:** 50 mg/m^2/cycle q4wks. Pre-hydrate w/ fluid 8-12h before therapy. **All Patients: Pretreatment Hydration/Repeat Course Parameters:** See PI.	⊕D ✿v Renal toxicity, ototoxicity, anaphylactoid reactions. **W** [3]

NAME	FORM/STRENGTH	DOSAGE	COMMENTS
Dasatinib (Sprycel)	**Tab:** 20 mg, 50 mg, 70 mg, 80 mg, 100 mg, 140 mg.	**Adults: Chronic Phase CML: Initial:** 100 mg qd. **Titrate:** If no response, increase to 140 mg qd. **Accelerated Phase CML/Myeloid or Lymphoid Blast Phase CML/Ph+ ALL: Initial:** 140 mg qd. **Titrate:** If no response, increase to 180 mg qd. **Concomitant Strong CYP3A4 Inducers:** Consider dose increase. **Concomitant Strong CYP3A4 Inhibitors:** Consider dose decrease to 20 mg qd (if taking 100 mg qd) or 40 mg qd (if taking 140 mg qd).	◉D ❄v Severe thrombocytopenia, neutropenia, anemia.
Degarelix (Firmagon)	**Inj:** 80 mg, 120 mg	**Adults: Initial:** 240 mg (as two SC injections of 120 mg) at 40 mg/ml conc. **Maint:** 80 mg SC q28 d at 20 mg/ml conc.	◉X ❄v
Erlotinib (Tarceva)	**Tab:** 25 mg, 100 mg, 150 mg	**Adults:** Take ≥1h ac or 2h pc. **Non-Small Cell Lung Cancer:** 150 mg qd. **Pancreatic Cancer:** 100 mg qd, in combination w/ gemcitabine. Continue until disease progression or unacceptable toxicity occurs.	◉D ❄v
Everolimus (Afinitor)	**Tab:** 2.5 mg, 5 mg, 7.5 mg, 10 mg	**Adults: Advanced Renal Cell Carcinoma/Progressive Neuroendocrine Tumors of Pancreatic Origin/Renal Angiomyolipoma w/ Tuberous Sclerosis Complex:** 10 mg qd. **Adults & Peds: ≥3 yo: Subependymal Giant Cell Astrocytoma: Initial: BSA: 0.5-1.2 m^2:** 2.5 mg qd. **1.3-2.1 m^2:** 5 mg qd. **≥2.2 m^2:** 7.5 mg qd. **Severe or Intolerable Adverse Reactions/Concomitant Moderate CYP3A4 or P-gp Inhibitors & CYP3A4 Inducers:** Refer to PI.	◉D ❄v H

Exemestane (Aromasin)	Tab: 25 mg	Advanced Breast Cancer in Postmenopausal Women/ Adjuvant Treatment in Early Breast Cancer: Adults: 25 mg qd pc. Concomitant Potent CYP3A4 Inducer: 50 mg qd pc.	⊡X ❋v
Imatinib Mesylate (Gleevec)	Tab: 100 mg, 400 mg	Adults: CML: Chronic Phase: 400 mg/d. Titrate: May increase to 600 mg qd. Accelerated Phase/Blast Crisis: 600 mg/d. Titrate: May increase to 400 mg bid. Relapsed/ Refractory Ph+ ALL: 600 mg/d. Myelodysplastic or Myeloproliferative Diseases/Aggressive Systemic Mastocytosis (ASM)/Hypereosinophilic Syndrome (HES) and/or Chronic Eosinophilic Leukemia (CEL): 400 mg/d. ASM w/ Eosinophilia/HEM or CEL w/ FIP1L1-PDGFRα: Initial: 100 mg/d. Titrate: May increase up to 400 mg/d. Dermatofibrosarcoma Protuberans: 800 mg/d (as 400 mg bid). GIST: 400 mg/d. Titrate: May increase up to 800 mg/d (as 400 mg bid). Peds: ≥2 yo: Ph+ CML: Newly Diagnosed: 340 mg/m²/d. Coadministration w/ Strong CYP3A4 Inducers: Increase dose by at least 50% & monitor carefully. Hepatotoxicity/Neutropenia/ Thrombocytopenia/Nonhematologic Adverse Reactions: See PI. Take w/ food & a large glass of water.	⊡D ❋v H R
Ixabepilone (Ixempra)	Inj: 15 mg, 45 mg	Adults: 40 mg/m² IV infusion over 3h q3wks. Adjust dose based on toxicities (see PI). Hepatic Impairment/Strong CYP3A4 Inhibitors/Strong CYP3A4 Inducers: See PI.	⊡D ❋v Monitor blood cell counts. H W [81]

NAME	FORM/STRENGTH	DOSAGE	COMMENTS
Lapatinib (Tykerb)	**Tab:** 250 mg	**HER2-Positive Metastatic Breast Cancer: Adults: Usual:** 1250 mg qd on Days 1-21 continuously w/ capecitabine 2000 mg/m^2/d on Days 1-14 in repeating 21d cycle. Continue treatment until disease progresses or unacceptable toxicity occurs. **Hormone Receptor Positive, HER2-Positive Metastatic Breast Cancer: Adults: Usual:** 1500 mg qd continuously w/ letrozole 2.5 mg qd. Take 1h before or after meals.	⊕D ❄v Hepatoxicity reported. **H**
Lenalidomide (Revlimid)	**Cap:** 2.5 mg, 5 mg, 10 mg, 15 mg, 25 mg	**Multiple Myeloma: Adults:** 25 mg qd w/ water. Administer as single dose on Days 1-21 of repeated 28-d cycles. Adjust dose based on platelet and/or neutrophil counts.	⊕X ❄v **W** [56]
Letrozole (Femara)	**Tab:** 2.5 mg	**Breast Cancer: Adults:** 2.5 mg qd. **Adjuvant Early Breast Cancer:** D/C at tumor relapse. **Advanced Breast Cancer:** Continue until tumor progression is evident.	⊕X ❄v **H**
Nilotinib (Tasigna)	**Cap:** 150 mg, 200 mg	**Adults: Newly Diagnosed Ph+ CML-CP:** 300 mg PO bid, 12h apart. **Resistant or Intolerant Ph+ CML-CP/CML-AP:** 400 mg PO bid, 12h apart. Avoid food for at least 2h before & 1h after dosing. Adjust dose based on toxicities, drug interactions, QT prolongation, & hepatic impairment (see PI).	⊕D ❄v May cause QT prolongation and sudden death. **H**
Paclitaxel (Taxol)	**Inj:** 6 mg/ml	**Adults: IV: Ovarian Carcinoma: Previously Untreated:** 175 mg/m^2 over 3h or 135 mg/m^2 over 24h q3wks followed by cisplatin 75 mg/m^2. **Treated:** 135 or 175 mg/m^2 over 3h q3wks. **Breast Cancer:** 175 mg/m^2 over 3h	⊕D ❄v Anaphylaxis & severe

		q3wks. **Non-Small Cell Lung Cancer:** 135 mg/m^2 over 24h q3wks. Do not repeat until neutrophil count ≥1500 cells/mm^3 and platelet count ≥100,000 cells/mm^3 (ovarian, breast, and NSCLC tumors). **Kaposi's Sarcoma:** 135 mg/ m^2 over 3h q3wks or 100 mg/m^2 over 3h q2wks. Do not give if baseline or subsequent neutrophil count <1000 cells/mm^3.	hypersensitivity reactions. **H W** [3]
Pemetrexed Disodium (Alimta)	**Inj:** 100 mg, 500 mg	**Adults:** Refer to PI for premedication regimen. **Combination w/ Cisplatin: Nonsquamous NSCLC/ Mesothelioma:** 500 mg/m^2 IV over 10 min on Day 1 of each 21-d cycle w/ cisplatin 75 mg/m^2 infused over 2h beginning 30 min after the end of administration. **Single-Agent Use: Nonsquamous NSCLC:** 500 mg/m^2 IV over 10 min on Day 1 of each 21-d cycle. Refer to PI for dose adjustments for hematologic, nonhematologic, and neurotoxicities.	⊕D ❄v R
Raloxifene HCl (Evista)	**Tab:** 60 mg	**Reduction of Breast Cancer in Postmenopausal Women w/ Osteoporosis & Postmenopausal Women at High Risk for Invasive Breast Cancer: Adults:** 60 mg qd.	⊕X ❄v

NAME	FORM/STRENGTH	DOSAGE	COMMENTS
Rituximab (Rituxan)	**Inj:** 10 mg/ml, 500 mg/ 50 ml	**Adults:** Premedicate & give as IV infusion. **Relapsed or Refractory, Low-Grade or Follicular, CD20-Positive, B-Cell NHL:** 375 mg/m² once wkly x 4 or 8 doses. **Retreatment:** 375 mg/m² once wkly x 4 doses. **Previously Untreated, Follicular, CD20-Positive, B-Cell NHL or Diffuse Large B-Cell NHL:** 375 mg/m² given on Day 1 of each chemo cycle x up to 8 doses. **Non-Progressing, Low-Grade, CD20-Positive, B-Cell NHL:** After completing 6-8 cycles of CVP chemo, give 375 mg/m² once wkly x 4 doses q6mths up to 16 doses. **CLL:** 375 mg/m² given on day prior to start of FC chemo cycle, then 500 mg/m² on Day 1 of cycles 2-6 (q28d). **Component of Zevalin:** See PI.	▣C ❄> W 65
Ruxolitinib (Jakafi)	**Tab:** 5 mg, 10 mg, 15 mg, 20 mg, 25 mg	**Intermediate- or High-Risk Myelofibrosis: Adults: Initial: Platelet Count >200 x 10⁹/L:** 20 mg bid. **Platelet Count 100-200 x 10⁹/L:** 15 mg bid. **Titrate:** Do not increase during 1st 4 wks of therapy. May increase in 5 mg bid increments not more frequently than q2wks. **Max:** 25 mg bid. D/C after 6 mths if no spleen size reduction or symptom improvement. If d/c for reasons other than thrombocytopenia, taper gradually. **W/ Strong CYP3A4 inhibitors: Initial: Platelet Count ≥100 x 10⁹/L:** 10 mg bid. Adjust dose based on thrombocytopenia and response; refer to PI.	▣C ❄v H R

Sipuleucel-T (Provenge)	Inj: 250 ml	**Metastatic (Hormone Refractory) Prostate Cancer:** **Adults:** 250 ml over 60 min q2wks x 3 doses. If unable to give scheduled infusion, additional leukapheresis is needed. Premedicate w/ PO APAP and antihistamine (eg, diphenhydramine) 30 min prior.	⊕N
Sorafenib (Nexavar)	Tab: 200 mg	**Advanced Renal Cell Carcinoma/Unresectable** **Hepatocellular Carcinoma: Adults:** 400 mg bid w/o food (1h ac or 2h pc). Continue until no clinical benefit or unacceptable toxicity. Temporary interruption or reduction to 400 mg qd or qod if serious adverse events suspected.	⊕D ❀v
Sunitinib Maleate (Sutent)	Cap: 12.5 mg, 25 mg, 50 mg	**Adults: Advanced Renal Cell Carcinoma (RCC)/** **Gastrointestinal Stromal Tumor (GIST):** 50 mg qd; 4 wks on, 2 wks off. **Advanced Pancreatic Neuroendocrine Tumor (pNET):** 37.5 mg qd; continuously w/o scheduled off-treatment. **Max:** 50 mg/d. Dose increase/reduction in 12.5-mg increments is recommended. **Concomitant Strong CYP3A4 Inhibitors:** Consider dose reduction to minimum of 37.5 mg qd (GIST & RCC) or 25 mg qd (pNET). **Concomitant CYP3A4 Inducer:** Consider dose increase to max of 87.5 mg qd (GIST & RCC) or 62.5 mg qd (pNET).	⊕D ❀v

NAME	FORM/STRENGTH	DOSAGE	COMMENTS
Temozolomide (Temodar)	**Cap:** 5 mg, 20 mg, 100 mg, 140 mg, 180 mg, 250 mg; **Inj:** 100 mg	**Adults: IV/PO:** Adjust according to nadir neutrophil & platelet counts of previous cycle & at time of initiating next cycle. **Glioblastoma Multiforme:** 75 mg/m² qd w/ focal radiotherapy. **Maint· Cycle 1 (28d):** 150 mg/m² qd x 5d. See PI for dosing for Cycles 2-6 (28d). **Anaplastic Astrocytoma: Initial:** 150 mg/m² qd x 5d (consecutive) per 28-d cycle. If ANC ≥1.5 x 10⁹/L & platelets ≥100 x 10⁹/L for both nadir & Day 29 (Day 1 of next cycle), may increase to 200 mg/m²/d x 5d (consecutive) per 28-d cycle. See PI for more details.	▣D ❄v
Vandetanib (Caprelsa)	**Tab:** 100 mg, 300 mg	**Symptomatic or Progressive Medullary Thyroid Cancer: Adults: Usual:** 300 mg PO qd. **Maint:** Continue until no longer benefiting from treatment or unacceptable toxicity occurs. CrCl <50 ml/min: **Initial:** 200 mg. Refer to PI for dose adjustments for toxicity & for corrected QT interval.	▣D ❄v QT prolongation, torsades de pointes, and sudden death reported. **H R**
Vorinostat (Zolinza)	**Cap:** 100 mg	**Cutaneous T-Cell Lymphoma: Adults:** 400 mg qd w/ food. **Intolerant to Therapy:** May reduce dose to 300 mg qd w/ food. If necessary, may further reduce dose to 300 mg qd w/ food x 5d (consecutive) each wk.	▣D ❄v

Angina
BETA BLOCKERS

Atenolol (Tenormin)	**Tab:** 25 mg, 50 mg, 100 mg	**Adults: Initial:** 50 mg qd. **Titrate:** May increase to 100 mg qd after 1 wk. **Max:** 200 mg/d.	⊕D ❄>R
Metoprolol Succinate (Toprol-XL)	**Tab,ER:** 25 mg, 50 mg, 100 mg, 200 mg	**Adults: Initial:** 100 mg qd. **Titrate:** May increase wkly. **Max:** 400 mg/d.	⊕C ❄>W [18]
Metoprolol Tartrate (Lopressor)	**Tab:** 50 mg, 100 mg	**Adults: Initial:** 50 mg bid. **Titrate:** May increase wkly. **Usual:** 100-400 mg/d. **Max:** 400 mg/d.	⊕C ❄>W [18]
Nadolol (Corgard)	**Tab:** 20 mg, 40 mg, 80 mg	**Adults: Initial:** 40 mg qd. **Titrate:** Increase by 40-80 mg q3-7d. **Usual:** 40-80 mg qd. **Max:** 240 mg/d.	⊕C ❄v R W [18]
Propranolol HCl	**Tab:** 10 mg, 20 mg, 40 mg, 60 mg, 80 mg	**Adults: Usual:** 80-320 mg/d given bid-qid.	⊕C ❄>W [18]

CALCIUM CHANNEL BLOCKER/HMG COA REDUCTASE INHIBITOR

Amlodipine Besylate/ **Atorvastatin Calcium** (Caduet)	**Tab:** 2.5-10 mg, 2.5-20 mg, 2.5-40 mg, 5-10 mg, 5-20 mg, 5-40 mg, 5-80 mg, 10-10 mg, 10-20 mg, 10-40 mg, 10-80 mg	Dosing is based on appropriate combination of recommendations for monotherapies. **Chronic Stable Angina/Vasospastic Angina/CAD: Adults: Amlodipine:** 5-10 mg qd. **Elderly:** Give the lower dose. **Atorvastatin:** See under Antilipidemic Agents for dosing.	⊕X ❄v H

NAME	FORM/STRENGTH	DOSAGE	COMMENTS
CALCIUM CHANNEL BLOCKERS (DIHYDROPYRIDINE)			
Amlodipine Besylate (Norvasc)	**Tab:** 2.5 mg, 5 mg, 10 mg	**Chronic Stable/Vasospastic Angina/CAD: Adults:** 5-10 mg qd. **Elderly:** Give lower dose.	⊙C ❄v H
Nicardipine HCl	**Cap:** 20 mg, 30 mg	**Chronic Stable Angina: Adults: Initial:** 20 mg tid. Allow at least 3d before increasing dose. **Usual:** 20-40 mg tid.	⊙C ❄v H R
Nifedipine (Nifedical XL, Procardia XL)	**Tab,ER:** (Nifedical XL) 30 mg, 60 mg; (Procardia XL) 30 mg, 60 mg, 90 mg	**Vasospastic/Chronic Stable: Adults:** Adjust dosage according to patient's needs. **Initial:** 30-60 mg qd. **Titrate:** May increase over 7-14d. **Max:** 120 mg/d. Caution w/ dose >90 mg.	⊙C ❄>
CALCIUM CHANNEL BLOCKERS (NON-DIHYDROPYRIDINE)			
Diltiazem HCl (Cardizem CD, Cardizem LA, Cartia XT)	**Cap,ER:** (Cardizem CD/Cartia XT) 120 mg, 180 mg, 240 mg, 300 mg, (Cardizem CD) 360 mg; **Tab,ER:** (Cardizem LA) 120 mg, 180 mg, 240 mg, 300 mg, 360 mg, 420 mg	**Adults: Chronic Stable Angina/Angina Due to Coronary Artery Spasm: Cardizem CD/Cartia XT: Initial:** 120-180 mg qd. **Titrate:** Adjust at 1-2 wk intervals. **Max:** 480 mg/d. **Chronic Stable Angina: Cardizem LA: Initial:** 180 mg qd (am or pm). **Titrate:** Adjust at 1-2 wk intervals. **Max:** 360 mg.	⊙C ❄v
Diltiazem HCl (Cardizem)	**Tab:** 30 mg, 60 mg, 90 mg, 120 mg	**Chronic Stable Angina/Angina Due to Coronary Artery Spasm: Adults: Initial:** 30 mg qid (ac & qhs). **Titrate:** Adjust at 1-2d intervals. **Usual:** 180-360 mg/d.	⊙C ❄v

Diltiazem HCl (Dilacor XR, Diltia XT)	Cap,ER: (Dilacor XR) 240 mg; (Diltia XT) 120 mg, 180 mg, 240 mg	**Chronic Stable Angina: Adults: Initial** 120 mg qd. **Titrate:** Adjust over a 1-2 wk period. **Max:** 480 mg/d.	⊕C ❄v
Diltiazem HCl (Taztia XT, Tiazac)	Cap,ER: (Taztia XT/ Tiazac) 120 mg, 180 mg, 240 mg, 300 mg, 360 mg; (Tiazac) 420 mg	**Adults: Initial:** 120-180 mg qd. **Titrate:** Adjust over 7-14d. **Max:** 540 mg/d.	⊕C ❄v
Verapamil HCl (Calan)	Tab: 40 mg, 80 mg, 120 mg	**Vasospastic/Unstable/Chronic Stable: Adults: Usual:** 80-120 mg tid. **Patients w/ Increased Response to Verapamil (eg, Elderly, Decreased Hepatic Function): Initial:** 40 mg tid. **Titrate:** May increase by qd (unstable angina) or qwk intervals. **Max:** 480 mg/d.	⊕C ❄v **H R**
Verapamil (Covera-HS)	Tab,ER: 180 mg, 240 mg	**Adults: Initial:** 180 mg qhs. **Titrate:** Increase to 240 mg qhs, then 360 mg qhs, then 480 mg qhs.	⊕C ❄v **H**

VASODILATORS

Isosorbide Dinitrate (Dilatrate-SR)	Cap,ER: 40 mg	**Adults: Prevention: Usual:** 40 mg bid. Separate doses by 6h. **Max:** 160 mg/d. Should have at least 18h nitrate-free interval.	⊕C ❄>
Isosorbide Mononitrate	Tab,ER: 30 mg, 60 mg, 120 mg	**Prevention: Adults: Initial:** 30 mg (single tab or 1/2 of 60-mg tab) or 60-mg (single tab) qam. **Titrate:** May increase to 120 mg/d. **Elderly:** Start at low end of dosing range.	⊕B ❄>

NAME	FORM/STRENGTH	DOSAGE	COMMENTS
Nitroglycerin (Nitrostat)	Tab,SL: 0.3 mg, 0.4 mg, 0.6 mg	**Treatment:** 1 tab SL or in buccal pouch at onset of attack. May repeat q5min until relief is obtained. If pain persists after a total of 3 tabs/15 min or pain is different than typically experienced, prompt medical attention recommended. **Prophylaxis:** Take 5-10 min before precipitating activity.	◐C ✿>CI w/ early MI, severe anemia, increased ICP, w/ PDE-5 inhibitors.
Nitroglycerin (Nitro-Bid)	Oint: 2% (15 mg/inch)	**Prevention: Initial:** 0.5 inch qam & 6h later. **Titrate:** May increase to 1 inch bid, then to 2 inches bid. Should have 10-12h nitrate-free period.	◐C ✿>

MISCELLANEOUS

NAME	FORM/STRENGTH	DOSAGE	COMMENTS
Ranolazine (Ranexa)	Tab,ER: 500 mg, 1000 mg	**Chronic Angina: Adults: Initial:** 500 mg bid. **Titrate:** Increase to 1000 mg bid prn based on clinical symptoms. **Max:** 1000 mg bid. **Use W/ Moderate CYP3A Inhibitors/P-gp Inhibitors:** See PI.	◐C ✿v H

Antiarrhythmics
GROUP IA

NAME	FORM/STRENGTH	DOSAGE	COMMENTS
Disopyramide Phosphate (Norpace, Norpace CR)	Cap: 100 mg, 150 mg; Cap,ER: 100 mg, 150 mg	**Adults: <50 kg: Cap:** 100 mg q6h. **Cap,ER:** 200 mg q12h. **≥50 kg: Cap:** 150 mg q6h. **Cap,ER:** 300 mg q12h. **Peds: 12-18 yo:** 6-15 mg/kg/d. **4-12 yo:** 10-15 mg/kg/d. **1-4 yo:** 10-20 mg/kg/d. **<1 yo:** 10-30 mg/kg/d.	◐C ✿v H R W [5]

| Quinidine Sulfate | Tab,ER: 300 mg | **Adults: A-Fib/Flutter Conversion: Initial:** 300 mg q8-12h. **Titrate:** Increase cautiously if no result & levels w/in therapeutic range. **A-Fib/Flutter Relapse Reduction:** 300 mg q8-12h. **Titrate:** Increase cautiously if needed. **Ventricular Arrhythmia:** Dosing regimens not adequately studied. Generally similar to A-fib/flutter. | ⊕C ❄v H R |

GROUP IB

| Lidocaine HCl (Xylocaine Injection, Xylocaine-MPF) | Inj: 0.5%, 1%, 2% | **Adults: Initial:** 50-100 mg IV given 25-50 mg/min, may repeat after 5 min. **Max:** 200-300 mg/h. Following bolus, initiate w/ 1-4 mg/min continuous infusion. **Maint:** Adjust according to cardiac rhythm & toxicity. **Peds:** 1 mg/kg bolus, then 30 mcg/kg/min. | ⊕B ❄> |
| Mexiletine HCl | Cap: 150 mg, 200 mg, 250 mg | **Adults:** Individualize dose. **Initial:** 200 mg q8h. **Titrate:** Adjust in 50-100 mg increments up or down q2-3d. **Max:** 1200 mg/d. | ⊕C ❄v H W [5] |

GROUP IC

| Flecainide Acetate (Tambocor) | Tab: 50 mg, 100 mg, 150 mg | **Adults: PSVT/PAF: Initial:** 50 mg q12h. **Titrate:** Increase by 50 mg bid q4d. **Max:** 300 mg/d. **Sustained VT: Initial:** 100 mg q12h. **Titrate:** Increase by 50 mg bid q4d. **Max:** 400 mg/d. **Peds: Initial:** >6 mths: 100 mg/m²/d given bid-tid. <6 mths: 50 mg/m²/d given bid-tid. **Max:** 200 mg/m²/d. | ⊕C ❄> H R |

NAME	FORM/STRENGTH	DOSAGE	COMMENTS
Propafenone HCl (Rythmol SR)	Cap,ER: 225 mg, 325 mg, 425 mg	Adults: Initial: 225 mg q12h. Titrate: Individualize based on response and tolerance. May increase at a minimum of 5d interval to 325 mg q12h, then to 425 mg q12h if additional therapeutic effect needed.	⊞C ❄v H W [5]

GROUP II

NAME	FORM/STRENGTH	DOSAGE	COMMENTS
Acebutolol HCl (Sectral)	Cap: 200 mg, 400 mg	Ventricular Arrhythmia: Adults: Initial: 200 mg bid. Maint: Increase gradually to 600-1200 mg/d. Elderly: Max: 800 mg/d.	⊞B ❄v R W [18]
Esmolol HCl (Brevibloc)	Inj: 10 mg/ml, 20 mg/ml	Adults: SVT: Initial: 500 mcg/kg x 1 min, then 50 mcg/kg/min x 4 min. Maint: 50-200 (avg 100) mcg/kg/min. Max: 300 mcg/kg/min. Intra-/Post-Op Tachycardia: Initial: Rapid: 80 mg IVP, then 150 mcg/kg/min infusion. Gradual: LD: 500 mcg/kg/min x 1 min. Maint: 50 mcg/kg/min x 4 min. If inadequate response w/in 5 min, repeat LD & give maint 100 mcg/kg/min.	⊞C ❄>
Propranolol HCl	Inj: 1 mg/ml; Tab: 10 mg, 20 mg, 40 mg, 60 mg, 80 mg	Adults: PO: A-Fib: 10-30 mg tid-qid, given ac & qhs. IV: Life-Threatening Arrhythmias: 1-3 mg IV at ≤1 mg/min.	⊞C ❄> W [18]

Amiodarone HCl (Cordarone)	**Tab:** 200 mg	**Adults:** Give LD in hospital. **LD:** 800-1600 mg/d x 1-3 wks. Give in divided doses w/ meals for total daily dose ≥1000 mg or if GI intolerance. After control achieved or w/ prominent side effects, 600-800 mg/d x 1 mth. **Maint:** 400 mg/d (up to 600 mg/d if needed). May give as single dose or bid if severe GI intolerance. Use lowest effective dose. Take consistently w/ regard to meals. **Elderly:** Start at low end of dosing range.	⊕D ❋v W [5]
Dofetilide (Tikosyn)	**Cap:** 0.125 mg, 0.25 mg, 0.5 mg	**A-Fib/Flutter: Adults:** ≥18 yo: Individualize dose. Dose according to CrCl and QTc (if HR <60 bpm). See PI for dosing charts.	⊕C ❋v Should be inpatient at least 3d when initiated. Monitor ECG & CrCl. **R**
Dronedarone (Multaq)	**Tab:** 400 mg	**Adults:** 400 mg bid. Take 1 tab w/ am meal and 1 tab w/ pm meal.	⊕X ❋v CI w/ NYHA Class IV HF or symptomatic HF w/ a recent decompensation.

NAME	FORM/STRENGTH	DOSAGE	COMMENTS
Sotalol HCl (Betapace AF)	**Tab:** 80 mg, 120 mg, 160 mg	**Adults:** Individualize dose. Dose according to CrCl (see PI). **Peds:** ≥2 yo: **Initial:** 30 mg/m² tid. **Titrate:** Wait ≥36h between dose increases. Guide dose by response, HR & QT$_c$. **Max:** 60 mg/m². **<2 yo:** See dosing chart in PI. Reduce dose or d/c if QT$_c$ >550 msec.	⊙B ❄v Initiate or reinitiate only in equipped facility for at least 3d. Monitor ECG & CrCl. **R W** [5]
Sotalol HCl (Betapace)	**Tab:** 80 mg, 120 mg, 160 mg	**Adults:** Individualize dose. **Initial:** 80 mg bid. **Titrate:** Increase q3d prn to 120-160 mg bid. **Usual:** 160-320 mg/d given bid-tid. **Peds:** ≥2 yo: **Initial:** 30 mg/m² tid. **Titrate:** Wait ≥36h between dose increases. Guide dose by response, HR & QT$_c$. **Max:** 60 mg/m². **<2 yo:** See dosing chart in PI. Reduce dose or d/c if QT$_c$ >550 msec.	⊙B ❄v Initiate or reinitiate only in equipped facility for at least 3d. Monitor ECG & CrCl. **R W** [5]
GROUP IV			
Verapamil HCl (Calan)	**Tab:** 40 mg, 80 mg, 120 mg	**Adults:** A-Fib (Digitalized): **Usual:** 240-320 mg/d given tid-qid. **PSVT Prophylaxis (Non-Digitalized):** 240-480 mg/d given tid-qid. **Max:** 480 mg/d.	⊙C ❄v **H R**

Antilipidemic Agents

BILE ACID SEQUESTRANTS

Colesevelam HCl (WelChol)	**Tab:** 625 mg; **Susp:** 1.875 gm, 3.75 gm [pkt]	**Adults: Tab:** 3 tabs bid or 6 tabs qd. Take w/ meal & liquid. **Adults & Peds: 10-17 yo: Susp:** 1.875 gm bid or 3.75 gm qd. Take w/ meals.	⊞B ❋^
Colestipol HCl (Colestid)	**Granules:** 5 gm/pkt or scoopful; **Tab:** 1 gm	**Adults: Initial:** 2 gm (tabs) or 5 gm (1 pkt or scoopful) qd-bid. **Titrate:** Increase by 2 gm qd or bid at 1-2 mth intervals. **Usual:** 2-16 gm/d (tab) or 1-6 pkts or scoopfuls qd or in divided doses.	⊞N ❋>

CALCIUM CHANNEL BLOCKER/HMG COA REDUCTASE INHIBITOR

Amlodipine Besylate/ Atorvastatin Calcium (Caduet)	**Tab:** 2.5-10 mg, 2.5-20 mg, 2.5-40 mg, 5-10 mg, 5-20 mg, 5-40 mg, 5-80 mg, 10-10 mg, 10-20 mg, 10-40 mg, 10-80 mg	Dosing based on appropriate combination of recommendations for monotherapies. **Atorvastatin: Adults: Hyperlipidemia/Mixed Dyslipidemia: Initial:** 10-20 mg qd (or 40 mg qd for LDL-C reduction >45%). **Titrate:** Adjust dose as needed at 2-4 wk intervals. **Usual:** 10-80 mg qd. **Homozygous Familial Hypercholesterolemia:** 10-80 mg qd. **Concomitant Cyclosporine: Max:** 10 mg qd. **Concomitant Clarithromycin/Itraconazole/Ritonavir plus Saquinavir or Lopinavir:** Caution w/ >20 mg; use lowest dose necessary. **Peds: 10-17 yo (postmenarchal): Heterozygous Familial Hypercholesterolemia: Initial:** 10 mg/d. **Titrate:** Adjust dose at ≥4 wk intervals. **Max:**	⊞X ❋v H

Continued on Next Page

NAME	FORM/STRENGTH	DOSAGE	COMMENTS
Amlodipine Besylate/ Atorvastatin Calcium (Caduet)			Continued
		Amlodipine: See under Angina & Hypertension for dosing.	
		20 mg/d.	

CHOLESTEROL ABSORPTION INHIBITOR

NAME	FORM/STRENGTH	DOSAGE	COMMENTS
Ezetimibe (Zetia)	**Tab:** 10 mg	**Adults:** 10 mg qd. May give w/ a statin (primary hyperlipidemia) or w/ fenofibrate (mixed hyperlipidemia) for incremental effect. Give either 2h before or ≥4h after bile acid sequestrant.	**©**C **❉❉>**

CHOLESTEROL ABSORPTION INHIBITOR/HMG COA REDUCTASE INHIBITOR

NAME	FORM/STRENGTH	DOSAGE	COMMENTS
Ezetimibe/Simvastatin (Vytorin)	**Tab:** 10-10 mg, 10-20 mg, 10-40 mg, 10-80 mg	**Adults:** Take qd pm. **Initial:** 10-10 mg or 10-20 mg qd. **Usual:** 10 mg-10 mg to 10mg-40mg qd. **LDL Reduction >55%: Initial:** 10-40mg qd. **Titrate:** Adjust at ≥2 wks. **Restricted Dosing for 10-80 mg:** Use 10-80 mg only if 10-80 mg has been taken chronically (eg, ≥12 mths) w/o muscle toxicity. See PI. **Homozygous Familial Hypercholesterolemia:** 10-40 mg qd. **Concomitant Bile Acid Sequestrant:** Take either ≥2h before or ≥4h after bile acid sequestrant. **Concomitant Diltiazem/Verapamil: Max:** 10-10 mg/d. **Concomitant Amiodarone/Amlodipine/ Ranolazine: Max:** 10-20 mg/d. **Chinese Patients Taking Lipid-Modifying Doses (≥1gm/d) of Niacin:** Caution w/ >10-20 mg qd; avoid qd 10-80 mg.	**©**X **❉❉>** H R

DIPEPTIDYL PEPTIDASE-4 INHIBITOR/HMG-COA REDUCTASE INHIBITOR

Simvastatin/Sitagliptin (Juvisync)	Tab: 10-100 mg, 20-100 mg, 40-100 mg	Adults: Usual: 10-100 mg, 20-100 mg, or 40-100 mg qd. Take as single dose in pm. Initial: 40-100 mg/d. Patients on Simvastatin w/ or w/o Sitagliptin 100 mg/d: Initial: 100 mg sitagliptin and dose of simvastatin already taken. Concomitant Insulin/Insulin Secretagogue (eg, sulfonylurea): May need lower dose of insulin/insulin secretagogue. Concomitant Verapamil/Diltiazem: Max: 10-100 mg qd. Concomitant Amiodarone/Amlodipine/Ranolazine: Max: 20-100 mg qd. Homozygous Familial Hypercholesterolemia: Usual: 40-100 mg qd. Chinese Patients Taking Lipid-Modifying Doses (≥1 gm/d) of Niacin-Containing Products: Caution w/ 40-100 mg qd.	◉X ✿v H R

FIBRIC ACIDS

Fenofibrate (Tricor)	Tab: 48 mg, 145 mg	Adults: Primary Hypercholesterolemia/Mixed Hyperlipidemia: Initial: 145 mg/d. Severe Hypertriglyceridemia: Individualize dose. Initial: 48-145 mg/d. Titrate: Adjust dose if needed after repeat lipid determinations at 4-8 wk intervals. Max: 145 mg/d.	◉C ✿v H R
Gemfibrozil (Lopid)	Tab: 600 mg	Adults: 600 mg bid 30 min ac.	◉C ✿v H R

NAME	FORM/STRENGTH	DOSAGE	COMMENTS

HMG COA REDUCTASE INHIBITORS

NAME	FORM/STRENGTH	DOSAGE	COMMENTS
Atorvastatin Calcium (Lipitor)	**Tab:** 10 mg, 20 mg, 40 mg, 80 mg	**Adults: Hyperlipidemia/Mixed Dyslipidemia: Initial:** 10-20 mg qd (or 40 mg qd for LDL reduction >45%). **Titrate:** Adjust at 2-4 wk intervals. **Usual:** 10-80 mg qd. **Homozygous Familial Hypercholesterolemia:** 10-80 mg qd. **Peds: 10-17 yo (postmenarchal): Heterozygous Familial Hypercholesterolemia: Initial:** 10 mg/d. **Titrate:** Adjust at ≥4-wk intervals. **Max:** 20 mg/d.	⊕X ✿v
Fluvastatin Sodium (Lescol, Lescol XL)	**Cap:** (Lescol) 20 mg, 40 mg; **Tab,ER:** (Lescol XL) 80 mg	**Adults: ≥18 yo: Initial:** (LDL reduction ≥25%) 40 mg cap qpm or 80 mg XL tab qd or 40 mg cap bid. **Initial:** (LDL reduction <25%) 20 mg cap qpm. **Range:** 20-80 mg/d. **Peds: 10-16 yo (≥1 yr postmenarchal): Heterozygous Familial Hypercholesterolemia: Initial:** 20 mg cap. **Titrate:** Adjust dose at 6-wk intervals. **Max:** 40 mg cap bid or 80 mg XL tab qd. **W/ Cyclosporine/Fluconazole: Max:** 20 mg bid.	⊕X ✿v H
Lovastatin (Mevacor)	**Tab:** 10 mg, 20 mg, 40 mg; (Mevacor) 20 mg, 40 mg	**Adults:** Individualize dose. **Initial:** 20 mg qd w/ pm meal (10 mg/d if need LDL reduction <20%). **Titrate:** May adjust at intervals of ≥4 wks. **Usual:** 10-80 mg/d as qd-bid. **Max:** 80 mg/d. **Peds: 10-17 yo: Heterozygous Familial Hypercholesterolemia: Initial:** 20 mg qd (10 mg qd if need LDL reduction <20%). **Titrate:** Adjust at intervals of ≥4 wks. **Usual:** 10-40 mg/d. **Max:** 40 mg/d. Adjust w/	⊕X ✿v H R

		danazol, diltiazem, other fibrates, niacin, verapamil, or amiodarone; see PI.	
Pitavastatin (Livalo)	Tab: 1 mg, 2 mg, 4 mg	**Adults:** Initial: 2 mg qd. Usual: 1-4 mg qd. Max: 4 mg qd. Can take at any time of the day. Concomitant Erythromycin: Max: 1 mg qd. Concomitant Rifampin: Max: 2 mg qd.	◉X ❄v H R
Pravastatin Sodium (Pravachol)	Tab: 10 mg, 20 mg, 40 mg, 80 mg	**Adults: ≥18 yo:** Initial: 40 mg qd. Titrate: May increase to 80 mg qd if needed. Heterozygous Familial Hypercholesterolemia: Peds: 14-18 yo: 40 mg qd. 8-13 yo: 20 mg qd. Concomitant Immunosuppressives (eg, cyclosporine): Initial:10 mg qhs. Max: 20 mg/d. Take at least 1h before or 4h after resins.	◉X ❄v R
Rosuvastatin (Crestor)	Tab: 5 mg, 10 mg, 20 mg, 40 mg	**Adults: Hypercholesterolemia/Mixed Dyslipidemia/ Slowing Progression of Atherosclerosis/Primary Prevention CV Disease:** Initial: 10-20 mg qd (or 5 mg qd for Asian patients). Titrate: Adjust dose if needed at 2-4 wk intervals. Range: 5-40 mg qd. Homozygous Familial Hypercholesterolemia: 20 mg qd. Peds: 10-17 yo (≥1 yr postmenarchal): Heterozygous Familial Hypercholesterolemia: 5-20 mg qd. Max: 20 mg/d. Adjust w/ cyclosporine, gemfibrozil, lopinavir/ritonavir, & atazanavir/ritonavir.	◉X ❄v H R

NAME	FORM/STRENGTH	DOSAGE	COMMENTS
Simvastatin (Zocor)	Tab: 5 mg, 10 mg, 20 mg, 40 mg, 80 mg	**Adults: Initial:** 10-20 mg qpm. **Usual:** 5-40 mg/d. **High Risk for CHD Events: Initial:** 40 mg/d. Check lipids after 4 wks & periodically thereafter. **Restricted Dosing:** Use 80 mg only if 80 mg has been taken chronically (eg, ≥12 mths) w/o muscle toxicity. See PI. **Homozygous Familial Hypercholesterolemia:** 40 mg qpm. **Peds: 10-17 yo: Heterozygous Familial Hypercholesterolemia: Initial:** 10 mg qpm. **Usual:** 10-40 mg/d. **Titrate:** Adjust at ≥4 wk intervals. **Max:** 40 mg/d. **Concomitant Verapamil/ Diltiazem: Max:** 10 mg/d. **Concomitant Amiodarone/ Amlodipine/Ranolazine: Max:** 20 mg/d. **Chinese Patients Taking Lipid-Modifying Doses (≥1 gm/d) of Niacin:** Caution w/ >20 mg qd; avoid 80 mg.	⊕X ✳v H R

HMG COA REDUCTASE INHIBITORS/NICOTINIC ACID

NAME	FORM/STRENGTH	DOSAGE	COMMENTS
Lovastatin/Niacin (Advicor)	Tab, ER: 20-500 mg, 20-750 mg, 20-1000 mg, 40-1000 mg	**Adults: Not Currently on ER Niacin: Initial:** 20-500 mg qhs. **Titrate: ER Niacin:** Increase by no more than 500 mg qd q4wks. **Max:** 40-2000 mg qd. **Concomitant Danazol/ Diltiazem/Verapamil: Lovastatin: Initial:** 10 mg/d. **Max:** 20 mg/d. **Concomitant Amiodarone: Lovastatin: Max:** 40 mg/d. Take w/ low-fat snack. Refer to PI for further dosing information.	⊕X ✳v H R

| Niacin/Simvastatin (Simcor) | Tab,ER: 500-20 mg, 500-40 mg, 750-20 mg, 1000-20 mg, 1000-40 mg | **Adults:** Not Currently on ER Niacin or Switching from Non-ER Niacin: Initial: 500-20 mg qhs. **W/ Simvastatin 20-40 mg Needing Additional Lipid Level Management:** Initial: 500-40 mg qhs. **Titrate:** ER Niacin: Increase by ≤500 mg qd q4wks. After Wk 8, titrate to response & tolerance. **Maint:** 1000-20 mg to 2000-40 mg qhs. **Max:** 2000-40 mg qhs. **Concomitant Amlodipine/Ranolazine: Max:** 1000-20 mg/d. **Chinese Patients:** Caution w/ >1000-20 mg/d. Do not break, crush, or chew. Take w/ low-fat snack. | ⊙X ❀v H R |

NICOTINIC ACID

| Niacin (Niaspan) | Tab,ER: 500 mg, 750 mg, 1000 mg | **Adults & Peds: >16 yo:** Individualize dose. **Initial:** 500 mg qhs. **Titrate:** Increase by 500 mg q4wks. After Wk 8, titrate to patient response and tolerance. Do not increase daily dose by >500 mg in any 4-wk period. **Maint:** 1-2 gm qhs. **Max:** 2 gm/d. **W/ Lovastatin/Simvastatin: Initial:** (lovastatin/simvastatin): 20 mg qd. Adjust dose at intervals of ≥4 wks. **Max:** 2 gm niacin/40 mg lovastatin/simvastatin qd. May pretreat w/ ASA to reduce flushing. | ⊙C ❀v H |

MISCELLANEOUS

| Omega-3-Acid Ethyl Esters (Lovaza) | Cap: 1 gm | **Adults:** 4 gm/d (4 caps qd or 2 caps bid). | ⊙C ❀> |

NAME	FORM/STRENGTH	DOSAGE	COMMENTS

Coagulation Modifiers
ADP RECEPTOR/PLATELET AGGREGATION-ADHESION INHIBITORS

NAME	FORM/STRENGTH	DOSAGE	COMMENTS
Clopidogrel Bisulfate (Plavix)	Tab: 75 mg, 300 mg	**Adults: Recent MI/Stroke/Peripheral Arterial Disease:** 75 mg qd. **Acute Coronary Syndrome: Non-ST-Segment Elevation MI/Unstable Angina: LD:** 300 mg. **Maint:** 75 mg qd. Take w/ 75-325 mg ASA qd. **ST-Segment Elevation MI:** 75 mg qd. Take w/ 75-325 mg ASA qd & w/ or w/o LD.	⊕B ✽v W [108]
Prasugrel (Effient)	Tab: 5 mg, 10 mg	**Acute Coronary Syndrome: Adults: LD:** 60 mg PO single dose. **Maint:** 10 mg qd. **<60 kg:** Consider reducing to 5 mg qd. Take w/ 75-325 mg ASA qd.	⊕B ✽> W [105]
Ticagrelor (Brilinta)	Tab: 90 mg	**Acute Coronary Syndrome/Prevention of Stent Thrombosis: Adults: LD:** 180 mg w/ ASA (usually 325 mg). **Maint:** 90 mg bid w/ ASA (75-100 mg/day). ACS patients who have received LD of clopidogrel may start ticagrelor therapy.	⊕C ✽v H

DIRECT THROMBIN INHIBITOR

NAME	FORM/STRENGTH	DOSAGE	COMMENTS
Dabigatran Etexilate Mesylate (Pradaxa)	Cap: 75 mg, 150 mg	**Adults: CrCl >30 ml/min:** 150 mg bid. **CrCl 15-30 ml/min:** 75 mg bid. **Conversion from Warfarin:** D/C warfarin & start when INR is <2.0. **Conversion from Parenteral Anticoagulants:** Start 0-2h before next dose of parenteral drug was to have been administered or at the time of d/c of continuously administered parenteral drug. **Surgery &**	⊕C ✽> R

| | **Interventions:** D/C 1-2d (CrCl ≥50 ml/min) or 3-5d (CrCl <50 ml/min) before invasive or surgical procedures. Refer to PI for conversion to warfarin & parenteral anticoagulants. | |

GLYCOSAMINOGLYCAN

Drug	Dosage	Details	Rating
Heparin Sodium	**Inj:** 1000 U/ml, 5000 U/ml, 10,000 U/ml, 20,000 U/ml	**Adults:** Based on 68 kg: **Initial:** 5000 U IV, then 10,000-20,000 U SC. **Maint:** 8000-10,000 U q8h or 15,000-20,000 U q12h. **Intermittent IV Inj: Initial:** 10,000 U. **Maint:** 5000-10,000 U q4-6h. **Continuous IV Infusion: Initial:** 5,000 U. **Maint:** 20,000-40,000 U/d. **Peds: Initial:** 50 U/kg IV. **Maint:** 100 U/kg IV q4h or 20,000 U/m²/d continuous IV.	⊕C ❃^ (preservative-free only)

LOW MOLECULAR WEIGHT HEPARINS

Drug	Dosage	Details	Rating
Dalteparin Sodium (Fragmin)	**Inj:** (Syringe) 2500 IU/0.2 ml, 5000 IU/0.2 ml, 7500 IU/0.3 ml, 10,000 IU/0.4 ml, 10,000 IU/ml, 12,500 IU/0.5 ml, 15,000 IU/0.6 ml, 18,000 IU/0.72 ml; (MDV) 95,000 IU/3.8 ml, 95,000 IU/9.5 ml	**Adults: SC: Prophylaxis of Ischemic Complications in Unstable Angina/Non-Q-Wave MI:** 120 IU/kg, up to 10,000 IU q12h w/ 75-165 mg/d ASA until clinically stabilized (usual 5-8d). **Prophylaxis of VTE in Hip Surgery: Pre-Op (Starting Day of Surgery): Usual:** 2500 IU w/in 2h pre-op, then 2500 IU 4-8h post-op. **Pre-Op (Starting Evening Prior to Surgery): Usual:** 5000 IU 10-14h pre-op, then 5000 IU 4-8h post-op. **Post-Op Start: Usual:** 2500 IU 4-8h post-op. **Maint (Pre-/Post-Op):** 5000 IU qd x 5-10d	⊕B ❃> R W [6]

Continued on Next Page

NAME	FORM/STRENGTH	DOSAGE	COMMENTS
Dalteparin Sodium (Fragmin) *Continued*		post-op (up to 14d). **Abdominal Surgery: Initial:** 2500 IU 1-2h pre-op. **Maint:** 2500 IU qd x 5-10d post-op. **Abdominal Surgery w/ High Risk: Initial:** 5000 IU evening before surgery. **Maint:** 5000 IU qd x 5-10d post-op. **Abdominal Surgery w/ Malignancy: Initial:** 2500 IU 1-2h pre-op, then 2500 IU 12h later. **Maint:** 5000 IU qd x 5-10d post-op. **Severely Restricted Mobility During Acute Illness:** 5000 IU qd x 12-14d. **Symptomatic VTE in Cancer Patients:** 200 IU/kg x 1st 30d, then 150 IU/kg qd for mths 2-6. **Max:** 18,000 IU/d. Adjust dose based on platelet count & anti-Xa levels.	
Enoxaparin (Lovenox)	**Inj:** 30 mg/0.3 ml, 40 mg/0.4 ml, 60 mg/ 0.6 ml, 80 mg/0.8 ml, 100 mg/ml, 120 mg/ 0.8 ml, 150 mg/ml, 300 mg/3 ml	**Adults: SC: Hip/Knee Replacement Surgery:** 30 mg q12h 12-24h post-op x 7-10d (up to 14d). **Hip (alternative dosing):** 40 mg qd 9-15h pre-op, then 40 mg qd x 3 wks. **Abdominal Surgery:** 40 mg qd, 2h pre-op x 7-10d (up to 12d). **DVT Outpatient Treatment:** 1 mg/kg q12h w/ warfarin (goal INR 2-3) x 7d (up to 17d). **DVT/PE Inpatient Treatment:** 1 mg/kg q12h or 1.5 mg/kg qd w/ warfarin (goal INR 2-3) x 7d (up to 17d). **Unstable Angina/ Non-Q-Wave MI:** 1 mg/kg q12h w/ 100-325 mg/d ASA x 2-8d (up to 12.5d). **Acute Illness:** 40 mg qd x 6-11d (up to 14d). **Acute STEMI: <75 yo:** 30 mg single IV bolus plus a 1 mg/kg SC dose followed by 1 mg/kg q12h SC (max 100 mg for 1st 2 doses) w/ 75-325 mg/d ASA x ≥8d or until hospital discharge. **Acute STEMI: ≥75 yo:** No initial IV	▣B ❀v R W [6]

		bolus. 0.75 mg/kg SC q12h (max 75 mg for 1st 2 doses) w/ 75-325 mg/d ASA x ≥8d or until hospital discharge. **Concomitant Thrombolytic Therapy:** Give 15 min before or 30 min after start of fibrinolytic. **PCI:** If last dose given >8h before balloon inflation, give 0.3 mg/kg IV bolus.	
Tinzaparin (Innohep)	Inj: 20,000 IU/ml	**DVT/PE Treatment: Adults:** 175 IU/kg SC qd for at least 6d & until anticoagulated w/ warfarin.	⊛B ✿> **W** [6]

PHOSPHODIESTERASE/PLATELET AGGREGATION-ADHESION INHIBITORS

Anagrelide HCl (Agrylin)	Cap: 0.5 mg, 1 mg	**Thrombocythemia: Initial: Adults:** 0.5 mg qid or 1 mg bid x ≥1 wk. **Peds: Initial:** 0.5 mg qd-0.5 mg qid. **Titrate: Adults & Peds:** May increase by ≤0.5 mg/d qwk. Adjust based on platelet count. **Max:** 10 mg/d or 2.5 mg/dose.	⊛C ✿v **H**
Cilostazol (Pletal)	Tab: 50 mg, 100 mg	**Intermittent Claudication: Adults:** 100 mg bid, 1/2h before or 2h after am & pm meal. **Concomitant CYP 3A4/2C19 Inhibitors:** Consider 50 mg bid.	⊛C ✿v CI in CHF. **H R**
Dipyridamole/ASA (Aggrenox)	Cap,ER: 200-25 mg	**Risk Reduction of Stroke: Adults:** 1 cap qam & qpm.	⊛D ✿> Avoid if CrCl <10 ml/ min. **H R**

NAME	FORM/STRENGTH	DOSAGE	COMMENTS

PLATELET AGGREGATION-ADHESION INHIBITOR

| **Aspirin**
(Bayer Aspirin,
Bayer Aspirin Children's) | **Chewtab:** 81 mg;
Tab: 81 mg, 325 mg;
Tab,Delay: 81 mg,
325 mg, 500 mg | **Adults: Stroke/TIA:** 50-325 mg qd. **Suspected AMI:** **Initial:** 160-162.5 mg qd as soon as suspect MI. **Maint:** 160-162.5 mg x 30d post-infarct. **Prevention or Recurrent MI:** 75-325 mg qd. | ◎N
✲v Avoid use
during 3rd
trimester. **H R** |

SPECIFIC FACTOR XA INHIBITORS

| **Fondaparinux Sodium**
(Arixtra) | **Inj:** 2.5 mg/0.5 ml, 5 mg/
0.4 ml, 7.5 mg/0.6 ml,
10 mg/0.8 ml | **Adults: SC: DVT Prophylaxis for Hip Fracture or Replacement Surgery/Knee Replacement Surgery/ Abdominal Surgery:** 2.5 mg qd, starting no earlier than 6-8h post-op x 5-9d. **Hip Fracture Surgery:** Extended prophylaxis up to 24 additional days. **DVT/PE Treatment: <50 kg:** 5 mg qd. **50-100 kg:** 7.5 mg qd. **>100 kg:** 10 mg qd. Add concomitant warfarin ASAP (usually w/in 72h) & continue til INR=2-3. | ◎B
✲> **R W** [6] |
| **Rivaroxaban**
(Xarelto) | **Tab:** 10 mg, 15 mg,
20 mg | **Adults: Reduction of Stroke/Systemic Embolism Risk in Nonvalvular Atrial Fibrillation: CrCl >50 ml/min:** 20 mg qd w/ pm meal. **CrCl 15-50 ml/min:** 15 mg qd w/ pm meal. Refer to PI for information when switching from or to warfarin/anticoagulants. **Prophylaxis of DVT:** 10 mg qd. Give initial dose at least 6-10h after surgery once hemostasis is established. **Treatment Duration: Hip Replacement Surgery:** 35d. **Knee Replacement Surgery:** 12d. Refer to PI for surgery/intervention. | ◎C
✲v **H R W** [6] |

VITAMIN K-DEPENDENT COAGULATION FACTOR INHIBITOR

| **Warfarin Sodium**
(Coumadin, Jantoven) | **Inj:** (Coumadin) 5 mg;
Tab: (Coumadin, Jantoven) 1 mg, 2 mg, 2.5 mg, 3 mg, 4 mg, 5 mg, 6 mg, 7.5 mg, 10 mg | **Adults:** Adjust dose based on INR. IV dose is the same as PO dose. **CYP2C9 and VKORC1 Genotypes Unknown: Initial:** 2-5 mg qd. **Maint:** 2-10 mg qd. **Venous Thromboembolism (including DVT & PE)/Non-Valvular A-Fib:** Target INR 2.5 (INR Range, 2-3). **Mechanical or Bioprosthetic Heart Valve:** Refer to PI for target INR depending on type of heart valve. **Post-MI:** INR 2-3 w/ low-dose ASA (≤100 mg/d) x at least 3 mths after MI. **Valvular Disease Associated w/ A-Fib/Mitral Stenosis/Recurrent Systemic Embolism of Unknown Etiology:** INR 2-3. Refer to PI for recommended durations, conversion from heparin, and dosing recommendation w/ consideration of genotype. | ⊕D (mechanical heart valves)
⊕X (other pregnant populations)
❈> May cause major/fatal bleeding. **H** |

Heart Failure
ACE INHIBITORS

| **Captopril** | **Tab:** 12.5 mg, 25 mg, 50 mg, 100 mg | **Adults: CHF: Initial:** 25 mg tid. **Usual:** 50-100 mg tid. **Max:** 450 mg/d. **Left Ventricular Dysfunction Following MI: Initial:** 6.25 mg single dose, then 12.5 mg tid. **Titrate:** Increase to 25 mg tid over next several days, then to 50 mg tid over next several wks. **Usual:** 50 mg tid. | ⊕D
❈v **R W**[7] |

NAME	FORM/STRENGTH	DOSAGE	COMMENTS
Enalapril Maleate (Vasotec)	**Tab:** 2.5 mg, 5 mg, 10 mg, 20 mg	**Adults: Initial:** 2.5 mg qd. **Usual:** 2.5-20 mg bid. Titrate upward, as tolerated, over few days or wks. **Max:** 40 mg/d in divided doses. **Asymptomatic Left Ventricular Dysfunction: Initial:** 2.5 mg bid. **Titrate:** Increase as tolerated to 20 mg/d (in divided doses). **Hyponatremia or SrCr >1.6 mg/dl w/ HF: Initial:** 2.5 mg/d. **Titrate:** Increase to 2.5 mg bid, then 5 mg bid & higher prn, usually at intervals of ≥4d. **Max:** 40 mg/d.	⊕D ❄v R W [7]
Fosinopril Sodium (Monopril)	**Tab:** 10 mg, 20 mg, 40 mg	**Adults: Initial:** 10 mg qd. **Titrate:** Increase over several wks. **Usual:** 20-40 mg qd. **Max:** 40 mg/d.	⊕C (1st trimester) ⊕D (2nd/3rd trimester) ❄v R W [7]
Lisinopril (Prinivil)	**Tab:** 5 mg, 10 mg, 20 mg	**Adults: Initial:** 5 mg qd. **Usual:** 5-20 mg qd. **Hyponatremia or CrCl ≤30 ml/min or SrCr >3 mg/dl: Initial:** 2.5 mg qd.	⊕D ❄v R W [7]
Lisinopril (Zestril)	**Tab:** 2.5 mg, 5 mg, 10 mg, 20 mg, 30 mg, 40 mg	**Adults: Initial:** 5 mg qd. **Usual:** 5-40 mg qd. **Titrate:** Increase by 10 mg q2wks. **Max:** 40 mg/d. **Hyponatremia or CrCl ≤30 ml/min or SrCr >3 mg/dl: Initial:** 2.5 mg qd.	⊕D ❄v R W [7]
Quinapril HCl (Accupril)	**Tab:** 5 mg, 10 mg, 20 mg, 40 mg	**Adults: Initial:** 5 mg bid. **Titrate:** Increase at wkly intervals. **Usual:** 20-40 mg/d given bid.	⊕D ❄> R W [7]

Ramipril (Altace)	**Cap:** 1.25 mg, 2.5 mg, 5 mg, 10 mg	**Adults: CHF Post-MI: Initial:** 2.5 mg bid, or 1.25 mg bid if hypotensive. **Titrate:** Increase to 5 mg bid at 3-wk intervals after 1 wk of initial dose. **Renal Artery Stenosis/ Volume Depletion/Concomitant Diuretic: Initial:** 1.25 mg qd. Adjust according to BP response.	⊕D ❄v **H R W** [7]
Trandolapril (Mavik)	**Tab:** 1 mg, 2 mg, 4 mg	**Post-MI CHF/Left-Ventricular Dysfunction: Adults: Initial:** 1 mg qd. **Titrate:** Increase to target dose of 4 mg qd as tolerated.	⊕D ❄v **H R W** [7]
ALDOSTERONE BLOCKER			
Eplerenone (Inspra)	**Tab:** 25 mg, 50 mg	**CHF Post-MI: Adults: Initial:** 25 mg qd. **Titrate:** To 50 mg qd w/in 4 wks. **Maint:** 50 mg qd. **Adjust dose based on K⁺ level:** See PI.	⊕B ❄v **R**
ALPHA/BETA BLOCKERS			
Carvedilol (Coreg, Coreg CR)	**Cap,ER:** 10 mg, 20 mg, 40 mg, 80 mg; **Tab:** 3.125 mg, 6.25 mg, 12.5 mg, 25 mg	**Adults:** Individualize dose. **CHF: Tab: Initial:** 3.125 mg bid x 2 wks. **Titrate:** May double dose q2wks up to 25 mg bid as tolerated. **Max:** 50 mg bid if >85 kg. Reduce dose if HR <55 beats/min. **Cap,ER: Initial:** 10 mg qam x 2 wks. **Titrate:** May double dose q2wks up to 80 mg qd as tolerated. Reduce dose if HR <55 beats/min. **LVD Post-MI: Tab: Initial:** 6.25 mg bid x 3-10d. **Titrate:** May double dose q3-10d to target of 25 mg bid. May begin w/ 3.125 mg bid	⊕C ❄v **H W** [17,18]

Continued on Next Page

NAME	FORM/STRENGTH	DOSAGE	COMMENTS
Carvedilol (Coreg, Coreg CR) *Continued*		and/or slow up-titration rate if clinically indicated. **Cap,ER: Initial:** 20 mg qam x 3-10d. **Titrate:** May double dose q3-10d to target of 80 mg qd. May begin w/ 10 mg qd and/ or slow up-titration if clinically indicated.	

ANGIOTENSIN II RECEPTOR ANTAGONISTS

NAME	FORM/STRENGTH	DOSAGE	COMMENTS
Candesartan Cilexetil (Atacand)	**Tab:** 4 mg, 8 mg, 16 mg, 32 mg	**Adults: Initial:** 4 mg qd. **Titrate:** Double dose at 2-wk intervals, as tolerated. **Target:** 32 mg qd.	▣D ❋v H W [9]
Valsartan (Diovan)	**Tab:** 40 mg, 80 mg, 160 mg, 320 mg	**Adults: Initial:** 40 mg bid. **Titrate:** May increase to 80 mg or 160 mg bid (use highest dose tolerated). **Max:** 320 mg/d in divided doses.	▣D ❋v H R W [9]

BETA BLOCKERS

NAME	FORM/STRENGTH	DOSAGE	COMMENTS
Metoprolol Succinate (Toprol-XL)	**Tab,ER:** 25 mg, 50 mg, 100 mg, 200 mg	**Adults: Initial: Class II HF:** 25 mg qd x 2 wks. **Severe HF:** 12.5 mg qd x 2 wks. **Titrate:** Double dose q2wks as tolerated. **Max:** 200 mg/d.	▣C ❋> W [18]

DIURETICS (LOOP)

NAME	FORM/STRENGTH	DOSAGE	COMMENTS
Bumetanide	**Inj:** 0.25 mg/ml; **Tab:** 0.5 mg, 1 mg, 2 mg	**Adults: PO: Usual:** 0.5-2 mg qd. **Maint:** Give qod or q3-4d. **Max:** 10 mg/d. **IV/IM: Initial:** 0.5-1 mg, may repeat q2-3h x 2-3 doses. **Max:** 10 mg/d.	▣C ❋v W [8]

| Furosemide (Lasix) | (Generic) **Inj:** 10 mg/ml; **Sol:** 10 mg/ml, 40 mg/ 5 ml; (Generic, Lasix) **Tab:** 20 mg, 40 mg, 80 mg | **Adults: Edema: PO: Initial:** 20-80 mg as single dose. **Titrate:** May repeat or increase by 20-40 mg after 6-8h. **Max:** 600 mg/d. Dose on 2-4 consecutive days/wk. **IV/ IM: Initial:** 20-40 mg as single dose. **Titrate:** May repeat or increase by 20 mg after 2h. **Acute Pulmonary Edema: Initial:** 40 mg IV. May increase to 80 mg IV after 1h. **Peds: PO: Initial:** 2 mg/kg as single dose, may increase by 1-2 mg/kg after 6-8h. **Max:** 6 mg/kg. **IV/IM:** 1 mg/kg single dose. May increase by 1 mg/kg after 2h. **Max:** 6 mg/kg. **Premature Infants: Max:** 1 mg/kg/d. | ⊕C ❄> W [8] |
| Torsemide (Demadex) | **Inj:** 10 mg/ml; **Tab:** 5 mg, 10 mg, 20 mg, 100 mg | **Adults: Initial:** 10-20 mg qd. **Titrate:** Double dose until desired response. **Max:** 200 mg single dose. | ⊕B ❄> |

DIURETICS (POTASSIUM-SPARING)

| Spironolactone (Aldactone) | **Tab:** 25 mg, 50 mg, 100 mg | **Adults: Edema: Initial:** 100 mg/d in single or divided doses for ≥5d. May add 2nd diuretic if inadequate response after 5d. **Usual:** 25-200 mg/d. **Severe HF (Serum K⁺ ≤5.0 mEq/l, SrCr ≤2.5 mg/dl): Initial:** 25 mg qd. **Titrate:** May increase to 50 mg qd if tolerated or reduce to 25 mg qod if not tolerated. | ⊕C ❄v R W [16] |
| Triamterene (Dyrenium) | **Cap:** 50 mg, 100 mg | **Adults: Initial:** 100 mg bid. **Max:** 300 mg/d. | ⊕C ❄v W [88] |

NAME	FORM/STRENGTH	DOSAGE	COMMENTS
DIURETICS (POTASSIUM SPARING/THIAZIDE)			
Spironolactone/ Hydrochlorothiazide (Aldactazide)	**Tab:** 25-25 mg, 50-50 mg	**Adults:** Individually titrate components. **Maint:** 100 mg/d per component qd or in divided doses. **Range:** 25-200 mg/d per component.	⊙C ❋v Not for initial therapy. R W [16]
Triamterene/ Hydrochlorothiazide (Dyazide)	**Cap:** 37.5-25 mg	**Adults: Usual:** (37.5-25 mg) 1-2 caps qd.	⊙C ❋v
Triamterene/ Hydrochlorothiazide (Maxzide, Maxzide-25)	**Tab:** 37.5-25 mg, 75-50 mg	**Adults: Usual:** (37.5-25 mg) 1-2 tabs qd. (75-50 mg) 1 tab qd.	⊙C ❋v W [88]
DIURETICS (THIAZIDE)			
Chlorothiazide (Diuril)	**Inj:** (Sodium Diuril) 0.5 gm; **Susp:** (Diuril) 250 mg/5 ml; **Tab:** 250 mg, 500 mg	**Adults:** IV/PO: 0.5-1 gm qd-bid. May give qod or 3-5d/ wk. **Peds: PO: Usual:** 10-20 mg/kg/d given qd-bid. **Max: 2-12 yo:** 1 gm/d. **<2 yo:** 375 mg/d. **<6 mths:** Up to 30 mg/kg/d given bid.	⊙C ❋v
Hydrochlorothiazide	**Cap:** 12.5 mg; **Tab:** 12.5 mg, 25 mg, 50 mg	**Adults: Tab: Usual:** 25-100 mg/d given qd or in divided doses. May give qod or 3-5d/wk. **Peds: Diuresis:** 1-2 mg/kg/d given qd-bid. **Max: 2-12 yo:** 100 mg/d. **Infants up to 2 yo:** 37.5 mg/d. **<6 mths:** Up to 3 mg/kg/d given bid may be required.	⊙B ❋v

Nesiritide (Natrecor)	Inj: 1.5 mg	**Adults:** 2 mcg/kg IV bolus over 60 sec, then 0.01 mcg/kg/min IV infusion.	⊕C ✿>

Hypertension
ACE INHIBITORS

Benazepril HCl (Lotensin)	Tab: 5 mg, 10 mg, 20 mg, 40 mg	**Adults: Initial:** 10 mg qd or 5 mg qd if on diuretic. **Maint:** 20-40 mg/d given qd or bid. **Max:** 80 mg/d. **Peds: ≥6 yo: Initial:** 0.2 mg/kg qd. **Max:** 0.6 mg/kg or 40mg/d.	⊕D ✿> R W [7]
Captopril	Tab: 12.5 mg, 25 mg, 50 mg, 100 mg	**Adults: Initial:** 25 mg bid-tid. **Titrate:** Increase to 50 mg bid-tid after 1-2 wks. **Usual:** 25-150 mg bid-tid. **Max:** 450 mg/d.	⊕D ✿v R W [7]
Enalapril Maleate (Vasotec)	Tab: 2.5 mg, 5 mg, 10 mg, 20 mg	**Adults: Initial:** 5 mg qd; 2.5 if on diuretic. **Usual:** 10-40 mg/d as qd-bid. **Peds: 1 mth-16 yo: Initial:** 0.08 mg/kg (up to 5 mg) qd. **Titrate:** According to BP response. **Max:** 0.58 mg/kg/dose (or 40 mg/dose).	⊕D ✿v R W [7]
Enalaprilat	Inj: 1.25 mg/ml	**Adults: Usual:** 1.25 IV over 5 min q6h. **Max:** 20 mg/d. **Concomitant Diuretic: Initial:** 0.625 mg over 5 min, may repeat after 1h. **Maint:** An additional dose of 1.25 mg q6h. **PO/IV Conversion:** See PI.	⊕C (1st trimester) ⊕D (2nd/3rd trimester) ✿v R W [7]

NAME	FORM/STRENGTH	DOSAGE	COMMENTS
Fosinopril Sodium (Monopril)	**Tab:** 10 mg, 20 mg, 40 mg	**Adults:** Initial: 10 mg qd. **Usual:** 20-40 mg qd. **Max:** 80 mg/d. **Peds:** >50 kg: 5-10 mg qd.	●C (1st trimester) ●D (2nd/3rd trimester) ❊v W [7]
Lisinopril (Prinivil)	**Tab:** 5 mg, 10 mg, 20 mg	**Adults:** If possible, d/c diuretic 2-3d prior to therapy. **Initial:** 10 mg qd; 5 mg qd w/ diuretic. **Usual:** 20-40 mg qd. Resume diuretic if BP not controlled. **Max:** 80 mg/d. **Peds:** ≥6 yo: **Initial:** 0.07 mg/kg qd (up to 5 mg total). Adjust dose based on BP response. **Max:** 0.61 mg/kg qd (up to 40 mg).	●D ❊v R W [7]
Lisinopril (Zestril)	**Tab:** 2.5 mg, 5 mg, 10 mg, 20 mg, 30 mg, 40 mg	**Adults:** If possible, d/c diuretic 2-3d prior to therapy. **Initial:** 10 mg qd; 5 mg qd w/ diuretic. **Usual:** 20-40 mg qd. Resume diuretic if BP not controlled. **Max:** 80 mg/d. **Peds:** ≥6 yo: **Initial:** 0.07 mg/kg qd (up to 5 mg total). Adjust dose based on BP response. **Max:** 0.61 mg/kg qd (or 40 mg/d).	●D ❊v R W [7]
Quinapril HCl (Accupril)	**Tab:** 5 mg, 10 mg, 20 mg, 40 mg	**Adults:** If possible, d/c diuretic 2-3d prior to therapy. **Initial:** 10 or 20 mg qd; 5 mg qd if on diuretic. **Titrate:** May adjust dose based on BP at intervals of at least 2 wks. **Usual:** 20, 40, or 80 mg/d given qd-bid. **Elderly:** **Initial:** 10 mg qd. **Titrate:** Increase to optimal response.	●D ❊> R W [7]

| Ramipril
(Altace) | Cap: 1.25 mg, 2.5 mg,
5 mg, 10 mg | **Adults: Initial:** 2.5 mg qd. Adjust dosage according to BP. **Maint:** 2.5-20 mg/d given qd-bid. Add diuretic if BP not controlled. **Renal Artery Stenosis/Volume Depletion/Concomitant Diuretic: Initial:** 1.25 mg qd. Adjust according to BP response. | ⊕D
❄v **H R W** [7] |

ACE INHIBITORS/CALCIUM CHANNEL BLOCKERS

| Amlodipine Besylate/
Benazepril HCl
(Lotrel) | Cap: 2.5-10 mg,
5-10 mg, 5-20 mg,
5-40 mg, 10-20 mg,
10-40 mg | **Adults: Usual:** Dose qd. **Add-On:** If inadequate control w/ amlodipine (or another dihydropyridine) alone or benazepril (or another ACE inhibitor) alone. If adequate control w/ amlodipine but w/ unacceptable edema. **Replacement:** May substitute for titrated components. **Elderly: Initial:** 2.5 mg amlodipine. | ⊕D
❄v **H R W** [7, 24] |

ACE INHIBITORS/THIAZIDES

| Enalapril/Hydrochlorothiazide | Tab: 5-12.5 mg, 10-25 mg | **Adults:** BP Not Controlled w/ Enalapril or HCTZ **Monotherapy: Initial:** 5-12.5 mg or 10-25 mg qd. **Titrate:** May increase after 2-3 wks. **Max:** 20 mg enalapril/50 mg HCTZ per day. **Replacement Therapy:** Substitute combination for titrated components. | ⊕D
❄v **R W** [7, 24] |

NAME	FORM/STRENGTH	DOSAGE	COMMENTS
Lisinopril/ Hydrochlorothiazide (Prinzide)	**Tab:** 10-12.5 mg, 20-12.5 mg	**Adults: Not Controlled w/ Lisinopril or HCTZ Monotherapy: Initial:** 10-12.5 mg tab or 20-12.5 mg tab qd. **Titrate:** May increase HCTZ dose after 2-3 wks. **Controlled on 25 mg HCTZ/d w/ Hypokalemia:** 10-12.5 mg tab. **Max:** 80-50 mg. **Replacement Therapy:** Substitute combination for titrated components.	●D ❀v H R W [7, 24]
Lisinopril/ Hydrochlorothiazide (Zestoretic)	**Tab:** 10-12.5 mg, 20-25 mg	**Adults: Not Controlled w/ Lisinopril or HCTZ Monotherapy: Initial:** 10-12.5 mg or 20-12.5 mg qd. **Titrate:** May increase HCTZ dose after 2-3 wks. **Controlled on HCTZ 25 mg/d w/ Hypokalemia:** 10-12.5 mg qd. **Replacement Therapy:** Substitute combination for titrated components.	●D ❀v H R W [7, 24]
Quinapril/Hydrochlorothiazide (Accuretic)	**Tab:** 10-12.5 mg, 20-12.5 mg, 20-25 mg	**Adults: Not Controlled w/ Quinapril Monotherapy: Initial:** 10-12.5 mg or 20-12.5 mg tab qd. **Titrate:** May increase dose based on clinical response. May increase HCTZ after 2-3 wks. **Controlled w/ HCTZ 25 mg/d w/ Hypokalemia:** 10-12.5 mg or 20-12.5 mg tab qd. **Adequately Treated w/ 20 mg Quinapril and 25 mg HCTZ w/o Significant Electrolye Disturbances:** May switch to 20-25 mg tab qd.	●D ❀> H R W [7, 24]
ALDOSTERONE BLOCKER			
Eplerenone (Inspra)	**Tab:** 25 mg, 50 mg	**Adults: Initial:** 50 mg qd. May increase to 50 mg bid if inadequate effect. **W/ Weak CYP3A4 Inhibitors: Initial:** 25 mg qd.	●B ❀v R

ALPHA ADRENERGIC AGONIST

Clonidine HCl (Catapres, Catapres-TTS)	**Patch: (TTS)** 0.1 mg/24h, 0.2 mg/24h, 0.3 mg/24h; **Tab:** 0.1 mg, 0.2 mg, 0.3 mg	**Adults: Patch: Initial:** 0.1 mg/24h patch wkly. **Titrate:** May increase after 1-2 wks. **Max:** 0.6 mg/24h. **Tab: Initial:** 0.1 mg bid. **Titrate:** May increase by 0.1 mg wkly. **Usual:** 0.2-0.6 mg/d. **Max:** 2.4 mg/d.	⊕C ✿> R

ALPHA/BETA BLOCKERS

Carvedilol (Coreg, Coreg CR)	**Cap,ER:** 10 mg, 20 mg, 40 mg, 80 mg; **Tab:** 3.125 mg, 6.25 mg, 12.5 mg, 25 mg	**Adults:** Individualize dose. **Tab: Initial:** 6.25 mg bid x 7-14d. **Titrate:** May double dose q7-14d. **Max:** 50 mg/d. **Cap,ER: Initial:** 20 mg qam x 7-14d. **Titrate:** May double dose q7-14d as tolerated. **Max:** 80 mg/d.	⊕C ✿v H W [17, 18]
Labetalol HCl	**Inj:** 5 mg/ml; **Tab:** 100 mg, 200 mg, 300 mg	**Adults: PO: Initial:** 100 mg bid. **Titrate:** Increase by 100 mg bid q2-3d. **Maint:** 200-400 mg bid. **Max:** 2400 mg/d. **IV: Initial:** 20 mg over 2 min, then may give 40-80 mg q10 min until desired response. **Max:** 300 mg.	⊕C ✿>

ALPHA₁ RECEPTOR BLOCKERS

Doxazosin Mesylate (Cardura)	**Tab:** 1 mg, 2 mg, 4 mg, 8 mg	**Adults: Initial:** 1 mg qd. **Titrate:** Based on response may increase to 2 mg, then 4 mg, 8 mg, and 16 mg. **Max:** 16 mg/d.	⊕C ✿> Syncope w/ 1st dose.
Terazosin HCl	**Cap:** 1 mg, 2 mg, 5 mg, 10 mg	**Adults: Initial:** 1 mg qhs. **Usual:** 1-5 mg/d. Slowly increase dose or use bid regimen if substantially diminished response at 24h. **Max:** 40 mg/d.	⊕C ✿> Syncope w/ 1st dose.

NAME	FORM/STRENGTH	DOSAGE	COMMENTS

ANGIOTENSIN II RECEPTOR ANTAGONISTS

NAME	FORM/STRENGTH	DOSAGE	COMMENTS
Azilsartan Medoxomil (Edarbi)	**Tab:** 40 mg, 80 mg	**Adults: Usual:** 80 mg qd. **W/ High-Dose Diuretics: Initial:** 40 mg qd.	⊞D ✿v W [9]
Candesartan Cilexetil (Atacand)	**Tab:** 4 mg, 8 mg, 16 mg, 32 mg	**Adults: Initial:** 16 mg qd. **Usual:** 8-32 mg/d, given qd-bid. **Peds: 6-<17 yo: <50 kg: Initial:** 4-8 mg. **Usual:** 2-16 mg/d. **>50 kg: Initial:** 8-16 mg. **Usual:** 4-32 mg/d. **1-<6 yo: Initial:** 0.20 mg/kg as PO sus; see PI. **Usual:** 0.05-0.4 mg/kg/d. Give qd or divided into 2 equal doses. PO sus may be substituted for children that cannot swallow; see PI.	⊞D ✿v H W [9]
Eprosartan Mesylate (Teveten)	**Tab:** 400 mg, 600 mg	**Adults: Initial (Monotherapy & Not Volume-Depleted):** 600 mg qd. **Usual:** 400-800 mg/d, given qd-bid. **Max:** 800 mg/d.	⊞D ✿v R W [9]
Irbesartan (Avapro)	**Tab:** 75 mg, 150 mg, 300 mg	**Adults: Initial:** 150 mg qd. **Titrate:** May increase to 300 mg qd. May add low-dose diuretic if BP not controlled. **Max:** 300 mg qd. **Intravascular Volume/Salt Depletion: Initial:** 75 mg qd.	⊞D ✿v W [9]
Losartan Potassium (Cozaar)	**Tab:** 25 mg, 50 mg, 100 mg	**HTN: Adults: Initial:** 50 mg qd. **Intravascular Volume Depletion/History of Hepatic Impairment: Initial:** 25 mg qd. **Usual:** 25-100 mg/d, given qd-bid. **HTN w/LVH: Initial:** 50 mg qd. Add HCTZ 12.5 mg qd and/or increase losartan to 100 mg qd, followed by an increase in HCTZ to 25 mg	⊞C (1st trimester) ⊞D (2nd/3rd trimester) ✿v H R W [9]

		qd based on BP response. **Peds: ≥6 yo: Initial:** 0.7 mg/kg qd (up to 50 mg total). **Max:** 1.4 mg/kg/d (or 100 mg/d).	
Olmesartan Medoxomil (Benicar)	**Tab:** 5 mg, 20 mg, 40 mg	**Adults:** Individualize. **Monotherapy W/O Volume Contraction: Initial:** 20 mg qd. **Titrate:** May increase to 40 mg qd after 2 wks if needed. May add diuretic if BP not controlled. **Intravascular Volume Depletion (eg, treated w/ diuretics, particularly w/ impaired renal function):** Lower initial dose; monitor closely. **Peds:** Individualize. **6-16 yo: 20-<35 kg: Initial:** 10 mg qd. **Titrate:** May increase to 20 mg qd after 2 wks if needed. **Max:** 20 mg qd. **≥35 kg: Initial:** 20 mg qd. **Titrate:** May increase to 40 mg qd after 2 wks if needed. **Max:** 40 mg qd.	▣D ❃v W [9]
Telmisartan (Micardis)	**Tab:** 20 mg, 40 mg, 80 mg	**Adults: Initial:** 40 mg qd. **Usual:** 20-80 mg qd. If additional BP reduction is required beyond that achieved w/ 80 mg dose, a diuretic may be added.	▣D ❃v H W [9]
Valsartan (Diovan)	**Tab:** 40 mg, 80 mg, 160 mg, 320 mg	**Adults: Monotherapy w/o Volume Depletion: Initial:** 80 or 160 mg qd. **Titrate:** May increase to max of 320 mg qd or add diuretic. **Max:** 320 mg qd. **Peds: 6-16 yo: Initial:** 1.3 mg/kg qd (up to 40 mg total). Adjust dose according to BP response. **Max:** 2.7 mg/kg (up to 160 mg) qd. Refer to PI for susp preparation from tab. Adjust dose accordingly when switching dosage forms; exposure w/ susp is 1.6X greater than w/ tab.	▣D ❃v H R W [9]

NAME	FORM/STRENGTH	DOSAGE	COMMENTS
ANGIOTENSIN II RECEPTOR ANTAGONISTS/CALCIUM CHANNEL BLOCKERS/THIAZIDES			
Amlodipine/Valsartan/ Hydrochlorothiazide (Exforge HCT)	**Tab:** 5-160-12.5 mg, 5-160-25 mg, 10-160-12.5 mg, 10-160-25 mg, 10-320-25 mg	**Adults: Usual:** Dose qd. May increase after 2 wks. **Max:** 10-320-25 mg qd. **Add-On/Switch Therapy:** If inadequate control on any 2 of the following antihypertensive classes: calcium channel blockers, angiotensin receptor blockers, and diuretics. If w/ dose-limiting adverse reactions to any component on dual therapy, switch to triple therapy containing lower dose of that component. **Replacement Therapy:** May substitute for individually titrated components.	⊕D ❄v **W** [9]
Olmesartan Medoxomil/ Hydrochlorothiazide/ Amlodipine (Tribenzor)	**Tab:** 20-12.5-5 mg, 40-12.5-5 mg, 40-25-5 mg, 40-12.5-10 mg, 40-25-10 mg	**Adults: Usual:** Dose qd. May increase after 2 wks. **Max:** 40-25-10 mg. **Add-On/Switch Therapy:** May use if not adequately controlled on any 2 of the following antihypertensive classes: angiotensin receptor blockers, calcium channel blockers, and diuretics. W/ dose-limiting adverse reactions to any component on dual therapy, switch to triple therapy containing lower dose of that component. **Replacement Therapy:** May substitute for individually titrated components.	⊕D ❄v **H R W** [9, 24]

ANGIOTENSIN II RECEPTOR ANTAGONISTS/THIAZIDES

Azilsartan Medoxomil/ Chlorthalidone (Edarbyclor)	**Tab:** 40-12.5 mg, 40-25 mg	**Adults: Initial:** 40-12.5 mg qd. **Titrate:** May increase to 40-25 mg after 2-4 wks. **Max:** 40-25 mg. **Add-On Therapy:** Use if not adequately controlled on angiotensin receptor blocker or diuretic monotherapy. **Replacement Therapy:** May substitute for titrated components.	⊙D ✿v W [9]
Irbesartan/ Hydrochlorothiazide (Avalide)	**Tab:** 150-12.5 mg, 300-12.5 mg	**Adults: Initial:** 150-12.5 mg qd. **Titrate:** May increase after 1-2 wks to a max dose of 300-25 mg qd. **Not Controlled w/ Monotherapy:** Recommended doses in order of increasing mean effect are 150-12.5 mg, 300-12.5 mg, & 300-25 mg. **Replacement Therapy:** May substitute for titrated components.	⊙D ✿v H R W [9]
Losartan/Hydrochlorothiazide (Hyzaar)	**Tab:** 50-12.5 mg, 100-12.5 mg, 100-25 mg	**Adults: HTN: Usual:** 50-12.5 mg qd. **Max:** 100-25 mg qd. **Uncontrolled BP on Losartan Monotherapy or HCTZ Alone/Uncontrolled BP on 25 mg qd HCTZ/Controlled BP on 25 mg qd HCTZ w/ Hypokalemia:** 50-12.5 mg qd. **Titrate:** If uncontrolled after 3 wks, increase to 100-25 mg qd. **Uncontrolled BP on 100 mg Losartan Monotherapy:** 100-12.5 mg qd. **Titrate:** If uncontrolled after 3 wks, increase to 100-25 mg qd. **Severe HTN: Initial:** 50-12.5 mg qd. **Titrate:** If inadequate response after 2-4 wks, increase to 100-25 mg qd. **Max:** 100-25 mg qd. **HTN w/ Left Ventricular Hypertrophy: Initial:** Losartan	⊙C (1st trimester) ⊙D (2nd/3rd trimester) ✿v H R W [9, 24]

Continued on Next Page

NAME	FORM/STRENGTH	DOSAGE	COMMENTS
Losartan/Hydrochlorothiazide (Hyzaar) *Continued*		50 mg qd. If inadequate BP reduction, add 12.5 mg HCTZ or substitute losartan-HCTZ 50-12.5 mg. If additional BP reduction needed, substitute w/ losartan 100 mg & HCTZ 12.5 mg or losartan-HCTZ 100-12.5 mg, followed by losartan 100 mg & HCTZ 25 mg or losartan-HCTZ 100-25 mg. **Replacement Therapy:** Combination may be substituted for titrated components.	
Olmesartan Medoxomil/ Hydrochlorothiazide (Benicar HCT)	**Tab:** 20-12.5 mg, 40-12.5 mg, 40-25 mg	**Adults: Replacement Therapy:** Individualize dose. Combination may be substituted for titrated components. **Uncontrolled BP on Olmesartan or HCTZ Alone:** Switch to 1 tab qd of combination therapy: **Titrate:** May increase at intervals of 2-4 wks. **Max:** 1 tab/d.	⊕D ❄v W [9]
Telmisartan/ Hydrochlorothiazide (Micardis HCT)	**Tab:** 40-12.5 mg, 80-12.5 mg, 80-25 mg	**Adults: Initial** (if not controlled on 80 mg telmisartan, or 25 mg HCTZ/d, or controlled on 25 mg HCTZ/d but serum K⁺ decreased): 80-12.5 mg tab qd or 80-25 mg tab qd (for those not controlled on 25 mg HCTZ/d). **Max:** 160-25 mg/d. **Replacement Therapy:** Substitute combination for titrated components.	⊕D ❄v H R W [9, 24]
Valsartan/ Hydrochlorothiazide (Diovan HCT)	**Tab:** 80-12.5 mg, 160-12.5 mg, 160-25 mg, 320-12.5 mg, 320-25 mg	**Adults: Initial Therapy:** 160-12.5 mg qd. **Titrate:** May increase after 1-2 wks of therapy. **Max:** 320-25 mg qd. **Add-On Therapy:** If not adequately controlled w/ valsartan (or another angiotensin receptor blocker) alone or HCTZ alone. If dose-limiting adverse reactions w/ either component alone, switch to valsartan-HCTZ containing lower dose of that component. **Titrate:** May increase after	⊕D ❄v W [9]

3-4 wks of therapy if BP uncontrolled. **Max:** 320-25 mg.
Replacement Therapy: May substitute for titrated components.

BETA BLOCKERS

Atenolol (Tenormin)	**Tab:** 25 mg, 50 mg, 100 mg	**Adults: Initial:** 50 mg qd. **Titrate:** May increase after 1-2 wks. **Max:** 100 mg qd.	⊞D ❄️> R
Bisoprolol Fumarate (Zebeta)	**Tab:** 5 mg, 10 mg	**Adults: Initial:** 2.5-5 mg qd. **Usual:** 5-20 mg qd.	⊞C ❄️> H R W [17, 18]
Metoprolol Succinate (Toprol-XL)	**Tab,ER:** 25 mg, 50 mg, 100 mg, 200 mg	**Adults: Initial:** 25-100 mg qd. **Titrate:** Increase wkly. **Max:** 400 mg/d. **Peds:** ≥6 yo: 1mg/kg qd. **Max:** 50 mg/d.	⊞C ❄️> W [18]
Metoprolol Tartrate (Lopressor)	**Tab:** 50 mg, 100 mg	**Adults: Initial:** 100 mg qd or 50 mg bid. **Titrate:** May increase at wkly (or longer) intervals. **Usual:** 100-450 mg/d. **Max:** 450 mg/d.	⊞C ❄️> W [18]
Nadolol (Corgard)	**Tab:** 20 mg, 40 mg, 80 mg	**Adults: Initial:** 40 mg qd. **Titrate:** Increase by 40-80 mg. **Usual:** 40-80 mg qd. **Max:** 320 mg/d.	⊞C ❄️v R W [18]
Nebivolol (Bystolic)	**Tab:** 2.5 mg, 5 mg, 10 mg, 20 mg	**Adults: Monotherapy/Combination Therapy: Initial:** 5 mg qd. **Titrate:** May increase dose at 2-wk intervals if needed. **Max:** 40 mg.	⊞C ❄️v H R
Propranolol HCl	**Tab:** 10 mg, 20 mg, 40 mg, 60 mg, 80 mg	**Adults: Initial:** 40 mg bid. **Maint:** 120-240 mg/d.	⊞C ❄️> W [18]

NAME	FORM/STRENGTH	DOSAGE	COMMENTS

BETA BLOCKER/THIAZIDE

| Atenolol/Chlorthalidone (Tenoretic) | Tab: 50-25 mg, 100-25 mg | **Adults:** Individualize dose. **Initial:** 50-25 mg tab qd. **Titrate:** May increase to 100-25 mg tab qd. | ⊞D ❄> R |

CALCIUM CHANNEL BLOCKER (DIHYDROPYRIDINE)/RENIN INHIBITOR

| Amlodipine/Aliskiren (Tekamlo) | Tab: 5-150 mg, 10-150 mg, 5-300 mg, 10-300 mg | **Adults: Initial:** 5-150 mg qd. **Titrate:** If BP remains uncontrolled after 2-4 wks, may increase up to a max dose of 10-300 mg qd. **Max:** 10-300 mg qd. **Add-On Therapy:** May use if not controlled w/ individual components alone. W/ dose-limiting adverse reactions to either component alone, switch to amlodipine-aliskiren containing a lower dose of that component. **Replacement Therapy:** May substitute for individually titrated components. | ⊞D ❄v H W [9] |

CALCIUM CHANNEL BLOCKER (DIHYDROPYRIDINE)/THIAZIDE/RENIN INHIBITOR

| Aliskiren/Amlodipine/ Hydrochlorothiazide (Amturnide) | Tab: 150-5-12.5 mg, 300-5-12.5 mg, 300-5-25 mg, 300-10-12.5 mg, 300-10-25 mg | **Adults: Usual:** Dose qd. **Titrate:** May increase after 2 wks of therapy. **Max:** 300-10-25 mg. **Add-On/Switch Therapy:** If inadequate control on any 2 of the following: aliskiren, dihydropyridine calcium channel blockers, and thiazide diuretics. If w/ dose-limiting adverse reactions w/ any component on dual therapy, switch to triple therapy containing lower dose of that component. **Replacement Therapy:** May substitute for individually titrated components. | ⊞D ❄v W [9] |

CALCIUM CHANNEL BLOCKER/HMG COA REDUCTASE INHIBITOR

| Amlodipine Besylate/ Atorvastatin Calcium (Caduet) | Tab: 2.5-10 mg, 2.5-20 mg, 2.5-40 mg, 5-10 mg, 5-20 mg, 5-40 mg, 5-80 mg, 10-10 mg, 10-20 mg, 10-40 mg, 10-80 mg | Dosing based on appropriate combination of recommendations for monotherapies. **Amlodipine: Adults:** Initial: 5 mg qd. Titrate over 7-14d. **Max:** 10 mg qd. **Small/ Fragile/Elderly/Concomitant Antihypertensive Therapy: Initial:** 2.5 mg qd. **Peds: 6-17 yo:** 2.5-5 mg qd. **Max:** 5 mg/d. **Atorvastatin:** See under Antilipidemic Agents for dosing. | ◉X ❀v H |

CALCIUM CHANNEL BLOCKERS (DIHYDROPYRIDINE)

Amlodipine Besylate (Norvasc)	Tab: 2.5 mg, 5 mg, 10 mg	**Adults: Initial:** 5 mg qd. Titrate: Over 7-14d. Adjust dose according to patient's need. **Max:** 10 mg qd. **Small/Fragile/ Elderly/Concomitant Antihypertensives:** 2.5 mg qd. **Peds: 6-17 yo:** Usual: 2.5-5 mg qd. **Max:** 5 mg qd.	◉C ❀v H
Isradipine (DynaCirc CR)	Tab,ER: 5 mg, 10 mg	**Adults:** Individualize dose. **Initial:** 5 mg qd alone or w/ a thiazide diuretic. **Titrate:** Adjust in increments of 5 mg/d at 2-4 wk intervals. **Max:** 20 mg/d.	◉C ❀v
Nicardipine (Cardene SR)	Cap: 20 mg, 30 mg; Cap,ER: (SR) 30 mg, 45 mg, 60 mg	**Adults: Initial:** 20 mg tid. **Usual:** 20-40 mg tid. **Cap,ER: Initial:** 30 mg bid. **Usual:** 30-60 mg bid.	◉C ❀v H
Nifedipine (Nifedical XL, Procardia XL)	Tab,ER: (Nifedical XL) 30 mg, 60 mg; (Procardia XL) 30 mg, 60 mg, 90 mg	**Adults:** Adjust dosage according to patient's needs. **Initial:** 30-60 mg qd. **Titrate:** May increase over 7-14d. **Max:** 120 mg/d.	◉C ❀>

NAME	FORM/STRENGTH	DOSAGE	COMMENTS
CALCIUM CHANNEL BLOCKERS (NON-DIHYDROPYRIDINE)			
Diltiazem HCl (Cardizem CD, Cardizem LA, Cartia XT)	**Cap,ER:** (Cardizem CD/Cartia XT) 120 mg, 180 mg, 240 mg, 300 mg, (Cardizem CD) 360 mg; **Tab,ER:** (Cardizem LA) 120 mg, 180 mg, 240 mg, 300 mg, 360 mg, 420 mg	**Adults: Cardizem CD/Cartia XT: Initial: Monotherapy:** 180-240 mg qd. **Titrate:** Adjust to individual patient needs. **Usual:** 240-360 mg/d. **Max:** 480 mg/d. **Cardizem LA: Initial: Monotherapy:** 180-240 mg qd (am or hs). **Titrate:** Adjust to individual patient needs. **Range:** 120-540 mg qd. **Max:** 540 mg qd.	⊙C ✿v
Diltiazem HCl (Dilacor XR, Diltia XT)	**Cap,ER:** (Dilacor XR) 240 mg; (Diltia XT) 120 mg, 180 mg, 240 mg	**Adults: Initial:** 180-240 mg qd. **Usual:** 180-480 mg qd. **≥60 yo:** May respond to 120 mg qd. **Max:** 540 mg/d.	⊙C ✿v
Diltiazem HCl (Taztia XT, Tiazac)	**Cap,ER:** (Taztia XT/Tiazac) 120 mg, 180 mg, 240 mg, 300 mg, 360 mg; (Tiazac) 420 mg	**Adults: Initial:** 120-240 mg qd. **Titrate:** Adjust at 2-wk intervals. **Usual:** 120-540 mg qd. **Max:** 540 mg/d.	⊙C ✿v
Verapamil HCl (Calan SR)	**Tab,ER:** 120 mg, 180 mg, 240 mg	**Adults: Initial:** 180 mg qam. **Titrate:** Increase to 240 mg qam, then 180 mg bid (or 240 mg qam + 120 mg qpm), then 240 mg q12h. Take w/ food.	⊙C ✿v **H R**

Verapamil HCl (Calan)	Tab: 40 mg, 80 mg, 120 mg	Adults: Initial (Monotherapy): 80 mg tid. Usual: 360-480 mg/d. Elderly/Small Stature: Initial: 40 mg tid. Max: 480 mg/d.	⊛C ❀v H R
Verapamil (Covera-HS)	Tab, ER: 180 mg, 240 mg	Adults: Initial: 180 mg qhs. Titrate: Increase to 240 mg qhs, then 360 mg qhs, then 480 mg qhs.	⊛C ❀v H
Verapamil (Verelan PM)	Cap, ER: 100 mg, 200 mg, 300 mg	Adults: Initial: 200 mg qhs. Titrate: Increase to 300 mg qhs, then 400 mg qhs.	⊛C ❀v H
Verapamil (Verelan)	Cap, ER: 120 mg, 180 mg, 240 mg, 360 mg	Adults: Usual: 240 mg qam. Titrate: If inadequate response w/ 120 mg, increase to 180 mg qam, then 240 mg qam, then 360 mg qam, then 480 mg qam based on therapeutic efficacy and safety evaluated approx. 24h after dosing.	⊛C ❀v H

CALCIUM CHANNEL BLOCKERS/ANGIOTENSIN II RECEPTOR ANTAGONISTS

| Olmesartan Medoxomil/ Amlodipine (Azor) | Tab: 20-5 mg, 20-10 mg, 40-5 mg, 40-10 mg | Adults: Initial: 20-5 mg qd. Titrate: May increase dose after 1-2 wks to control BP. Max: 40-10 mg qd. Replacement Therapy: May substitute for individually titrated components. When substituting for individual components, the dose of 1 or both components may be increased if inadequate BP control. Add-On Therapy: May be used to provide additional BP lowering when not adequately controlled on amlodipine (or another dihydropyridine calcium channel blocker) or olmesartan (or another angiotensin receptor blocker) alone. | ⊛D ❀v W [9] |

NAME	FORM/STRENGTH	DOSAGE	COMMENTS
Telmisartan/Amlodipine (Twynsta)	**Tab:** 40-5 mg, 40-10 mg, 80-5 mg, 80-10 mg	**Adults: Initial:** 40-5 mg qd. **Patients Requiring Large BP Reduction: Initial:** 80-5 mg qd. **Titrate:** Adjust dose if needed after 2 wks. **Max:** 80-10 mg qd. **Patients ≥75 yo:** Not recommended for initial therapy. Titrate slowly. **Add-On:** May use if not adequately controlled on amlodipine (or another dihydropyridine calcium channel blocker) alone or telmisartan (or another angiotensin receptor blocker) alone. If experiencing adverse reactions w/ amlodipine 10 mg, may switch to 40-5 mg qd. **Replacement:** May substitute for individual components.	●D ❄v H W [9]
Valsartan/Amlodipine (Exforge)	**Tab:** 160-5 mg, 160-10 mg, 320-5 mg, 320-10 mg	**Adults: Initial:** 160-5 mg qd. **Titrate:** If inadequate control, may increase after 1-2 wks of therapy. **Max:** 320-10 mg qd. **Add-On:** If inadequate control w/ amlodipine (or another dihydropyridine calcium channel blocker) alone or valsartan (or another angiotensin II receptor blocker) alone. If dose-limiting adverse reactions w/ either component alone, switch to amlodipine-valsartan containing lower dose of that component. **Titrate:** If inadequate control after 3-4 wks of therapy, may increase dose. **Max:** 320-10 mg qd. **Replacement:** May be substituted for titrated components. **Elderly: Initial:** 2.5 mg amlodipine.	●D ❄v H R W [9]

DIURETICS (LOOP)

Furosemide (Lasix)	(Generic) **Inj:** 10 mg/ml; **Sol:** 10 mg/ml, 40 mg/ 5 ml; (Generic, Lasix) **Tab:** 20 mg, 40 mg, 80 mg	**Adults: Initial:** 40 mg bid PO. **Maint:** Adjust according to response. **Concomitant Antihypertensives:** Reduce dose of other agents by 50%.	⊕C ❄️> **W** [8]
Torsemide (Demadex)	**Inj:** 10 mg/ml; **Tab:** 5 mg, 10 mg, 20 mg, 100 mg	**Adults: Initial:** 5 mg qd. **Titrate:** May increase to 10 mg qd after 4-6 wks, then may add additional antihypertensive agent if needed.	⊕B ❄️>

DIURETICS (POTASSIUM-SPARING)

Spironolactone (Aldactone)	**Tab:** 25 mg, 50 mg, 100 mg	**Adults: Initial:** 50-100 mg/d as single or divided doses. **Maint:** After 2 wks, adjust by response.	⊕C ❄️v **R W** [16]
Triamterene (Dyrenium)	**Cap:** 50 mg, 100 mg	**Adults: Initial:** 100 mg bid. **Max:** 300 mg/d.	⊕C ❄️v **W** [88]

DIURETICS (POTASSIUM-SPARING/THIAZIDE)

Spironolactone/ Hydrochlorothiazide (Aldactazide)	**Tab:** 25-25 mg, 50-50 mg	**Adults:** Individually titrate components. 50-100 mg/d per component qd or in divided doses.	⊕C ❄️v Not for initial therapy. **R W** [16]
Triamterene/ Hydrochlorothiazide (Maxzide, Maxzide-25)	**Tab:** 37.5-25 mg, 75-50 mg	**Adults: Usual:** (37.5-25 mg) 1-2 tabs qd. (75-50 mg) 1 tab qd.	⊕C ❄️v **W** [88]

NAME	FORM/STRENGTH	DOSAGE	COMMENTS
DIURETIC (QUINAZOLINE)			
Metolazone (Zaroxolyn)	**Tab:** 2.5 mg, 5 mg, 10 mg	**Adults: Initial:** 2.5-5 mg qd. **Elderly:** Start at low end of dosing range.	●B ❀v Rapid & slow formulations not equivalent.
DIURETICS (THIAZIDE)			
Chlorothiazide (Diuril)	**Susp:** (Diuril) 250 mg/5 ml; **Tab:** 250 mg, 500 mg	**Adults: Initial:** 0.5-1 gm/d given qd or in divided doses. **Titrate:** Adjust based on BP. **Max:** 2 gm/d given in divided doses. **Peds: Usual:** 10-20 mg/kg/d given qd-bid. **Max: 2-12 yo:** 1 gm/d. **≤2 yo:** 375 mg/d. **<6 mths:** Up to 30 mg/kg/d given bid.	●C ❀v
Hydrochlorothiazide	**Cap:** 12.5 mg; **Tab:** 12.5 mg, 25 mg, 50 mg	**Adults: Cap: Initial:** 12.5 mg qd. **Max:** 50 mg/d. **Elderly: Initial:** 12.5 mg. **Titrate:** Increase by 12.5 mg/d increments if needed. **Tab: Initial:** 25 mg. **Titrate:** May increase to 50 mg/d given qd-bid. **Peds:** 1-2 mg/kg/d given qd-bid. **Max: 2-12 yo:** 100 mg/d. **Infants up to 2 yo:** 37.5 mg/d. **<6 mths:** Up to 3 mg/kg/d given bid may be required.	●B ❀v
PHOSPHODIESTERASE TYPE 5 INHIBITOR			
Tadalafil (Adcirca)	**Tab:** 20 mg	**Adults:** 40 mg qd. **Patients on Ritonavir For ≥1 Wk: Initial:** 20 mg qd. **Titrate:** May increase to 40 mg qd. D/C ≥24h before ritonavir initiation.	●B ❀> H R

RENIN INHIBITOR

Aliskiren (Tekturna)	Tab: 150 mg, 300 mg	Adults: Initial: 150 mg qd. Titrate: May increase to 300 qd if needed. Max: 300 mg/d.	⊙D ❄v W [9]

RENIN INHIBITOR/THIAZIDE

Aliskiren/Hydrochlorothiazide (Tekturna HCT)	Tab: 150-12.5 mg, 150-25 mg, 300-12.5 mg, 300-25 mg	Adults: Add-On/Initial Therapy: Initial: 150-12.5 mg qd. Titrate: May increase up to max of 300-25 mg qd if uncontrolled after 2-4 wks. Max: 300-25 mg qd. Replacement Therapy: May substitute for individually titrated components.	⊙D ❄v W [9]

DERMATOLOGY

Acne Preparations
ANTIBACTERIAL/KERATOLYTIC

Adapalene/Benzoyl Peroxide (Epiduo)	Gel: 0.1%-2.5%	Adults & Peds: ≥12 yo: Apply pea-sized amt to affected area(s) of face or trunk qd after washing.	⊙C ❄>

ANTI-INFECTIVES AND COMBINATIONS

Benzoyl Peroxide/ Clindamycin (Duac)	Gel: 5%-1%	Acne Vulgaris: Adults & Peds: ≥12 yo: Apply qpm or ud.	⊙C ❄v

NAME	FORM/STRENGTH	DOSAGE	COMMENTS
Clindamycin Phosphate/ Benzoyl Peroxide (Acanya)	Gel: 1.2-2.5%	**Adults & Peds: ≥12 yo:** Apply pea-sized amt to face qd. Minimize sun exposure.	▣C ❄v
Clindamycin Phosphate/ Tretinoin (Ziana)	Gel: 1.2%-0.025%	**Adults & Peds: ≥12 yo:** Apply pea-sized amt to entire face qd at hs. Avoid eyes, mouth, angles of nose, or mucous membranes.	▣C ❄>
Clindamycin Phosphate (Evoclin)	Foam: 1%	**Adults & Peds: ≥12 yo:** Apply to affected area(s) qd.	▣B ❄v
Minocycline HCl (Solodyn)	Tab,ER: 45 mg, 55 mg, 65 mg, 80 mg, 90 mg, 105 mg, 115 mg, 135 mg	**Adults & Peds: ≥12 yo:** 1 mg/kg qd x 12 wks.	▣D ❄v R
Tetracycline HCl (Sumycin)	Cap: 250 mg, 500 mg; Susp: 125 mg/5 ml	**Severe Acne: Adults & Peds: >8 yo:** 1 gm/d in divided doses. **Maint:** After improvement, 125-500 mg/d.	▣D ❄v R

RETINOID-LIKE AGENT

NAME	FORM/STRENGTH	DOSAGE	COMMENTS
Adapalene (Differin)	Cre, Lot: 0.1%; Gel: 0.1%, 0.3%	**Adults & Peds: ≥12 yo:** Apply to affected area(s) qhs. Avoid eyes, lips & mucous membranes.	▣C ❄>

RETINOIDS

NAME	FORM/STRENGTH	DOSAGE	COMMENTS
Isotretinoin (Amnesteem, Claravis, Sotret)	Cap: 10 mg, 20 mg, 40 mg; (Claravis, Sotret) 30 mg	**Adults & Peds: ≥12 yo: Initial:** 0.5-1 mg/kg/d given bid x 15-20 wks w/ food. Repeat if needed after 2 mths off of drug.	▣X ❄v W [52]

| Tretinoin (Retin-A, Retin-A Micro) | **Cre:** 0.025%, 0.05%, 0.1%; **Gel:** 0.01%, 0.025%, (Micro) 0.04%, 0.1%; **Sol:** 0.05% | **Retin-A: Adults:** Apply to affected area(s) qhs. **Retin-A Micro: Adults & Peds: ≥12 yo:** Apply to affected area(s) qhs. | ◉C ❄> |

Anti-Infective Agents
ANTIBACTERIALS

Gentamicin Sulfate	**Cre, Oint:** 0.1%	**Adults & Peds: >1 yo:** Apply to lesions tid-qid.	◉N ❄>
Metronidazole (MetroGel)	**Gel:** (Generic) 0.75%, 1%	**Rosacea: Adults:** Wash affected area before application. Apply and rub in a thin film to the entire affected area(s) bid, am and pm (0.75%) or qd (1%).	◉B ❄v
Mupirocin Calcium (Bactroban Nasal)	**Oint:** 2%	**Nasal Colonization w/ MRSA: Adults & Peds: ≥12 yo:** Apply 1/2 tube per nostril bid x 5d.	◉B ❄v
Mupirocin (Bactroban)	**Cre, Oint:** 2%	***S. aureus/S. pyogenes: Adults & Peds ≥2 mths: Oint:** Apply tid. **≥3 mths: Cre:** Apply tid x 10d.	◉(Cre) B, (Oint) ◉N ❄>
Polymyxin B Sulfate/ Bacitracin Zinc/Neomycin (Neosporin Ointment)	**Oint:** 5,000 U-400 U-3.5 mg/gm	**Prevent Infection in Minor Cuts, Scrapes, & Burns: Adults & Peds:** Apply to affected area(s) qd-tid.	◉N ❄>
Retapamulin (Altabax)	**Oint:** 1%	**Impetigo: Adults & Peds: ≥9 mths:** Apply thin layer (up to 100 cm^2 in total area for adults or 2% total BSA for peds) bid x 5d. May cover w/ sterile bandage or gauze.	◉B ❄>

NAME	FORM/STRENGTH	DOSAGE	COMMENTS
ANTIFUNGALS			
Butenafine (Mentax)	Cre: 1%	**Adults & Peds: ≥12 yo: Interdigital Tinea Pedis:** Apply bid x 7d or qd x 4 wks. **Tinea Corporis/Tinea Cruris/Tinea Versicolor:** Apply qd x 2 wks.	Ⓑ ☼
Ciclopirox (Loprox TS)	Cre, Gel: 0.77%; Shampoo: 1%; Susp: (TS) 0.77%	**Seborrheic Dermatitis: Adults:** (Shampoo) Apply about 5 ml (up to 10 ml for long hair) to wet scalp. Lather & rinse off after 3 min. Repeat twice weekly x 4 wks, at least 3d apart. **Tinea Pedis/Tinea Cruris/Tinea Corporis/Cutaneous Candidiasis/Tinea Versicolor: Adults:** (Cre/Gel/Susp) Massage affected & surrounding area(s) bid (am & pm) up to 4 wks. **Peds: ≥10 yo:** (Cre/Susp) Massage affected & surrounding area(s) bid (am & pm) up to 4 wks. Gel or shampoo not recommended in peds <16 yo.	Ⓑ ☼
Ketoconazole (Extina)	Foam: 2%	**Seborrheic Dermatitis: Adults & Peds: ≥12 yo:** Apply to affected area(s) bid x 4 wks.	Ⓒ ☼
Naftifine (Naftin)	Cre, Gel: 1%	**Tinea Pedis/Tinea Cruris/Tinea Corporis: Adults: Cre:** Apply qd. **Gel:** Apply qam & qpm.	Ⓑ ☼
Oxiconazole (Oxistat)	Cre, Lot: 1%	**Adults: Tinea Curis/Tinea Corporis: Cre/Lot:** Apply qd-bid x 2 wks. **Tinea Pedis: Cre/Lot:** Apply qd-bid x 4 wks. **Tinea Versicolor: Cre:** Apply qd x 2 wks. **Peds: ≥12 yo: Cre:** Same as adult dose.	Ⓑ ☼
Sertaconazole Nitrate (Ertazo)	Cre: 2%	**Interdigital Tinea Pedis: Adults & Peds: ≥12 yo:** Apply bid x 4 wks. Re-evaluate if no improvement after 2 wks.	Ⓒ ☼

ANTI-INFECTIVES AND COMBINATIONS

Doxycycline (Oracea)	**Cap:** 40 mg (30 mg IR/10 mg DR)	**Rosacea: Adults:** 40 mg qd in am. Take on empty stomach.	◙D ✿v

ANTIVIRALS

Acyclovir (Zovirax Cream)	**Cre:** 5%	**Herpes Labialis: Adults & Peds:** ≥12 yo: Apply 5X/d x 4d.	◙B ✿>
Acyclovir (Zovirax Ointment)	**Oint:** 5%	**Genital Herpes/Mucocutaneous Herpes: Adults:** Apply q3h, 6X/d x 7d. Initiate w/ 1st sign/symptom.	◙B ✿>
Penciclovir (Denavir)	**Cre:** 1%	**Recurrent Herpes Labialis (Cold Sores): Adults:** Apply q2h w/a w x 4d. Start w/ earliest sign or symptom.	◙B ✿v
Podofilox (Condylox)	**Gel, Sol:** 0.5%	**External Genital Warts (Condyloma Acuminata) (Gel/ Sol), Perianal Warts (Gel): Adults:** Apply q12h x 3d, then withhold x 4d. May repeat up to 4 treatment cycles. **Max:** 0.5 gm/d or 0.5 ml/d & <10 cm² of wart tissue.	◙C ✿v

Anti-Infective Combinations
ANTIBIOTIC/ANTI-INFLAMMATORY AGENTS

Clotrimazole/Betamethasone (Lotrisone)	**Cre, Lot:** 1-0.05%	**Adults:** ≥17 yo: **Tinea Cruris/Tinea Corporis:** Apply bid x 2 wks. **Tinea Pedis:** Apply bid x 4 wks.	◙C ✿>
Hydrocortisone/Iodoquinol (Alcortin)	**Gel:** 2-1%	**Adults & Peds:** ≥12 yo: Apply to affected area(s) tid-qid or ud.	◙C ✿>

NAME	FORM/STRENGTH	DOSAGE	COMMENTS
Neomycin/Polymyxin B/ Bacitracin/Hydrocortisone (Cortisporin)	**Oint:** 3.5 mg-5,000 U-400 U-10 mg/gm	**Adults:** Apply to affected area(s) bid-qid up to 7d.	▣C ❄>

Antipruritics/Anti-Inflammatory Agents
HISTAMINE RECEPTOR BLOCKER & COMBINATION

NAME	FORM/STRENGTH	DOSAGE	COMMENTS
Doxepin HCl (Zonalon)	**Cre:** 5%	**Adults:** Apply thin film qid up to 8d. Wait at least 3-4h between applications. Avoid occlusive dressings.	▣B ❄v

MISCELLANEOUS

NAME	FORM/STRENGTH	DOSAGE	COMMENTS
Pimecrolimus (Elidel)	**Cre:** 1%	**Adults & Peds:** ≥2 yo: Apply bid. D/C upon resolution. Reevaluate if signs & symptoms persist beyond 6 wks.	▣C ❄v
Tacrolimus (Protopic)	**Oint:** 0.03%, 0.1%	**Moderate-Severe Atopic Dermatitis: Adults:** ≥16 yo: **0.03%/0.1%:** Apply bid. **Peds: 2-15 yo: 0.03%:** Apply bid.	▣C ❄v

Psoriasis
IMMUNOSUPPRESSIVES

NAME	FORM/STRENGTH	DOSAGE	COMMENTS
Alefacept (Amevive)	**Inj:** 15 mg	**Adults:** 15 mg IM once wkly x 12 wks. May retreat x 12 wks if >12-wk interval since 1st course. Adjust dose, d/c, and/or retreat, based on CD4+ count.	▣B ❄v CI w/ HIV.

Cyclosporine (Neoral)	**Cap:** 25 mg, 100 mg; **Sol:** 100 mg/ml	**Adults: Initial:** 2.5 mg/kg/d given bid x 4 wks. **Maint:** If no improvement, increase q2wks by 0.5 mg/kg/d. **Max:** 4 mg/kg/d.	▣C ❄v W [90]

MONOCLONAL ANTIBODIES

Infliximab (Remicade)	**Inj:** 100 mg	**Adults: Induction:** 5 mg/kg IV at 0, 2, & 6 wks. **Maint:** 5 mg/kg q8wks.	▣B ❄v Hepatosplenic T-cell lymphoma & other malignancies reported. **W** [86]
Ustekinumab (Stelara)	**Inj:** 45 mg/0.5 ml, 90 mg/ml	**Adults: ≤100 kg:** 45 mg SC and 4 wks later, followed by 45 mg q12wks. **>100 kg:** 90 mg SC and 4 wks later, followed by 90 mg q12wks.	▣B ❄> W [86]

MONOCLONAL ANTIBODY/TNF-BLOCKER

Adalimumab (Humira)	**Inj:** 20 mg/0.4 ml, 40 mg/0.8 ml	**Adults: Initial:** 80 mg SC. **Maint:** 40 mg qow starting 1 wk after 1st dose.	▣B ❄v W [86]

NAME	FORM/STRENGTH	DOSAGE	COMMENTS
PSORALENS			
Methoxsalen (Oxsoralen-Ultra)	Cap: 10 mg	**Adults: Initial:** <30 kg: 10 mg; 30-50 kg: 20 mg; 51-65 kg: 30 mg; 66-80 kg: 40 mg; 81-90 kg: 50 mg; 91-115 kg: 60 mg; >115 kg: 70 mg. Take 1.5-2h before UVA exposure w/ a low-fat meal or milk. **Titrate:** May increase by 10 mg after 15th treatment under certain conditions. **Max:** Do not treat more often than qod.	◘© ❋ **W** [21]
RETINOID			
Tazarotene (Tazorac)	Cre, Gel: 0.05%, 0.1%	**Adults & Peds: ≥18 yo:** (Cre) Start w/ 0.05% cre, increase to 0.1% if tolerated and medically indicated. Apply to lesions qpm. (Gel) Start w/ 0.05% gel, increase to 0.1% if tolerated and medically indicated. Apply to lesions qpm. **≥12 yo:** (Gel) Start w/ 0.05% gel, increase to 0.1% if tolerated and medically indicated. Apply to lesions qpm. Apply gel to no more than 20% of BSA.	◘© X ❋
STEROIDS, TOPICAL			
Clobetasol Propionate (Clobex)	Lot, Shampoo, Spr: 0.05%	**Adults: ≥18 yo: Lot:** Apply bid for up to 2 consecutive wks. May repeat for additional 2 wks. Limit treatment to 4 wks. **Max:** 50 gm/wk. **Shampoo:** Apply thin film qd to dry scalp on affected area(s) only for up to 4 consecutive wks. Leave x 15 min before lathering & rinsing. **Spr:** Spr on affected area(s) bid. Reassess after 2 wks. Limit treatment to 4 wks. **Max:** 26 spr/application (52 spr/d) or 50 gm/wk x 4 wks.	◘© ❋

Fluocinonide (Vanos)	Cre: 0.1%	Adults & Peds: ≥12 yo: Apply qd-bid ud. Max: 60 gm/wk. Do not use >2 wks.	⊕C ❄v

TUMOR NECROSIS FACTOR RECEPTOR BLOCKER

Etanercept (Enbrel)	Inj: 25 mg, 50 mg	Plaque Psoriasis: Adults: Initial: 50 mg SC biw x 3 mths. May begin w/ 25-50 mg/wk. Maint: 50 mg/wk.	⊕B ❄v W [86]

Miscellaneous
ALPHA-REDUCTASE INHIBITOR

Finasteride (Propecia)	Tab: 1 mg	Androgenetic Alopecia: Adults: 1 mg qd.	⊕X ❄v

IMMUNE CELL ACTIVATOR

Imiquimod (Aldara)	Cre: 5%	Adults: Actinic Keratosis: Apply 2X/wk qhs to area(s) on face/scalp (but not both concurrently). Wash off after 8h. Max: 36 pkts for 16 wks of therapy. Adults & Peds: ≥12 yo: Genital/Perianal Warts (Condyloma Acuminata): Apply 3X/wk qhs. Wash off after 6-10h. Use until warts clear. Max: 16 wks of therapy. Do not occlude treatment area.	⊕C ❄>

NAME	FORM/STRENGTH	DOSAGE	COMMENTS

EENT/NASAL PREPARATIONS

Anticholinergic

NAME	FORM/STRENGTH	DOSAGE	COMMENTS
Ipratropium Bromide (Atrovent Nasal)	Spr: (0.03%) 21 mcg/spr, (0.06%) 42 mcg/spr	**Rhinorrhea w/ Common Cold: Adults & Peds: ≥12 yo:** (0.06%) 2 spr/nostril tid-qid for ≤4d. **5-11 yo:** (0.06%) 2 spr/nostril tid for ≤4d. **Rhinorrhea w/ Seasonal Allergic Rhinitis: Adults & Peds: ≥5 yo:** (0.06%) 2 spr/nostril qid for ≤3 wks. **Rhinorrhea w/ Allergic/Nonallergic Perennial Rhinitis: Adults & Peds: ≥6 yo:** (0.03%) 2 spr/nostril bid-tid.	▣B ❄>

Antihistamine/Corticosteroid Combination

NAME	FORM/STRENGTH	DOSAGE	COMMENTS
Azelastine HCl/ Fluticasone Propionate (Dymista)	Spr: 137 mcg/spr-50 mcg/spr	**Adults & Peds: ≥12 yo:** 1 spr/nostril bid.	▣C ❄v

Corticosteroids

NAME	FORM/STRENGTH	DOSAGE	COMMENTS
Beclomethasone Dipropionate (Qnasl)	Spr: 80 mcg/spr	**Seasonal/Perennial Allergic Rhinitis: Adults & Peds: ≥12 yo: Usual:** 2 spr/nostril qd. **Max:** 4 spr/d.	▣C ❄>

Beclomethasone (Beconase, Beconase AQ)	**Spr:** 42 mcg/spr	**Allergic/Nonallergic (Vasomotor) Rhinitis: Beconase AQ:** **Adults & Peds:** ≥6 yo: 1-2 spr/nostril bid. **Beconase: Adults & Peds:** ≥12 yo: 1 spr/nostril bid-qid. **6-12 yo:** 1 spr/nostril tid.	◉C ❄v
Budesonide (Rhinocort Aqua)	**Spr:** 32 mcg/spr	**Seasonal/Perennial Rhinitis: Adults & Peds:** ≥6 yo: **Initial:** 1 spr/nostril qd. **Max:** ≥12 yo: 4 spr/nostril qd. **6-<12 yo:** 2 spr/nostril qd.	◉B ❄>
Ciclesonide (Omnaris)	**Spr:** 50 mcg/spr	**Perennial Allergic Rhinitis: Adults & Peds:** ≥12 yo: 2 spr/nostril qd. **Max:** 2 spr/nostril/d (200 mcg/d). **Seasonal Allergic Rhinitis: Adults & Peds:** ≥6 yo: 2 spr/nostril qd. **Max:** 2 spr/nostril/d (200 mcg/d). **Elderly:** Start at low end of dosing range.	◉C ❄>
Fluticasone Furoate (Veramyst)	**Spr:** 27.5 mcg/spr	**Seasonal/Perennial Allergic Rhinitis: Adults & Peds:** ≥12 yo: **Initial:** 2 spr/nostril qd. **Maint:** 1 spr/nostril qd. **2-11 yo: Initial:** 1 spr/nostril qd. **Titrate:** If inadequate response, may increase to 2 spr/nostril, then return to initial dose when controlled.	◉C ❄>
Fluticasone Propionate (Flonase)	**Spr:** 50 mcg/spr	**Seasonal & Perennial Allergic/Nonallergic Rhinitis:** **Adults: Initial:** 2 spr/nostril qd or 1 spr/nostril bid. **Maint:** 1 spr/nostril qd. **Peds:** ≥4 yo: **Initial:** 1-2 spr/nostril qd. **Maint:** 1 spr/nostril qd. **Max:** 2 spr/nostril/d. **Seasonal Allergic Rhinitis: Adults & Peds:** ≥12 yo: May also dose as 2 spr/nostril qd prn.	◉C ❄>

NAME	FORM/STRENGTH	DOSAGE	COMMENTS
Mometasone Furoate Monohydrate (Nasonex)	Spr: 50 mcg/spr	**Treatment & Prevention of Seasonal Allergic Rhinitis/ Nasal Congestion/Treatment of Perennial Allergic Rhinitis: Adults & Peds: ≥12 yo:** 2 spr/nostril qd. **Treatment of Seasonal/Perennial Allergic Rhinitis/Nasal Congestion: Peds: 2-11 yo:** 1 spr/nostril qd. **Nasal Polyps: Adults: ≥18 yo:** 2 spr/nostril qd-bid.	▣C ❅>
Triamcinolone Acetonide (Nasacort AQ)	Spr: 55 mcg/spr	**Seasonal/Perennial Allergic Rhinitis: Adults & Peds: ≥12 yo: Initial/Max:** 2 spr/nostril qd. **Maint:** 1 spr/nostril qd. **6-12 yo: Initial:** 1 spr/nostril qd. **Max:** 2 spr/nostril qd. **2-5 yo: Initial/Max:** 1 spr/nostril qd.	▣C ❅>

EENT/OPHTHALMOLOGY

Antibiotic Agents

NAME	FORM/STRENGTH	DOSAGE	COMMENTS
Azithromycin (Azasite)	Sol: 1%	**Bacterial Conjunctivitis: Adults & Peds: ≥1 yo: Initial:** 1 gtt bid, 8-12h apart x first 2d. **Maint:** 1 gtt qd x next 5d.	▣B ❅>
Ciprofloxacin HCl (Ciloxan)	Oint, Sol: 0.3%	**Adults & Peds: ≥1 yo: Bacterial Conjunctivitis: Sol:** 1-2 gtts q2h w/a x 2d, then 1-2 gtts q4h w/a x 5d. **Adults & Peds: ≥2 yo: Oint:** 1/2 inch tid x 2d, then bid x 5d. **Adults & Peds: ≥2 yo: Corneal Ulcers: Sol:** 2 gtts q15min x 6h, then 2 gtts q30min on Day 1, then 2 gtts q1h on Day 2, then 2 gtts q4h on Days 3-14.	▣C ❅>
Gatifloxacin (Zymar)	Sol: 0.3%	**Bacterial Conjunctivitis: Adults & Peds: ≥1 yo:** 1 gtt q2h w/a, up to 8x/d for 2d; then 1 gtt up to qid w/a for 5d.	▣C ❅>

Gatifloxacin (Zymaxid)	Sol: 0.5%	**Bacterial Conjunctivitis: Adults & Peds: ≥1 yo: Day 1:** 1 gtt q2h w/a, up to 8X/d. **Days 2-7:** 1 gtt bid-qid w/a.	◉C ❄>
Levofloxacin (Iquix)	Sol: 1.5%	**Adults & Peds: ≥6 yo: Corneal Ulcer: Days 1-3:** 1-2 gtts q30min-2h w/a & 4-6h after retiring. **Day 4-Completion:** 1-2 gtts q1-4h w/a.	◉C ❄>
Levofloxacin (Quixin)	Sol: 0.5%	**Bacterial Conjunctivitis: Adults & Peds: ≥1 yo: Days 1-2:** 1-2 gtts q2h w/a up to 8X/d. **Days 3-7:** 1-2 gtts q4h w/a up to qid.	◉C ❄>
Moxifloxacin HCl (Moxeza)	Sol: 0.5%	**Bacterial Conjunctivitis: Adults & Peds: ≥4 mths:** 1 gtt bid x 7d.	◉C ❄>
Moxifloxacin HCl (Vigamox)	Sol: 0.5%	**Adults & Peds:** 1 gtt tid x 7d.	◉C ❄>
Tobramycin (Tobrex)	Oint: 0.3%; Sol: 0.3%	**Adults: Usual:** 1/2 inch bid-tid or 1-2 gtts q4h. **Severe Infection:** 1/2 inch q3-4h or 2 gtts q1h until improvement.	◉B ❄v

Antibiotic/Corticosteroid Combinations

Prednisolone Acetate/ Sulfacetamide Sodium (Blephamide, Blephamide S.O.P.)	Oint, Susp: 0.2-10%	**Adults & Peds: ≥6 yo: Initial: Oint:** Apply 1/2 inch 3-4X/d & 1-2X/qpm. **Susp:** Instill 2 gtts q4h in am & pm. **Max:** Do not prescribe >20 ml or 8 gm initially. Reduce dose when condition improves.	◉C ❄v
Tobramycin/Dexamethasone (TobraDex, TobraDex ST)	Oint: 0.1-0.3%; Susp: 0.1-0.3%; ST: 0.05-0.3%	**Adults & Peds: ≥2 yo: Oint:** Apply 1/2 inch up to tid-qid. **Susp:** 1-2 gtts q4-6h. **ST:** 1 gtt q4-6h. **Titrate:** May increase 1-2 gtts (susp) or 1 gtt (ST) q2h for 1st 24-48h.	◉C ❄>

NAME	FORM/STRENGTH	DOSAGE	COMMENTS

Corticosteroids

NAME	FORM/STRENGTH	DOSAGE	COMMENTS
Loteprednol Etabonate (Alrex)	Susp: 0.2%	Adults: 1 gtt into the affected eye(s) qid.	▣C ❀>
Prednisolone Acetate (Pred Forte)	Susp: 1%	Adults: 1-2 gtts bid-qid. May increase frequency during 1st 24-48h.	▣C ❀v
Prednisolone Acetate (Pred Mild)	Susp: 0.12%	Adults: 1-2 gtts bid-qid. May increase frequency during 1st 24-48h.	▣C ❀v

Fungal Infection

NAME	FORM/STRENGTH	DOSAGE	COMMENTS
Natamycin (Natacyn)	Susp: 5%	Adults: Keratitis: 1 gtt q1-2h x 3-4d, then 1 gtt 6-8X/d x 14-21d. Blepharitis/Conjunctivitis: 1 gtt 4-6x/d.	▣C ❀>

Glaucoma
ADRENERGIC AGONIST

NAME	FORM/STRENGTH	DOSAGE	COMMENTS
Dipivefrin HCl (Propine)	Sol: 0.1%	Adults: Usual: 1 gtt q12h.	▣B ❀>

BETA BLOCKERS

NAME	FORM/STRENGTH	DOSAGE	COMMENTS
Betaxolol (Betoptic S)	Susp: 0.25%	Adults & Peds: 1 gtt bid.	▣C ❀>

Carteolol HCl (Ocupress)	Sol: 1%	**Adults:** 1 gtt bid.	⊙C ❄>
Levobunolol HCl (Betagan)	Sol: 0.25%, 0.5%	**Adults: Usual:** (0.5%) 1-2 gtts qd. (0.25%) 1-2 gtts bid. **Severe/Uncontrolled:** (0.5%) 1-2 gtts bid.	⊙C ❄>
Metipranolol (Optipranolol)	Sol: 0.3%	**Adults:** 1 gtt bid.	⊙C ❄v
Timolol Maleate (Timoptic, Timoptic Ocudose, Timoptic-XE)	Sol: 0.25%, 0.5%; Sol, Gel-Forming: (XE) 0.25%, 0.5%	**Adults: Timoptic/Timoptic Ocudose: Initial:** 1 gtt 0.25% bid, may increase to 1 gtt 0.5% bid. **Maint:** 1 gtt 0.25%/0.5% qd. **Max:** 1 gtt (0.5%) bid. **Timoptic-XE: Initial:** 1 gtt 0.25%/0.5% qd. **Max:** 1 gtt 0.5% qd.	⊙C ❄v

CARBONIC ANHYDRASE INHIBITOR/BETA BLOCKER

Dorzolamide HCl/ Timolol Maleate (Cosopt)	Sol: 2-0.5%	**Adults & Peds: ≥2 yo:** 1 gtt bid.	⊙C ❄v

CARBONIC ANHYDRASE INHIBITORS

Brinzolamide (Azopt)	Susp: 1%	**Adults:** 1 gtt tid.	⊙C ❄v
Dorzolamide (Trusopt)	Sol: 2%	**Adults & Peds:** 1 gtt tid.	⊙C ❄v

NAME	FORM/STRENGTH	DOSAGE	COMMENTS
CHOLINERGIC AGONISTS			
Pilocarpine HCl (Isopto Carpine)	Sol: 1%, 2%, 4%	**Adults & Peds: ≥2 yo: Elevated IOP in Open-Angle Glaucoma/Ocular HTN:** 1 gtt 1%, 2%, or 4% sol up to qid. Start pilocarpine-naive patients on 1% sol. **Acute Angle-Closure Glaucoma: Initial:** 1 gtt 1%, 2%, or 4% sol up to 3X over 30 min. Refer to PI if used with laser iridoplasty/iridomy. **Prevention of Elevated IOP After Laser Surgery:** 1 gtt 1%, 2%, or 4% sol (or 2 gtts 5 min apart) 15-60 min prior to surgery. **Induction of Miosis:** 1 gtt 1%, 2%, or 4% sol (or 2 gtts 5 min apart). **<2 yo: Usual:** 1 gtt 1% sol bid. **Peds: Miosis Induction Prior to Goniotomy/Trabeculotomy:** 1 gtt 1% or 2% sol 15-60 min prior to surgery. **Use with Other Topical Ophthalmic Medications:** Give at least 5 min apart.	▣Ⓒ ✿<
Pilocarpine HCl (Pilopine HS)	Gel: 4%	**Adults:** Apply 1/2 inch ribbon in the lower conjunctival sac of the affected eye(s) qd at hs.	▣Ⓒ ✿<
PROSTAGLANDIN ANALOGUES			
Bimatoprost (Lumigan)	Sol: 0.01%, 0.03%	**Adults & Peds: ≥16 yo: Usual/Max:** 1 gtt qpm.	▣Ⓒ ✿<
Latanoprost (Xalatan)	Sol: 0.005%	**Adults: Usual:** 1 gtt qpm. **Max:** Once daily dosing.	▣Ⓒ ✿<

Travoprost (Travatan Z)	Sol: 0.004%	Adults & Peds: ≥16 yo: 1 gtt qpm.	◉C ❀>

SYMPATHOMIMETIC/BETA-BLOCKER

Brimonidine Tartrate/ Timolol Maleate (Combigan)	Sol: 2-5 mg/ml	Adults & Peds: ≥2 yo: 1 gtt bid (q12h). Instill other topical ophthalmic products ≥5 min apart.	◉C ❀v

SYMPATHOMIMETIC

Brimonidine Tartrate (Alphagan P)	Sol: 0.1%, 0.15%	Adults & Peds: ≥2 yo: 1 gtt tid (q8h).	◉B ❀v

NSAIDs

Bromfenac (Bromday)	Sol: 0.09%	Adults: 1 gtt qd in affected eye(s) 1d prior to surgery, the day of surgery, and continue x 2 wks.	◉C ❀>
Flurbiprofen Sodium (Ocufen)	Sol: 0.03%	Inhibit Intraoperative Miosis: Adults: 2 gtts q30min x 4 doses, beginning 2h prior to surgery.	◉C ❀v
Ketorolac Tromethamine (Acular LS, Acular PF)	Sol: (LS) 0.4% ; PF (preservative free) 0.5%	Pain/Burning/Stinging: (LS) Adults & Peds: ≥3 yo: 1 gtt qid post-op PRN x 4d. Pain/Photophobia: (PF) Adults & Peds: ≥3 yo:1 gtt qid post-op PRN x 3d	◉C ❀>
Nepafenac (Nevanac)	Susp: 0.1%	Cataract Surgery: Adults & Peds: ≥10 yo: 1 gtt tid, start 24h prior to surgery, continue on day of surgery & x 2 wks postop.	◉C ❀>

NAME	FORM/STRENGTH	DOSAGE	COMMENTS

Ocular Decongestant/Allergic Conjunctivitis

H. RECEPTOR ANTAGONISTS

NAME	FORM/STRENGTH	DOSAGE	COMMENTS
Alcaftadine (Lastacaft)	Sol: 0.25%	Adults & Peds: ≥2 yo: 1 gtt in each eye qd.	●B ❀>
Azelastine HCl (Optivar)	Sol: 0.05%	Adults & Peds: ≥3 yo: 1 gtt bid.	●C ❀>
Bepotastine besilate (Bepreve)	Sol: 1.5%	Allergic Conjunctivitis: Adults & Peds: ≥2 yo: 1 gtt bid in affected eye(s).	●C ❀>
Epinastine HCl (Elestat)	Sol: 0.05%	Adults & Peds: ≥2 yo: 1 gtt bid in each eye. Continue treatment throughout the period of exposure, even when symptoms are absent.	●C ❀>

MAST CELL STABILIZERS

NAME	FORM/STRENGTH	DOSAGE	COMMENTS
Nedocromil Sodium (Alocril)	Sol: 2%	Adults & Peds: ≥3 yo: 1-2 gtts bid.	●B ❀>
Pemirolast Potassium (Alamast)	Sol: 0.1%	Adults & Peds: ≥3 yo: 1-2 gtts qid in affected eye.	●C ❀>

Androgens

Methyltestosterone CIII (Testred)	**Cap:** 10 mg	**Adults: Androgen-Deficient Males:** 10-50 mg/d. **Breast Cancer in Females:** 50-200 mg/d. **Peds: Delayed Puberty:** Use lower range of 10-50 mg/d x 4-6 mths.	⊙X ✿v
Testosterone CIII (Androderm)	**Patch:** 2 mg/24h, 4 mg/ 24h	**Adults: Initial:** Apply one 4 mg/d system qhs on back, abdomen, upper arm, or thigh. **Maint:** 2-6 mg/d.	⊙X ✿v
Testosterone CIII (Androgel)	**Gel:** 1%, 1.62%	**Adults: Initial:** (Gel 1%) Apply 5 gm qd to shoulders & upper arms and/or abdomen. **Titrate:** May increase to 7.5 gm qd, then 10 gm qd. (Gel 1.62%) Apply 40.5 mg qd to shoulders & upper arms. May adjust dose between 20.25-81 mg. **Titrate:** Based on pre-dose am serum testosterone concentration at 14d & 28d after start of therapy or following dose change.	⊙X ✿v W [104]
Testosterone CIII (Striant)	**Tab, Buccal:** 30 mg	**Adults:** 30 mg q12h to gum region above incisor tooth on either side of mouth. Rotate sites w/ each application. Hold in place for 30 sec.	⊙X ✿v
Testosterone CIII (Axiron)	**Sol:** 30 mg	**Adults: Usual:** 60 mg (30 mg to each axilla) qam. **Titrate: Serum Concentration <300 ng/dl:** May increase from 60 to 90 mg or from 90 to 120 mg. **Serum Concentration >1050 ng/dl:** Decrease from 60 to 30 mg. D/C if consistently >1050 ng/dl at lowest qd dose of 30 mg.	⊙X ✿v W [104]

NAME	FORM/STRENGTH	DOSAGE	COMMENTS
Testosterone CIII (Fortesta Gel)	**Gel:** 10 mg/actuation	**Adults: Initial:** Apply 40 mg (4 pump actuations) qam to thighs. May adjust between 10-70 mg based on drug level from blood draw 2h after application, 14d, & 35d after start or after dose adjustment. **Max:** 70 mg. **Serum Concentration: ≥2500 ng/dl:** Decrease by 20 mg. **≥1250-<2500 ng/dl:** Decrease by 10 mg. **≥500-<1250 ng/dl:** Continue on current dose. **<500 ng/dl:** Increase by 10 mg.	▣X ❄v **W** [104]

Antidiabetic Agents
BIGUANIDE/MEGLITINIDE

NAME	FORM/STRENGTH	DOSAGE	COMMENTS
Metformin HCl/Repaglinide (Prandimet)	**Tab:** 500-1 mg, 500-2 mg	**Adults:** Individualize dose. Give bid-tid up to 1000-4 mg/meal. Take dose w/in 15-30 min ac. **Max:** 2500-10 mg/d. **Inadequately Controlled w/ Metformin Monotherapy: Initial:** 500-1 mg bid. **Titrate:** Gradually escalate dose to reduce risk of hypoglycemia. **Inadequately Controlled w/ Meglitinide Monotherapy: Initial:** 500 mg of metformin component bid. **Titrate:** Gradually escalate dose to reduce GI side effects. **Concomitant Use of Repaglinide/ Metformin:** Initiate at dose of repaglinide & metformin similar to (not exceeding) current doses. Titrate to max daily dose as necessary.	▣C ❄v May cause lactic acidosis. **H R**

BIGUANIDES

Metformin HCl (Glucophage, Glucophage XR, Riomet)	**Sol:** (Riomet) 500 mg/ 5 ml; **Tab:** (Glucophage) 500 mg, 850 mg, 1000 mg; **Tab,ER:** (Glucophage XR) 500 mg, 750 mg	**Adults: Sol/Tab: Initial:** 500 mg bid or 850 mg qd w/ meals. **Titrate:** Increase by 500 mg qwk, or 850 mg q2wks, or from 500 mg bid to 850 mg bid after 2 wks. **Max:** 2550 mg/d. **W/ Insulin: Initial:** 500 mg qd. **Titrate:** 500 mg qwk. **Max:** 2500 mg/d. Decrease insulin dose by 10-25% when FPG <120 mg/dl. **Tab,ER: Glucophage XR: W/ W/o Insulin: Initial:** 500 mg qd w/ pm meal. **Titrate:** Increase by 500 mg qwk. **Max:** 2000 mg/d. **Peds: 10-16 yo: Sol/ Tab: Initial:** 500 mg bid w/ meals. **Titrate:** Increase by 500 mg qwk. **Max:** 2000 mg/d in divided doses.	⊕B ❋v Lactic acidosis reported (rare). **H R**
Metformin HCl (Fortamet)	**Tab,ER:** 500 mg, 1000 mg	**Adults: Initial:** 500-1000 mg qd w/ pm meal. **W/ Insulin: Initial:** 500 mg qd. **Titrate:** May increase by 500 mg/wk. **Max:** 2500 mg/d. Decrease insulin dose by 10-25% when FPG <120 mg/dl.	⊕B ❋v Lactic acidosis reported (rare). **H R**
Metformin HCl (Glumetza)	**Tab,ER:** 500 mg, 1000 mg	**Adults: Initial:** 500 mg qd w/ pm meal. **Titrate:** May increase by 500 mg/wk. **Max:** 2000 mg/d.	⊕B ❋v Lactic acidosis reported (rare). **H R**

BILE ACID SEQUESTRANTS

Colesevelam HCl (WelChol)	**Tab:** 625 mg; **Susp:** 1.875 gm, 3.75 gm [pkt]	**Adults: Improve Glycemic Control: Tab:** 3 tabs bid or 6 tabs qd. Take w/ meal & liquid. **Susp:** 1.875 gm bid or 3.75 gm qd. Take w/ meals.	⊕B ❋^

NAME	FORM/STRENGTH	DOSAGE	COMMENTS

DIPEPTIDYL PEPTIDASE-4 INHIBITOR/HMG-COA REDUCTASE INHIBITOR

NAME	FORM/STRENGTH	DOSAGE	COMMENTS
Simvastatin/Sitagliptin (Juvisync)	Tab: 10-100 mg, 20-100 mg, 40-100 mg	**Adults: Usual:** 10-100 mg, 20-100 mg, or 40-100 mg qd. Take as single dose in pm. **Initial:** 40-100 mg/d. **Patients on Simvastatin w/ or w/o Sitagliptin 100 mg/d: Initial:** 100 mg sitagliptin and dose of simvastatin already taken. **Concomitant Insulin/Insulin Secretagogue (eg, sulfonylurea):** May need lower dose of insulin/insulin secretagogue. **Concomitant Verapamil/Diltiazem: Max:** 10-100 mg qd. **Concomitant Amiodarone/Amlodipine/Ranolazine: Max:** 20-100 mg qd. **Homozygous Familial Hypercholesterolemia: Usual:** 40-100 mg qd. **Chinese Patients Taking Lipid-Modifying Doses (≥1 gm/d) of Niacin-Containing Products:** Caution w/ 40-100 mg qd.	■X ❖v H R

DIPEPTIDYL PEPTIDASE-4 INHIBITORS

NAME	FORM/STRENGTH	DOSAGE	COMMENTS
Linagliptin (Tradjenta)	Tab: 5 mg	**Adults:** 5 mg qd.	■B ❖>
Saxagliptin (Onglyza)	Tab: 2.5 mg, 5 mg	**Adults:** 2.5 mg or 5 mg qd. **Concomitant Strong CYP3A4/5 Inhibitors:** 2.5 mg qd.	■B ❖> R
Sitagliptin (Januvia)	Tab: 25 mg, 50 mg, 100 mg	**Adults:** 100 mg qd.	■B ❖> R

DIPEPTIDYL PEPTIDASE-4 INHIBITORS/BIGUANIDE

Linagliptin/Metformin HCl (Jentadueto)	**Tab:** 500-2.5 mg, 850-2.5 mg, 1000-2.5 mg	**Adults:** Individualize dose. Take bid w/ meals. **Initial: Not Currently on Metformin:** 500-2.5 mg bid. **On Metformin:** 2.5 mg linagliptin & current metformin dose taken at each of the 2 daily meals. **On Individual Components:** May be switched to strength w/ same doses of each component. **Titrate:** Increase gradually to reduce GI side effects of metformin. **Max:** 1000-2.5 mg bid. **W/ Insulin Secretagogue:** May require lower dose of insulin secretagogue.	▣B ✹v Lactic acidosis reported (rare). **H R**
Saxagliptin/Metformin HCl (Kombiglyze XR)	**Tab,ER:** 500-5 mg, 1000-5 mg, 1000-2.5 mg	**Adults:** Individualize dose. Take qd w/ pm meal. **On Metformin:** Dose should provide metformin at the dose already being taken, or the nearest therapeutically appropriate dose. **Need 5 mg of Saxagliptin & Not Currently Treated w/ Metformin: Initial:** 5 mg saxagliptin-500 mg metformin ER. **Need 2.5 mg of Saxagliptin in Combination w/ Metformin ER: Initial:** 2.5 mg saxagliptin-1000 mg metformin ER. **Need 2.5 mg of Saxagliptin & Are Metformin-Naive/Require a Dose of Metformin >1000 mg:** Use individual components. **Max:** 5 mg saxagliptin & 2000 mg metformin ER. **W/ Strong CYP3A4/5 Inhibitors: Max:** 2.5 mg saxagliptin-1000 mg metformin ER qd.	▣B ✹> Lactic acidosis reported (rare). **H R**

NAME	FORM/STRENGTH	DOSAGE	COMMENTS
Sitagliptin/Metformin HCl (Janumet XR)	**Tab,ER:** 500-50 mg, 1000-50 mg, 1000-100 mg	**Adults:** Individualize dose. Take qd w/ meal, preferably in pm. **Not Currently on Metformin: Initial:** 1000-100 mg; if metformin dose is inadequate to achieve glycemic control, titrate gradually (to reduce GI side effects of metformin) up to max recommended daily dose. **On Metformin: Initial:** 100 mg sitagliptin and previously prescribed metformin dose. **On Metformin Immediate-Release (IR) 850 mg bid or 1000 mg bid: Initial:** Two 1000-50 mg tabs taken together qd. **Max Daily Dose:** 2000-100 mg. Please refer to PI for additional dosing recommendations.	▣B ❄> Lactic acidosis reported (rare). **H R**
Sitagliptin/Metformin HCl (Janumet)	**Tab:** 50-500 mg, 50-1000 mg	**Adults:** Individualize dose. Take bid w/ meals w/ gradual dose increase to reduce GI side effects. **Not Currently on Metformin: Initial:** 50 mg/500 mg bid. **On Metformin: Initial:** 50 mg bid of sitagliptin and current metformin dose. **On Metformin 850 mg bid: Initial:** 50 mg/1000 mg bid. **Max:** 100 mg/2000 mg.	▣B ❄> Lactic acidosis reported (rare). **H R**
GLUCOSIDASE INHIBITORS			
Acarbose (Precose)	**Tab:** 25 mg, 50 mg, 100 mg	**Adults:** Individualize dose. **Initial:** 25 mg tid w/ meals. **Titrate:** Adjust at 4-8 wk intervals. **Maint:** 50-100 mg tid. **Max: ≤60 kg:** 50 mg tid. **>60 kg:** 100 mg tid.	▣B ❄v **R**

Miglitol (Glyset)	Tab: 25 mg, 50 mg, 100 mg	Adults: Initial: 25 mg tid w/ meals. Titrate: Increase after 4-8 wks to 50 mg tid x approx. 3 mths, then may further increase to 100 mg tid. Maint: 50-100 mg tid. Max: 100 mg tid.	⊛B ❄v R

INCRETIN MIMETICS

Exenatide (Byetta)	Inj: 250 mcg/ml	Adults: Initial: 5 mcg SC bid, w/in 60 min before two main meals, approx. 6h or more apart. Titrate: May increase to 10 mcg bid after 1 mth. Consider reduction of sulfonylurea dose to reduce risk of hypoglycemia.	⊛C ❄v R W [35]
Liraglutide (rDNA Origin) (Victoza)	Inj: 6 mg/ml	Adults: Initial: 0.6 mg SC qd x 1 wk. Titrate: Increase to 1.2 mg after 1 wk, then to 1.8 mg if acceptable glycemic control not achieved. Reinitiate at 0.6 mg if >3d have elapsed since the last dose and titrate ud. W/ Insulin Secretagogues/Insulin: Consider reducing dose of insulin secretagogues or insulin.	⊛C ❄v Risk of thyroid tumors.

MEGLITINIDES

Nateglinide (Starlix)	Tab: 60 mg, 120 mg	Adults: 120 mg tid 1-30 min ac. May use 60 mg tid for near goal HbA1c. Skip dose if meal is skipped.	⊛C ❄v

NAME	FORM/STRENGTH	DOSAGE	COMMENTS
Repaglinide (Prandin)	Tab: 0.5 mg, 1 mg, 2 mg	Adults: Take dose w/in 15-30 min ac (bid-qid in response to changes in meal pattern). Initial: Treatment-Naive or HbA1c <8%: 0.5 mg ac. Previous Therapy w/ Blood Glucose-Lowering Drugs & HbA1c ≥8%: 1-2 mg ac. Titrate: May double preprandial dose up to 4 mg at no less than 1-wk intervals until response is achieved. Maint: 0.5-4 mg ac. Max: 16 mg/d. Occurrence of Hypoglycemia w/ Metformin or Thiazolidinedione (TZD) Combination: Reduce repaglinide dose. Replacement Therapy of Other Oral Hypoglycemic Agents: Start repaglinide on the day after final dose is given. Combination Therapy w/ Metformin or TZD: Starting dose and dose adjustments same as repaglinide monotherapy.	●C ✥V H R
SULFONYLUREAS/BIGUANIDE			
Glipizide/Metformin HCl (Metaglip)	Tab: 2.5-250 mg, 2.5-500 mg, 5-500 mg	Adults: Initial: 2.5-250 mg pd qd w/ meals. If FBG 280-320 mg/d, give 2.5-500 mg bid. Titrate: Increase by ≤5-500 mg or ≤5-500 mg bid w/ meals. Max: 10-2000 mg/d. 2nd-Line Therapy: 1 tab/d q2wks. Max: 20-2000 mg/d.	●C ✥V Lactic acidosis reported (rare). H R
Glyburide/Metformin HCl (Glucovance)	Tab: 1.25-250 mg, 2.5-500 mg, 5-500 mg	Adults: Inadequate Glycemic Control on Diet/Exercise Alone: Initial: 1.25-250 mg qd-bid w/ meals. If HbA1c<9% or FPG 200-200 mg/d, give bid w/meals. Titrate: Increase by ≤1.25-250 mg q2wks. Max: 20-2000 mg/d. Inadequate Glycemic Control on Sulfonylurea and/or Metformin: Initial: 2.5-500 mg or	●B ✥V Lactic acidosis reported (rare). H R

5-500 mg bid w/ meals. Do not exceed daily doses of glyburide or metformin already being taken. **Titrate:** Increase by ≤5-500 mg/d. **Max:** 20-2000 mg/d.

SULFONYLUREAS-2ND GENERATION

Glimepiride (Amaryl)	**Tab:** 1 mg, 2 mg, 4 mg	**Adults: Initial:** 1-2 mg qd w/ breakfast. **Titrate:** Increase by 1 mg or 2 mg at 1-2 wk intervals. **Max:** 8 mg/d.	⊙C ❀v R
Glipizide (Glucotrol, Glucotrol XL)	**Tab:** 5 mg, 10 mg; **Tab,ER:** 2.5 mg, 5 mg, 10 mg	**Adults: Glucotrol XL: Initial/Combination Therapy:** 5 mg qd w/ breakfast. **Usual:** 5-10 mg qd. **Max:** 20 mg/d. **Glucotrol: Initial:** 5 mg qd 30 min ac. **Titrate:** Increase by 2.5-5 mg; divide if above 15 mg. **Max:** 15 mg qd or 40 mg/d.	⊙C ❀v H R
Glyburide (Glynase PresTab)	**Tab:** 1.5 mg, 3 mg, 6 mg	**Adults: Initial:** 1.5-3 mg qd w/ breakfast. **Titrate:** Increase by no more than 1.5 mg at wkly intervals; may give >6 mg bid. **Maint:** 0.75-12 mg/d. **Max:** 12 mg/d.	⊙B ❀v H R
Glyburide (Diabeta)	**Tab:** 1.25 mg, 2.5 mg, 5 mg	**Adults: Initial:** 2.5-5 mg qd w/ breakfast. **Titrate:** Increase by no more than 2.5 mg at wkly intervals. **Maint:** 1.25-20 mg given qd or in divided doses. **Max:** 20 mg/d. May give bid if dose >10 mg/d.	⊙C ❀v H R

NAME	FORM/STRENGTH	DOSAGE	COMMENTS
THIAZOLIDINEDIONES			
Pioglitazone (Actos)	**Tab:** 15 mg, 30 mg, 45 mg	**Adults: W/o CHF: Initial:** 15 or 30 mg qd. **W/ CHF: Initial:** 15 mg qd. **Titrate:** By 15 mg increments. **Max:** 45 mg/d. **Combination Therapy w/ Insulin Secretagogue:** Decrease insulin secretagogue dose if hypoglycemic. **Combination Therapy w/ Insulin:** Decrease insulin by 10-25% if hypoglycemic. **W/ Strong CYP2C8 Inhibitor: Max:** 15 mg qd.	▣C ❄v H W [79]
Rosiglitazone Maleate (Avandia)	**Tab:** 2 mg, 4 mg, 8 mg	**Adults: Initial:** 2 mg bid or 4 mg qd. **Titrate:** May increase to 8 mg/d after 8-12 wks if response to treatment is inadequate. **Max:** 8 mg/d.	▣C ❄v H W [82]
THIAZOLIDINEDIONE/BIGUANIDE			
Pioglitazone HCl Metformin HCl/ (Actoplus Met, Actoplus Met XR)	**Tab:** (Actoplus Met) 500-15 mg, 850-15 mg; (Actoplus Met XR) 1000-15 mg, 1000-30 mg	**Adults:** Individualize dose. Titrate gradually prn based on response. **Actoplus Met: Initial:** 500-15 mg or 850-15 mg qd-bid w/ food. **Max:** 2550-45 mg/d in divided doses w/ food. **Actoplus Met XR: Initial:** 1000-15 mg or 1000-30 mg qd w/ pm meal. **Max:** 2000-45 mg qd w/pm meal. **Elderly/Debilitated/Malnourished:** Conservative dosing; do not titrate to max dose.	▣C ❄v Lactic acidosis reported (rare). **H R W** [79]

| Rosiglitazone Maleate/ Metformin HCl (Avandamet) | Tab: 2-500 mg, 4-500 mg, 2-1000 mg, 4-1000 mg | Adults: Initial: Rosiglitazone: Lowest recommended dose. Prior Metformin Therapy of 1000 mg/d: Initial: 2-500 mg tab bid. Prior Metformin Therapy of 2000 mg/d: Initial: 2-1000 mg tab bid. Prior Rosiglitazone Therapy of 4 mg/d: Initial: 2-500 mg tab bid. Prior Rosiglitazone Therapy of 8 mg/d: 4-500 mg tab bid. Titrate: May increase by increments of 4 mg rosiglitazone and/ or 500 mg metformin. Max: 8-2000 mg/d. Elderly/ Debilitated/Malnourished: Do not titrate to max dose. Take w/ meals. | ⊕C ✿v Lactic acidosis reported (rare). H R W [82] |

THIAZOLIDINEDIONES/SULFONYLUREA

| Pioglitazone HCl/Glimepiride (Duetact) | Tab: 30-2 mg, 30-4 mg | Adults: Individualize dose. Base recommended starting dose on current regimen of pioglitazone and/or sulfonylurea. Give w/ 1st meal of day. Current Glimepiride Monotherapy or Prior Therapy of Pioglitazone plus Glimepiride Separately: Initial: 30-2 mg or 30-4 mg qd. Current Pioglitazone or Different Sulfonylurea Monotherapy or Combination of Both: Initial: 30-2 mg qd. Adjust dose based on response. Max: Once-daily at any dosage strength. Elderly/Debilitated/Malnourished: Initial: 1 mg glimepiride prior to prescribing Duetact. Systolic Dysfunction: Initial: Give lowest approved dose only after titration from 15-30 mg of pioglitazone is safely tolerated. | ⊕C ✿v H R W [79] |

NAME	FORM/STRENGTH	DOSAGE	COMMENTS
Rosiglitazone Maleate/ Glimepiride (Avandaryl)	**Tab:** 4-1 mg, 4-2 mg, 4-4 mg, 8-2 mg, 8-4 mg	**Adults: Initial:** 4-1 mg qd w/ 1st meal of day. **Already Treated w/ Sulfonylurea or Rosiglitazone: Initial:** 4-2 mg qd. **Switching from Prior Combination Therapy as Separate Tab:** Same dose of each component. **Switching from Current Rosiglitazone Monotherapy:** Increase glimepiride by ≤2 mg if inadequate after 1-2 wks; titrate Avandaryl if inadequate after 1-2 wks. **Switching from Current Sulfonylurea Monotherapy:** Titrate rosiglitazone if inadequate after 8-12 wks; titrate Avandaryl if inadequate after 2-3 mths. **Max:** 8-4 mg/day. **Elderly/Debilitated/ Malnourished/Adrenal Insufficiency: Initial:** 4-1 mg qd.	◨C ✿v H R W [82]

Antithyroid Agents

NAME	FORM/STRENGTH	DOSAGE	COMMENTS
Methimazole (Tapazole)	**Tab:** 5 mg, 10 mg	**Adults: Initial:** 5 mg q8h for mild hyperthyroidism; 30-40 mg/d given q8h for moderately severe hyperthyroidism, 20 mg q8h for severe hyperthyroidism. **Maint:** 5-15 mg/d. **Peds: Initial:** 0.4 mg/kg/d divided q8h. **Maint:** 1/2 of initial dose.	◨D ✿v CI in nursing.
Propylthiouracil	**Tab:** 50 mg	**Adults: Initial:** 100 mg q8h. May give 400 mg/d divided q8h for severe hyperthyroidism/large goiters, and up to 600-900 mg/d if needed. **Maint:** 100-150 mg/d if divided q8h. **Peds: ≥6 yo: Initial:** 50 mg/d divided q8h. **Maint:** Determine dose by response.	◨D ✿> W [41]

Gout

URICOSURIC

Probenecid	**Tab:** 500 mg	**Adults:** 250 mg bid x 1 wk. **Titrate:** Increase by 500 mg q4wks. **Maint:** 500 mg bid. **Max:** 2 gm/d.	⊕N ❄> R

XANTHINE OXIDASE INHIBITORS

Allopurinol (Zyloprim)	**Tab:** 100 mg, 300 mg	**Adults: Reduction of Flare-Up of Acute Gouty Attacks: Initial:** 100 mg/d. **Titrate:** Increase qwk by 100 mg until serum uric acid ≤6 mg/dl. **Mild Gout: Usual:** 200-300 mg/d in single or divided doses. **Moderate-Severe Gout: Usual:** 400-600 mg/d in divided doses. **Max:** 800 mg/d.	⊕C ❄> R
Febuxostat (Uloric)	**Tab:** 40 mg, 80 mg	**Hyperuricemia w/ Gout: Adults: Initial:** 40 mg qd. **Serum Uric Acid ≥6 mg/dl after 2 Wks at 40 mg:** 80 mg qd.	⊕C ❄>

MISCELLANEOUS

Colchicine (Colcrys)	**Tab:** 0.6 mg	**Adults & Peds: >16 yo: Prophylaxis of Gout Flares:** 0.6 mg qd or bid. **Max:** 1.2 mg/d. **Adults: Treatment of Gout Flares:** 1.2 mg at first sign of gout flare, then 0.6 mg given 1h later. **Max:** 1.8 mg/h. May administer for treatment of gout flare during prophylaxis; wait 12h then resume prophylactic dose. See PI for dose modifications w/ concomitant drugs.	⊕C ❄> H R

NAME	FORM/STRENGTH	DOSAGE	COMMENTS
Pegloticase (Krystexxa)	Inj: 8 mg/ml	**Adults:** 8 mg IV infusion q2wks. Do not administer as IV push or bolus.	◉C ❖v Anaphylaxis & infusion reactions reported. Monitor serum uric acid levels.
Probenecid/Colchicine	Tab: 500-0.5 mg	**Adults: Initial:** 1 tab qd x 1 wk, then 1 tab bid. **Titrate:** May increase by 1 tab/d q4wks. **Max:** 4 tabs/d. Not for acute gouty attacks. May reduce dose by 1 tab q6mths if acute attacks absent ≥6 mths.	◉N ❖> CI in pregnancy. R

Osteoporosis
BISPHOSPHONATES AND COMBINATIONS

NAME	FORM/STRENGTH	DOSAGE	COMMENTS
Alendronate Sodium/ Cholecalciferol (Fosamax Plus D)	Tab: 70 mg-2800 IU, 70 mg-5600 IU	**Treatment in Postmenopausal Women/Bone Mass Increase in Men: Adults:** 1 tab qwk. **Usual:** 70 mg-5600 IU qwk. Take ≥30 min before 1st food, beverage, or med of day. Take tab w/ 6-8 oz water. Do not lie down x ≥30 min after dose & until after 1st food of day.	◉C ❖> R
Alendronate Sodium (Fosamax)	Sol: 70 mg/75 ml; Tab: 5 mg, 10 mg, 35 mg, 40 mg, 70 mg	**Adults: Treatment in Females/Bone Mass Increase in Men:** 10 mg qd or 70 mg qwk. **Prevention: Females:** 5 mg qd or 35 mg qwk. **Glucocorticoid-Induced: Men/Women:** 5 mg qd. **Postmenopausal Women Not Receiving Estrogen:** 10 mg qd. Take ≥30 min before 1st food, beverage, or med of day. Take tab w/ 6-8 oz water. Take ≥2	◉C ❖> R

		oz water after oral sol. Do not lie down x ≥30 min after dose & until after 1st food of day.	
Risedronate Sodium (Actonel)	Tab: 5 mg, 30 mg, 35 mg, 150 mg	**Adults: Postmenopausal Osteoporosis Prevention/ Treatment:** 5 mg qd, or 35 mg once wkly, or 150 mg once mthly. **Glucocorticoid-Induced Osteoporosis Prevention/Treatment:** 5 mg qd. **Increase Bone Mass in Men w/ Osteoporosis:** 35 mg once wkly. **Paget's Disease:** 30 mg qd x 2 mths. May retreat after 2 mths. Take ≥30 min before 1st food or drink of day other than water. Swallow in upright position w/ 6-8 oz water. Do not lie down x 30 min after dose.	◉C ❁v R
Risedronate Sodium (Atelvia)	Tab, Delay: 35 mg	**Treatment in Postmenopausal Women:** 35 mg qwk. Take in am immediately following breakfast. Swallow in upright position & w/ at least 4 oz of water. Do not lie down x 30 min after dose.	◉C ❁v R
CALCITONIN			
Calcitonin-Salmon (rDNA origin) (Fortical)	Nasal Spr: 200 IU/spr	**Treatment: Adults: Female: Intranasal:** 1 spr (200 IU) qd intranasally. Alternate nostrils daily.	◉C ❁v
Calcitonin-Salmon (Miacalcin)	Inj: 200 IU/ml; Spr: 200 IU/spr	**Treatment: Adults: Postmenopausal: Spr:** 200 IU (1 spr) qd intranasally, alternate nostrils daily. **Inj:** 100 IU IM/ SC qod.	◉C ❁v

NAME	FORM/STRENGTH	DOSAGE	COMMENTS
ESTROGEN/PROGESTIN COMBINATION			
Estradiol/Levonorgestrel (Climara Pro)	**Patch:** 0.045-0.015 mg/d	**Adults: Prevention:** Apply 1 patch qwk to lower abdomen (avoid breasts/waistline). Rotate application site; allow 1 wk between applications to same site.	●N ❄>CI in pregnancy. **H W** [4, 28]
Medroxyprogesterone Acetate/Conjugated Estrogens (Premphase, Prempro)	**Tab:** (Premphase) 0.625 mg (conjugated estrogens), 5-0.625 mg; (Prempro) 1.5-0.3 mg, 1.5-0.45 mg, 2.5-0.625 mg, 5-0.625 mg	**Adults: Prevention: Female: Premphase:** 0.625-mg tab qd on Days 1-14 & 5-0.625 mg tab qd on Days 15-28. **Prempro:** 1 tab qd. Reevaluate treatment need periodically.	●N ❄v CI in pregnancy. **H W** [4, 28]
Norethindrone Acetate/ Estradiol (Activella)	**Tab:** 0.5-1 mg, 0.1-0.5 mg	**Prevention: Adults: Female:** 1 tab qd. Reevaluate treatment need periodically (eg, 3-6 mth intervals).	●N ❄>CI in pregnancy. **W** [28]
Norethindrone Acetate/ Ethinyl Estradiol (femhrt)	**Tab:** 0.5 mg-2.5 mcg, 1 mg-5 mcg	**Prevention: Adults:** 1 tab qd.	●N ❄> **H W** [4, 28]
ESTROGENS			
Conjugated Estrogens (Premarin Tablets)	**Tab:** 0.3 mg, 0.45 mg, 0.625 mg, 0.9 mg, 1.25 mg	**Prevention: Adults: Female: Initial:** 0.3 mg qd given continuously or cyclically (25d on, 5d off).	●N ❄v CI in pregnancy. **W** [4, 28]

Estradiol (Estrace)	**Tab:** 0.5 mg, 1 mg, 2 mg	**Prevention: Adults: Female:** Use lowest effective dose. Reevaluate treatment need periodically (eg, 3-6 mth intervals).	⊡X (Tab), CI in pregnancy (Cre). ❋v **W** [4, 10, 28]
Estradiol (Alora)	**Patch:** 0.025 mg/d, 0.05 mg/d, 0.075 mg/d, 0.1 mg/d	**Prevention: Adults: Female:** Apply 0.025 mg/d patch twice wkly. **Titrate:** May increase depending on bone mineral density & adverse events.	⊡X ❋> **W** [4, 28]
Estradiol (Climara)	**Patch:** 0.025 mg/d, 0.0375 mg/d, 0.05 mg/d, 0.06 mg/d, 0.075 mg/d, 0.1 mg/d	**Prevention: Adults: Female:** Apply 0.025 mg/d patch qwk (minimum effective dose).	⊡X ❋> **W** [4, 28]
Estradiol (Menostar)	**Patch:** 14 mcg/d	**Prevention: Adults: Female:** Apply 1 patch (14 mcg/d) qwk.	⊡N ❋> **W** [4, 28]
Estropipate	**Tab:** 0.75 mg, 1.5 mg, 3 mg	**Prevention: Adults: Female:** 0.75 mg qd x 25d of 31d cycle/mth.	⊡X ❋> **W** [4, 28]

MONOCLONAL ANTIBODIES

Denosumab (Prolia)	**Inj:** 60 mg/ml	**Treatment: Postmenopausal Women/Women Receiving Adjuvant Aromatase Inhibitors for Breast Cancer/ Men Receiving Androgen Deprivation Therapy for Nonmetastatic Prostate Cancer: Adults:** 60 mg SC q6mths in upper arm, upper thigh, or abdomen. Give missed dose when patient is available & schedule inj q6mths from date of last inj.	⊡X ❋v

NAME	FORM/STRENGTH	DOSAGE	COMMENTS

SERM (SELECTIVE ESTROGEN RECEPTOR MODULATOR)

NAME	FORM/STRENGTH	DOSAGE	COMMENTS
Raloxifene HCl (Evista)	**Tab:** 60 mg	**Treatment/Prevention: Adults: Female:** 60 mg qd.	◯X ✲v

Thyroid Agents
THYROID HORMONES

NAME	FORM/STRENGTH	DOSAGE	COMMENTS
Levothyroxine Sodium (Levoxyl)	**Tab:** 0.025 mg, 0.05 mg, 0.075 mg, 0.088 mg, 0.1 mg, 0.112 mg, 0.125 mg, 0.137 mg, 0.15 mg, 0.175 mg, 0.2 mg	**Adults & Peds (Growth/Puberty Complete): Hypothyroidism:** 1.7 mcg/kg/d. >200 mcg/d seldom required. **>50 yo or <50 yo w/ Underlying Cardiac Disease: Initial:** 25-50 mcg/d. **Titrate:** Increase by 12.5-25 mcg increments q6-8 wks as needed. **Elderly w/ Cardiac Disease: Initial:** 12.5-25 mcg/d. **Titrate:** Increase by 12.5-25 mcg increments q4-6 wks until euthyroid. **Severe Hypothyroidism: Initial:** 12.5-25 mcg/d. **Titrate:** Increase by 25 mcg/d q2-4 wks until TSH normalized. **Peds: >12 yo (Growth/Puberty Incomplete):** 2-3 mcg/kg/d. **6-12 yo:** 4-5 mcg/kg/d. **1-5 yo:** 5-6 mcg/kg/d. **6-12 mths:** 6-8 mcg/kg/d. **3-6 mths:** 8-10 mcg/kg/d. **0-3 mths:** 10-15 mcg/kg/d. **Infants at Risk for Cardiac Failure:** Use lower dose (eg, 25 mcg/d). **Titrate:** Increase q4-6 wks as needed. **Infants w/ Serum T4 <5 mcg/dl: Initial:** 50 mcg/d. **Chronic/Severe Hypothyroidism: Children: Initial:** 25 mcg/d. **Titrate:** Increase by 25 mcg increments q2-4 wks until desired effect. **Adults: Pituitary TSH**	◯A ✲>

		Suppression in Well-Differentiated Thyroid Cancer and Thyroid Nodules: Individualize; see PI.	
Levothyroxine Sodium (Synthroid)	Tab: 0.025 mg, 0.05 mg, 0.075 mg, 0.088 mg, 0.1 mg, 0.112 mg, 0.125 mg, 0.137 mg, 0.15 mg, 0.175 mg, 0.2 mg, 0.3 mg	**Adults & Peds (Growth/Puberty Complete): Hypothyroidism:** 1.7 mcg/kg/d. >200 mcg/d seldom required. **>50 yo or <50 yo w/ Underlying Cardiac Disease: Initial:** 25-50 mcg/d. **Titrate:** Increase by 12.5-25 mcg increments q6-8 wks as needed. **Elderly w/ Cardiac Disease: Initial:** 12.5-25 mcg/d. **Titrate:** Increase by 12.5-25 mcg increments q4-6 wks until euthyroid. **Severe Hypothyroidism: Initial:** 12.5-25 mcg/d. **Titrate:** Increase by 25 mcg/d q2-4 wks until TSH normalized. **Peds: >12 yo (Growth/Puberty Incomplete):** 2-3 mcg/kg/d. **6-12 yo:** 4-5 mcg/kg/d. **1-5 yo:** 5-6 mcg/kg/d. **6-12 mths:** 6-8 mcg/kg/d. **3-6 mths:** 8-10 mcg/kg/d. **0-3 mths:** 10-15 mcg/kg/d. **Infants at Risk for Cardiac Failure:** Use lower dose (eg, 25 mcg/d). **Titrate:** Increase q4-6 wks as needed. **Infants w/ Serum T4 <5 mcg/dl: Initial:** 50 mcg/d. **Chronic/Severe Hypothyroidism: Children: Initial:** 25 mcg/d. **Titrate:** Increase by 25 mcg increments q2-4 wks until desired effect. **Adults: Pituitary TSH Suppression in Well-Differentiated Thyroid Cancer and Thyroid Nodules:** Individualize; see PI.	▣A ✽>

NAME	FORM/STRENGTH	DOSAGE	COMMENTS
Levothyroxine Sodium, T4 (Levothroid)	**Tab:** 0.025 mg, 0.05 mg, 0.075 mg, 0.088 mg, 0.1 mg, 0.112 mg, 0.125 mg, 0.137 mg, 0.15 mg, 0.175 mg, 0.2 mg, 0.3 mg	**Adults <50 yo or >50 yo & Recently Treated for Hyperthyroidism or Hypothyroid for Short Time & Peds >12 yo (Growth/Puberty Complete): Hypothyroidism:** 1.7 mcg/kg/d. >200 mcg/d seldom required. **>50 yo or <50 yo w/ Underlying Cardiac Disease: Initial:** 25-50 mcg/d until TSH normalized. **Severe Hypothyroidism/Elderly w/ Cardiac Disease: Initial:** 12.5-25 mcg/d until TSH normalized. **Peds: >12 yo (Growth/Puberty Incomplete):** 2-3 mcg/kg/d. **6-12 yo:** 4-5 mcg/kg/d. **1-5 yo:** 5-6 mcg/kg/d. **6-12 mths:** 6-8 mcg/kg/d. **3-6 mths:** 8-10 mcg/kg/d. **0-3 mths:** 10-15 mcg/kg/d. **Adults: Pituitary TSH Suppression: Thyroid Cancer, Well-Differentiated: Adjunct:** TSH suppression to <0.1 mU/l usually requires >2 mcg/kg/d. **High-Risk Tumors:** Target TSH suppression may be <0.01 mU/l. **Benign Nodules/Nontoxic Multinodular Goiter:** Target TSH suppression of 0.1-1 mU/l.	▣A ❃>
Liothyronine, T3 (Cytomel)	**Tab:** 0.005 mg, 0.025 mg, 0.05 mg	**Adults:** Individualize dose. **Mild Hypothyroidism: Initial:** 25 mcg qd. **Titrate:** May increase up to 25 mcg qd q1-2wks. **Maint:** 25-75 mcg qd. **Myxedema: Initial:** 5 mcg qd. **Titrate:** May increase by 5-10 mcg qd q1-2wks up to 25 mcg qd, then increase by 5-25 mcg qd q1-2wks until desired response. **Maint:** 50-100 mcg/d. **Simple (Non-Toxic) Goiter: Initial:** 5 mcg/d. **Titrate:** May increase	▣A ❃>

		by 5-10 mcg qd q1-2wks up to 25 mcg qd, then by 12.5-25 mcg qd q1-2wks. **Maint:** 75 mcg qd. **Elderly/ Angina Pectoris/Coronary Artery Disease: Initial:** 5 mcg qd. **Titrate:** Increase by no more than 5 mcg qd at 2-wk intervals. **Peds: Congenital Hypothyroidism: Initial:** 5 mcg qd. **Titrate:** Increase by 5 mcg qd q3-4d until desired response. **Maint: >3 yo:** 25-75 mcg/d. **1-3 yo:** 50 mcg qd. **<1 yo:** 20 mcg qd.	
Thyroid, Desiccated (Armour Thyroid)	**Tab:** 15 mg, 30 mg, 60 mg, 90 mg, 120 mg, 180 mg, 240 mg, 300 mg	**Adults: Initial:** 30 mg qd (15 mg qd w/ long-standing myxedema). **Titrate:** Increase by 15 mg q2-3wks. **Maint:** 60-120 mg/d. **Peds: >12 yo:** 1.2-1.8 mg/kg/d. **6-12 yo:** 2.4-3 mg/kg/d. **1-5 yo:** 3-3.6 mg/kg/d. **6-12 mths:** 3.6-4.8 mg/kg/d. **0-6 mths:** 4.8-6 mg/kg/d.	⊙A ❄>

Miscellaneous
BONE RESORPTION INHIBITORS

Pamidronate Disodium (Aredia)	**Inj:** 30 mg, 90 mg	**Adults: Moderate Hypercalcemia:** 60-90 mg IV single dose over 2-24h. **Severe Hypercalcemia:** 90 mg IV single dose over 2-24h. **Retreatment:** May repeat after 7d. **Paget's Disease:** 30 mg qd IV over 4h x 3d. **Osteolytic Bone Lesions of Multiple Myeloma:** 90 mg IV over 4h once mthly. **Osteolytic Bone Metastases of Breast Cancer:** 90 mg IV over 2h q3-4wks. **Max:** 90 mg/single dose for all indications.	⊙D ❄> R

NAME	FORM/STRENGTH	DOSAGE	COMMENTS
Zoledronic Acid (Reclast)	Inj: 5 mg/100 ml	**Adults: Paget's Disease:** 5 mg IV via separate vented infusion line over ≥15 min at constant infusion rate. Hydrate prior to administration.	⊕D ❄v R
Zoledronic Acid (Zometa)	Inj: 4 mg/5 ml, 4 mg/100 ml	**Adults: IV: Hypercalcemia of Malignancy: Max:** 4 mg infused over no less than 15 min. **Retreatment (if necessary):** Wait ≥7d from initial dose. **Multiple Myeloma/Bone Metastases:** 4 mg infused over 15 min q3-4wks. Take w/ PO calcium 500 mg/d & vitamin D 400 IU/d.	⊕D ❄v R

ENZYME INHIBITOR

NAME	FORM/STRENGTH	DOSAGE	COMMENTS
Miglustat (Zavesca)	Cap: 100 mg	**Mild-Moderate Type 1 Gaucher Disease: Adults:** 100 mg tid at regular intervals. May reduce to 100 mg qd or bid for adverse effects. **Elderly:** Start at low end of dosing range.	⊕X ❄v R

GROWTH HORMONE RELEASING FACTOR

NAME	FORM/STRENGTH	DOSAGE	COMMENTS
Tesamorelin (Egrifta)	Inj: 1 mg	**Lipodystrophy HIV-Patients: Adults:** 2 mg SC in the abdomen qd.	⊕X ❄v

URIC ACID AGENTS

NAME	FORM/STRENGTH	DOSAGE	COMMENTS
Allopurinol Sodium (Aloprim)	Inj: 500 mg	**Elevated Serum/Urinary Uric Acid Levels: Adults: Initial:** 200-400 mg/m²/d IV as qd or in divided doses every 6, 8, or 12h. **Max:** 600 mg/d. **Peds: Initial:** 200 mg/m²/d IV as qd or in divided doses every 6, 8, or 12h.	⊕C ❄> R

| Allopurinol
(Zyloprim) | Tab: 100 mg, 300 mg | **Prevention of Uric Acid Nephropathy w/ Chemo: Adults:** Usual: 600-800 mg/d x 2-3d w/ high fluid intake. | ●C
❋> R |
| Rasburicase
(Elitek) | Inj: 1.5 mg, 7.5 mg | **Anticipated Chemo-Related Hyperuricemia: Adults & Peds: ≥1 mth:** 0.2 mg/kg IV infusion over 30 min qd for up to 5d. | ●C
❋v W [39] |

GASTROINTESTINAL AGENTS

Antidiarrheal Agents

Diphenoxylate HCl/ Atropine CV (Lomotil)	Liq: 0.025-2.5 mg/5 ml; Tab: 0.025-2.5 mg	**Adults: Initial:** 2 tabs or 10 ml qid. **Maint:** 2 tabs or 10 ml tid. **Max:** 20 mg diphenoxylate/d. **Peds: 13-16 yo: Initial:** 2 tabs or 10 ml qd. **2-12 yo: Initial:** 0.3-0.4 mg/kg/d given qid. **Maint:** 1/4 of initial daily dose.	●C ❋>
Nitazoxanide (Alinia)	Susp: 100 mg/5 ml; Tab: 500 mg	*G.lamblia* **Diarrhea: Adults & Peds: ≥12 yo:** 500 mg q12h x 3d. Take w/ food. *C.parvum/G.lamblia* **Diarrhea: Peds: 1-3 yo:** 100 mg (5 ml) q12h x 3d. **4-11 yo:** 200 mg (10 ml) q12h x 3d.	●B ❋>
Rifaximin (Xifaxan)	Tab: 200 mg, 550 mg	**Travelers' Diarrhea: Adults & Peds: ≥12 yo:** 200 mg tid x 3d.	●C ❋v

NAME	FORM/STRENGTH	DOSAGE	COMMENTS

Antiemetics

5-HT₃ ANTAGONISTS

NAME	FORM/STRENGTH	DOSAGE	COMMENTS
Dolasetron Mesylate (Anzemet)	**Inj:** 20 mg/ml; **Tab:** 50 mg, 100 mg	**Adults: Prevent Chemo N/V:** 100 mg PO w/in 1h before chemo. **Peds: 2-16 yo:** 1.8 mg/kg PO w/in 1h before chemo. **Max:** 100 mg. **Adults: Prevention/Treatment Postop N/V:** 12.5 mg IV. **Prevention:** 100 mg PO. **Peds: 2-16 yo:** 0.35 mg/kg IV, up to 12.5 mg IV; or 1.2 mg/kg PO, up to 100 mg PO. Give PO w/in 2h pre-op, IV 15 min before anesthesia cessation (prevention) or at start of N/V (treatment).	●B ❄>
Granisetron HCl	**Inj:** 0.1 mg/ml, 1mg/ml; **Tab:** 1 mg	**Prevent Chemo N/V: Adults:** PO: 2 mg qd up to 1h before chemo or 1 mg bid (up to 1h before chemo & 12h later). IV: 10 mcg/kg over 30 sec (undiluted) or 5 min (diluted), w/in 30 min before chemo. **Peds: 2-16 yo:** IV: 10mcg/kg w/in 30 min before chemo. **Prevent Radiation N/V: Adults:** PO: 2 mg qd w/in 1h of radiation.	●B ❄>
Granisetron HCl (Granisol)	**Sol:** 2 mg/10 ml	**Adults: Prevent Chemo N/V:** 2 mg PO qd up to 1h before chemo or 1 mg PO bid up to 1h before chemo & 12h later. **Prevent Radiation N/V:** 2 mg PO qd w/in 1h of radiation.	●B ❄>
Granisetron (Sancuso)	**Patch:** 3.1 mg/24h	**Adults:** Apply single patch to upper outer arm a minimum of 24h before chemo. May be applied up to max of 48h before chemo. Remove patch minimum of 24h after completion of chemo. Patch may be worn for up to 7d depending on duration of chemo regimen.	●B ❄>

| **Ondansetron HCl** (Zofran) | **Inj:** 2 mg/ml; **Sol:** 4 mg/ 5 ml; **Tab:** 4 mg, 8 mg; **Tab,Dissolve:** (ODT) 4 mg, 8 mg | **Prevent Chemo N/V: Adults: (Inj):** Three 0.15-mg/kg IV doses; give 1st dose 30 min (over 15 min) before chemo w/ subsequent doses given 4h & 8h after 1st dose. **Max:** 16mg/dose. **Peds: 6 mths-18 yo: (Inj):** Three 0.15-mg/kg IV doses. Infuse over 15 min; give 1st dose 30 min before chemo w/ subsequent doses given 4h & 8h after 1st dose. **Max:** 16mg/dose. **Prevent Highly Emetogenic Chemo N/V: Adults: (Tab):** Three 8-mg tabs (24 mg) PO 30 min before chemo. **Prevent Moderately Emetogenic Chemo N/V: Adults & Peds: ≥12 yo: (PO):** 8 mg bid; given 30 min before chemo, then 8h after 1st dose, then 8 mg q12h x 1-2d after complete therapy. **4-11 yo:** 4 mg tid 30 min before chemo, then 4h & 8h after 1st dose, then 4 mg q8h x 1-2d. **Prevent Postop N/V: Adults: (PO):** 16 mg 1h before anesthesia. **(Inj): Adults:** 4 mg IV/IM immediately before anesthesia or postop. **Peds: 1 mth-12 yo: ≤40 kg:** 0.1 mg/kg IV single dose. **>40 kg:** 4 mg IV single dose over 2-5 min prior to or after anesthesia or postop. Infuse over 2-5 min prior to or after anesthesia or postop. **≥12 yo:** 4 mg IV/IM immediately before anesthesia or postop. **Prevent Radiation N/V: Adults: (PO): Usual:** 8 mg tid. **Total Body Irradiation: (PO):** 8 mg 1-2h before therapy daily. **Single High-Dose Therapy to Abdomen: (PO):** 8 mg 1-2h before therapy then q8h after 1st dose x 1-2d after | ▣B ✿> H |

Continued on Next Page

NAME	FORM/STRENGTH	DOSAGE	COMMENTS
Ondansetron HCl (Zofran) *Continued*		complete therapy. **Daily Fractionated Therapy to Abdomen: (PO):** 8 mg 1-2h before therapy then q8h after 1st dose of each day therapy is given.	
Ondansetron (Zuplenz)	Film,Oral: 4 mg, 8 mg	**Adults: Prevent Highly Emetogenic Chemo N/V:** 24 mg 30 min before chemo. **Adults & Peds: ≥12 yo: Prevent Moderately Emetogenic Chemo N/V:** 8 mg 30 min before chemo, then 8h after 1st dose, then q12h x 1-2d after chemo completion. **Peds: 4-11 yo:** 4 mg 30 min before chemo, then 4 & 8h after 1st dose, then q8h x 1-2d after chemo completion. **Adults: Prevent Radiation N/V: Usual:** 8 mg tid. **Total Body Irradiation:** 8 mg 1-2h before therapy daily. **Single High-Dose Therapy to Abdomen:** 8 mg 1-2h before therapy then q8h after 1st dose x 1-2d after complete therapy. **Daily Fractionated Therapy to Abdomen:** 8 mg 1-2h before therapy then q8h after 1st dose for each day of therapy. **Adults: Prevent Postop N/V:** 16 mg 1h before anesthesia.	●B ✦> H
Palonosetron HCl (Aloxi)	Inj: 0.25 mg/5 ml, 0.075 mg/1.5 ml	**Adults: Prevent Chemo-Induced N/V:** 0.25 mg IV single dose over 30 sec. Dosing should occur approx. 30 min before start of chemo. **Prevent Postop N/V:** 0.075 mg IV single dose over 10 sec immediately before induction of anesthesia.	●B ✦v

ANTICHOLINERGICS

| Scopolamine (Transderm Scop) | Patch: 1.5 mg | **Adults: Motion Sickness N/V:** 1 patch at least 4h before the antiemetic effect is required. Replace patch after 3d if therapy is required for >3d. **Postop N/V:** 1 patch on the evening before surgery or 1h prior to cesarean section. Remove patch 24h following surgery. Apply to the hairless area behind one ear. | ⊕C ✿> |

ANTIHISTAMINES

Hydroxyzine HCl	Inj: 25 mg/ml, 50 mg/ml	**N/V: Adults:** 25-100 mg IM. **Peds:** 0.5 mg/lb IM.	⊕N ✿v CI in early pregnancy.
Meclizine HCl (Antivert)	Tab: 12.5 mg, 25 mg, 50 mg	**Adults & Peds: ≥12 yo: Vertigo: Usual:** 25-100 mg/d in divided doses. **Motion Sickness: Initial:** 25-50 mg 1h before trip/departure; repeat q24h prn.	⊕B ✿>
Meclizine HCl (Zentrip)	Strip, Oral: 25 mg	**Adults & Peds: ≥12 yo:** Dissolve 1-2 strips on tongue qd or ud. **Prevention:** ≥1h prior to travel.	⊕N ✿>
Prochlorperazine	Inj: (edisylate) 5 mg/ml; Tab: (maleate) 5 mg, 10 mg	**N/V: Adults: Tab:** 5-10 mg tid-qid. **IM:** 5-10 mg 3-4h prn. **Max:** 40 mg/d. **IV:** 2.5-10 mg. **Max:** 10 mg single dose; 5 mg/min rate; 40 mg/d. **Peds: ≥2 yo & >20 lbs: IM:** 0.06 mg/lb. **Tab: 20-29 lbs:** 2.5 mg qd-bid. **Max:** 7.5 mg/d. **30-39 lbs:** 2.5 mg bid-tid. **Max:** 10 mg/d. **40-85 lbs:**	⊕N ✿> W [30]

Continued on Next Page

NAME	FORM/STRENGTH	DOSAGE	COMMENTS
Prochlorperazine *Continued*		2.5 mg tid or 5 mg bid. **Max:** 15 mg/d. **N/V w/ Surgery: Adults:** IM: 5-10 mg 1-2h before induction of anesthesia, or during or after surgery; repeat once if needed. **IV:** 5-10 mg 15-30 min before anesthesia, or during or after surgery; repeat once if needed. **Max:** 10 mg single dose; 5 mg/min rate; 40 mg/d.	
Promethazine HCl (Phenadoz, Promethazine, Promethegan)	**Sup:** (Phenadoz, Promethazine) 12.5 mg, 25 mg, (Promethegan) 50 mg; **Syr:** 6.25 mg/5 ml; **Tab:** (Promethazine) 12.5 mg, 25 mg, 50 mg	**Adults: Prevent N/V & Post-Op N/V: PO/PR: Usual:** 25 mg, then 12.5-25 mg q4-6h prn. **Peds:** ≥2 yo: **PO/PR: Usual:** 0.5 mg/lb or 25 mg, then 12.5-25 mg q4-6h prn. **Adults: Motion Sickness: PO/PR: Initial:** 25 mg 30-60 min before travel; repeat after 8-12h prn. **Maint:** 25 mg bid. **Peds:** ≥2 yo: **PO/PR:** 12.5-25 mg bid.	▣C ❧v Potential for fatal respiratory depression; not for use in peds <2 yo. **R**
DOPAMINE ANTAGONIST/PROKINETIC			
Metoclopramide (Reglan)	**Inj:** 5 mg/ml	**Adults: Prevent Chemo N/V:** 1-2 mg/kg IV infusion over ≥15 min, 30 min before chemo, then q2h x 2 doses, then q3h x 3 doses. **Prevent Postop N/V:** 10-20 mg IM near end of surgery.	▣B ❧> May cause tardive dyskinesia. **R**

SUBSTANCE P/NEUROKININ 1 RECEPTOR ANTAGONIST

Aprepitant (Emend)	Cap: 40 mg, 80 mg, 125 mg; BiPack (two 80 mg); TriPack (one 125 mg & two 80 mg caps)	**Adults: Prevention of Chemo-Induced N/V: Day 1:** 125 mg 1h prior to chemo. **Days 2 & 3:** 80 mg qam. Regimen should include a corticosteroid & 5-HT₃ antagonist. Refer to PI for dosing w/ dexamethasone or methylprednisolone. **Prevention of Postop N/V:** 40 mg w/in 3h prior to induction of anesthesia.	◉B ✿v

MISCELLANEOUS

Dronabinol CIII (Marinol)	Cap: 2.5 mg, 5 mg, 10 mg	**Adults & Peds: Prevent Chemo N/V: Initial:** 5 mg/m² 1-3h before chemo, then q2-4h after chemo, up to 4-6 doses/d. **Titrate:** May increase dose by 2.5 mg/m² increments. **Max:** 15 mg/m²/dose.	◉C ✿v
Nabilone CII (Cesamet)	Cap: 1 mg	**Adults: Usual:** 1 or 2 mg bid. **Day of Chemotherapy: Initial:** Administer 1-3h before chemotherapy. Start w/ lower dose & increase prn. 1 or 2 mg the night before may be useful to minimize side effects. May be given bid or tid during the chemotherapy cycle & prn for 48h after the last dose of each cycle. **Max:** 6 mg/d given in divided doses tid. **Elderly:** Start at the low end of dosing range.	◉C ✿v

NAME	FORM/STRENGTH	DOSAGE	COMMENTS

Antispasmodics

NAME	FORM/STRENGTH	DOSAGE	COMMENTS
Clidinium Bromide/ Chlordiazepoxide HCl (Librax)	Cap: 2.5-5 mg	Adults: Usual: 1-2 caps tid-qid ac & hs.	⊕N ❄>
Dicyclomine HCl (Bentyl)	Cap: 10 mg; Inj: 10 mg/ml; Syr: 10 mg/ 5 ml; Tab: 20 mg	Adults: Initial: PO: 20 mg qid. Maint: 40 mg qid if tolerated after 1 wk of initial dose. D/C if no improvement after 2 wks or if doses ≥80 mg/d not tolerated. Inj: 20 mg IM qid x 1-2d, followed by PO dose. Not for IV use.	⊕B ❄v
Hyoscyamine Sulfate (Levbid)	Tab,ER: 0.375 mg	Adults & Peds: ≥12 yo: 1-2 tabs q12h. Max: 4 tabs/24h. Do not crush or chew.	⊕C ❄>
Scopolamine Hydrobromide/ Hyoscyamine Sulfate/ Atropine Sulfate/ Phenobarbital (Donnatal Extentabs)	Tab/Eli (per 5 ml): 0.0194-0.1037-16.2- 0.0065 mg	Adults: 1-2 tabs or 5-10 ml tid-qid. Peds: 100 lbs: 5 ml q4h or 7.5 ml q6h. 75 lbs: 3.75 ml q4h or 5 ml q6h. 50 lbs: 2.5 ml q4h or 3.75 ml q6h. 30 lbs: 1.5 ml q4h or 2 ml q6h. 20 lbs: 1 ml q4h or 1.5 ml q6h. 10 lbs: 0.5 ml q4h or 0.75 ml q6h.	⊕C ❄> H

Antiulcer Agents
DUODENAL ULCER ADHERENT COMPLEX

NAME	FORM/STRENGTH	DOSAGE	COMMENTS
Sucralfate (Carafate)	Susp: 1 gm/10 ml; Tab: 1 gm	Active Duodenal Ulcer: Adults: Sus/Tab: 1 gm qid x 4-8 wks unless healing is demonstrated. Maint: Tab: 1 gm bid.	⊕B ❄>

H₂ ANTAGONISTS

Drug	Forms	Dosing	
Cimetidine (Tagamet)	**Sol:** 300 mg/5 ml; **Tab:** 200 mg, 300 mg, 400 mg, 800 mg	**Adults & Peds: ≥16 yo: Active DU:** 800 mg qhs or 300 mg qid or 400 mg bid x 4-6 wks. **Maint:** 400 mg qhs. **Active Benign GU:** 800 mg qhs or 300 mg qid x 6 wks.	⊕B ✿v R
Famotidine (Pepcid)	**Inj:** (Generic) 20 mg/50 ml, 10 mg/ml; **Susp:** (Pepcid) 40 mg/5 ml; **Tab:** 20 mg, 40 mg	**Adults: DU: PO:** 20 mg bid or 40 mg qhs x 4-8 wks. **Maint:** 20 mg qhs. **IV:** 20 mg q12h. Switch to PO when possible. **GU: PO:** 40 mg qhs. **IV:** 20 mg q12h. Switch to PO when possible. **Peds 1-16 yo: DU/GU: PO:** 0.5 mg/kg/d qhs or divided bid. **Max:** 40 mg/d. **IV:** 0.25 mg/kg q12h. **Max:** 40 mg/d.	⊕B ✿v R
Nizatidine (Axid)	**Cap:** 150 mg, 300 mg; **Sol:** 15 mg/ml	**Adults: GU/DU: Healing:** 150 mg bid or 300 mg qhs x up to 8 wks. **DU Maint:** 150 mg qhs x up to 1 yr.	⊕B ✿v R
Ranitidine HCl (Zantac)	**Inj:** 1 mg/ml, 25 mg/ml; **Syr:** 15 mg/ml; **Tab:** 150 mg, 300 mg; **Tab,Eff:** 25 mg	**Adults: GU/DU: PO: Healing:** 150 mg bid or (DU) 300 mg after evening meal or qhs. **Maint:** 150 mg qhs. **IV/IM:** 50 mg q6-8h. May adjust as needed. **Continuous IV:** 6.25 mg/h. **Max:** 400 mg/d. **Peds: 1 mth-16 yo: GU/DU: PO: Healing:** 2-4 mg/kg bid. **Max:** 300 mg/d. **Maint:** 2-4 mg/kg qd. **Max:** 150 mg/d. **IV:** 2-4 mg/kg/d divided and given q6-8h. **Max:** 50 mg q6-8h. **<1 mth: IV Bolus:** 2 mg/kg q12-24h. **Continuous IV:** 2 mg/kg/d.	⊕B ✿> R

PROSTAGLANDIN E₁ ANALOG

Drug	Forms	Dosing	
Misoprostol (Cytotec)	**Tab:** 100 mcg, 200 mcg	**NSAID Ulcer Prevention: Adults:** 200 mcg qid w/ food. May use 100 mcg dose if 200 mcg not tolerated.	⊕X ✿v Abortifacient.

NAME	FORM/STRENGTH	DOSAGE	COMMENTS
PROTON PUMP INHIBITORS AND COMBINATIONS			
Amoxicillin/Clarithromycin/ Lansoprazole (Prevpac)	**Cap:** (Amoxicillin) 500 mg, **Tab:** (Clarithromycin) 500 mg, **Cap,Delay:** (Lansoprazole) 30 mg	**DU/*H. pylori* Eradication for Risk Reduction of DU Recurrence: Adults:** 1 gm amoxicillin, 500 mg clarithromycin & 30 mg lansoprazole, all bid (am & pm) before meals x 10 or 14d. Swallow each pill whole.	⊞C ❄v H R
Esomeprazole Magnesium (Nexium)	**Cap,Delay:** 20 mg, 40 mg; **Susp,Delay:** 2.5 mg, 5 mg, 10 mg, 20 mg, 40 mg (granules/ pkt)	**Adults: Risk Reduction of NSAID-Associated GU:** 20 mg or 40 mg qd up to 6 mths. ***H. pylori* Triple Therapy:** 40 mg qd + amoxicillin 1000 mg bid + clarithromycin 500 mg bid, all for 10d.	⊞B ❄v H
Lansoprazole (Prevacid, Prevacid SoluTab)	**Cap,Delay:** 15 mg, 30 mg; **Tab,Delay,Dissolve:** (SoluTab) 15 mg, 30 mg	**Adults: DU Treatment:** 15 mg qd x 4 wks. **DU Maint:** 15 mg qd. **Benign GU:** 30 mg qd x up to 8 wks. **NSAID-Associated GU: Healing:** 30 mg qd x 8 wks. **Risk Reduction:** 15 mg qd x up to 12 wks.	⊞B ❄v H
Omeprazole (Prilosec)	**Cap,Delay:** 10 mg, 20 mg, 40 mg; **Sus,Delay:** 2.5 mg, 10 mg (granules/pkt)	**Adults: DU:** 20 mg qd x 4 wks; may require additional 4 wks. ***H. pylori* Eradication: Triple Therapy:** Omeprazole 20 mg + clarithromycin 500 mg + amoxicillin 1000 mg bid x 10d; if ulcer present at treatment initiation, give omeprazole 20 mg qd for an additional 18d. **Dual Therapy:** Omeprazole 40 mg qd + clarithromycin 500 mg tid x 14d; if ulcer present at treatment initiation, give omeprazole 20 mg qd for an additional 14d. **GU:** 40 mg qd x 4-8 wks.	⊞C ❄v H

Rabeprazole Sodium (Aciphex)	Tab,Delay: 20 mg	**Adults: DU Treatment:** 20 mg qd x up to 4 wks. Take after am meal. **_H. pylori_ Triple Therapy:** 20 mg + clarithromycin 500 mg + amoxicillin 1 gm, all bid w/ am & pm meals x 7d.	●B ❀v
Sodium Bicarbonate/ Omeprazole (Zegerid)	**Cap:** 1100-20 mg, 1100-40 mg; **Susp:** 1680-20 mg/pkt, 1680-40 mg/pkt	**Adults: Cap/Susp: DU:** 20 mg qd x 4-8 wks. **GU:** 40 mg qd x 4-8 wks. **Susp (1680-40 mg): Risk Reduction of Upper GI Bleeding in Critically Ill Patients: Initial:** 40 mg, followed by 40 mg 6-8h later. **Maint:** 40 mg qd x 14d. **Asian Population:** Consider dose reduction.	●C ❀v H

GERD

DOPAMINE ANTAGONISTS/PROKINETICS

Metoclopramide (Reglan)	(Generic) **Sol:** 5 mg/5 ml; (Reglan) **Tab:** 5 mg, 10 mg	**Adults:** 10-15 mg up to qid 30 min ac & qhs. **Max:** 12 wks of therapy. **Intermittent Symptoms:** Up to 20 mg single dose prior to provoking situation. If esophageal lesions are present, 15 mg qid. **Sensitive to Metoclopramide/Elderly:** 5 mg/dose.	●B ❀> May cause tardive dyskinesia. R
Metoclopramide HCl (Metozolv ODT)	Tab,Dissolve: 5 mg, 10 mg	**Adults:** 10-15 mg up to qid on empty stomach ≥30 min ac and qhs. **Max:** 12 wks of therapy. **Intermittent Symptoms:** ≤20 mg as single dose prior to the symptoms. If esophageal lesions are present, 15 mg qid.	●B ❀v May cause tardive dyskinesia. R

NAME	FORM/STRENGTH	DOSAGE	COMMENTS
H₂ ANTAGONISTS			
Cimetidine (Tagamet)	**Sol:** 300 mg/5 ml; **Tab:** 200 mg, 300 mg, 400 mg, 800 mg	**Adults & Peds:** ≥16 yo: 400 mg qid or 800 mg bid x 12 wks. **Max:** 12 wks.	▣B ❄v R
Famotidine (Pepcid)	**Inj:** (Generic) 20 mg/ 50 ml, 10 mg/ml; **Susp:** (Pepcid) 40 mg/5 ml; **Tab:** 20 mg, 40 mg	**Adults:** PO: 20 mg bid x up to 6 wks. **Peds: 1-16 yo: PO:** 0.5 mg/kg PO bid x. **Max:** 40 mg bid. IV: 0.25 mg/kg q12h. **Max:** 40 mg/d. **3 mths-1 yo:** PO: 0.5 mg/kg bid x up to 8 wks. **<3 mths:** PO: 0.5 mg/kg qd x up to 8 wks. **Erosive Esophagitis: Adults:** PO: 20-40 mg bid x up to 12 wks.	▣B ❄v R
Nizatidine (Axid)	**Cap:** 150 mg, 300 mg; **Sol:** 15 mg/ml	**Adults:** 150 mg bid x up to 12 wks. **Peds: ≥12 yo: Erosive Esophagitis/GERD: Sol:** 150 mg bid x up to 8 wks. **Max:** 300 mg/d.	▣B ❄v R
Ranitidine HCl (Zantac)	**Inj:** 1 mg/ml, 25 mg/ml; **Syr:** 15 mg/ml; **Tab:** 150 mg, 300 mg; **Tab,Eff:** 25 mg	**Adults:** PO: Symptomatic GERD: 150 mg bid. **Erosive Esophagitis:** 150 mg qid. **Maint:** 150 mg bid. IV/IM: 50 mg q6-8h. **Continuous IV:** 6.25 mg/h. **Max:** 400 mg/d. **Peds: 1 mth-16 yo: Symptomatic GERD/Erosive Esophagitis:** 2.5-5 mg/kg PO bid. **IV:** 2-4 mg/kg/d divided and given q6-8h. **Max:** 50 mg q6-8h. **<1 mth:** IV Bolus: 2 mg/kg q12-24h. **Continuous IV:** 2 mg/kg/d.	▣B ❄> R

PROTON PUMP INHIBITORS AND COMBINATIONS

Dexlansoprazole (Dexilant)	**Cap, Delay:** 30 mg, 60 mg	**Adults: Healing of Erosive Esophagitis:** 60 mg qd x up to 8 wks. **Maint:** 30 mg qd x up to 6 mths. **Symptomatic Non-Erosive GERD:** 30 mg qd x 4 wks.	⊕B ❀v H
Esomeprazole Magnesium (Nexium)	**Cap, Delay:** 20 mg, 40 mg; **Susp, Delay:** 2.5 mg, 5 mg, 10 mg, 20 mg, 40 mg (granules/pkt)	**Adults: Symptomatic GERD:** 20 mg qd x 4 wks. May repeat x 4 wks if needed. **Erosive Esophagitis: Healing:** 20 mg or 40 mg qd x 4-8 wks. May repeat x 4-8 wks if needed. **Maint:** 20 mg qd x up to 6 mths. **Peds: Symptomatic GERD: 12-17 yo:** 20 mg or 40 mg qd x up to 8 wks. **1-11 yo:** 10 mg qd x up to 8 wks. **Max:** 1 mg/kg/d. **Erosive Esophagitis: 1-11 yo: <20 kg:** 10 mg qd x 8 wks. **≥20 kg:** 10 mg or 20 mg qd x 8 wks. **Max:** 1 mg/kg/d. **Erosive Esophagitis Due to Acid-Mediated GERD: 1 mth-<1 yo: 3-5 kg:** 2.5 mg qd x up to 6 wks. **>5-7.5 kg:** 5 mg qd x up to 6 wks. **>7.5-12 kg:** 10 mg qd x up to 6 wks. **Max:** 1.33 mg/kg/d.	⊕B ❀v H
Esomeprazole Sodium (Nexium IV)	**Inj:** 20 mg, 40 mg	**Adults:** 20 or 40 mg IV qd for up to 10d. **Peds: 1-17 yo: ≥55 kg:** 20 mg IV qd. **<55 kg:** 10 mg IV qd. **1 mth-<1 yo:** 0.5 mg/kg IV qd. D/C as soon as patient can resume PO therapy.	⊕B ❀v H

NAME	FORM/STRENGTH	DOSAGE	COMMENTS
Lansoprazole (Prevacid, Prevacid SoluTab)	**Cap,Delay:** 15 mg, 30 mg; **Tab,Delay,Dissolve:** (SoluTab) 15 mg, 30 mg	**Adults: Symptomatic GERD:** 15 mg qd x up to 8 wks. **Erosive Esophagitis (EE):** 30 mg qd x up to 8 wks. May repeat x 8 wks if needed. If recurrence, may consider additional 8 wks. **Maint:** 15 mg qd. **Peds: 12-17 yo: Symptomatic GERD: Nonerosive GERD:** 15 mg qd x up to 8 wks. **EE:** 30 mg qd x up to 8 wks. **1-11 yo: Symptomatic GERD/EE: ≤30 kg:** 15 mg qd x up to 12 wks; may increase up to 30 mg bid after ≥2 wks if symptomatic. **>30 kg:** 30 mg qd x up to 12 wks; may increase up to 30 mg bid after ≥2 wks if symptomatic.	●B ❄v H
Omeprazole (Prilosec)	**Cap,Delay:** 10 mg, 20 mg, 40 mg; **Sus,Delay:** 2.5 mg, 10 mg (granules/pkt)	**Adults: Symptomatic GERD:** 20 mg qd x up to 4 wks. **Erosive Esophagitis (EE):** 20 mg qd x 4-8 wks. **Maint:** 20 mg qd x up to 12 mths. **Peds: 1-16 yo: GERD/EE: ≥20 kg:** 20 mg qd. **10-<20 kg:** 10 mg qd. **5-<10 kg:** 5 mg qd.	●C ❄v H
Pantoprazole Sodium (Protonix, Protonix IV)	**Inj:** 40 mg; **Susp,Delay:** 40 mg (granules/pkt); **Tab,Delay:** 20 mg, 40 mg	**Adults: Erosive Esophagitis (EE): PO:** 40 mg qd x up to 8 wks. May repeat x 8 wks if needed. **Maint:** 40 mg qd. **GERD: IV:** 40 mg qd x 7-10d. Switch to PO when possible. **Peds: ≥5 yo: EE: PO: ≥15 kg-<40 kg:** 20 mg qd x up to 8 wks. **≥40 kg:** 40 mg qd x up to 8 wks.	●B ❄v
Rabeprazole Sodium (Aciphex)	**Tab,Delay:** 20 mg	**Adults: Erosive/Ulcerative GERD: Healing:** 20 mg qd x 4-8 wks. May repeat x 8 wks if needed. **Maint:** 20 mg qd. **Symptomatic GERD:** 20 mg qd x 4 wks. May repeat if needed. **Peds: ≥12 yo: Symptomatic GERD:** 20 mg qd x up to 8 wks.	●B ❄v

| Sodium Bicarbonate/ Omeprazole (Zegerid) | Cap: 1100-20 mg, 1100-40 mg; Susp: 1680-20 mg/pkt, 1680-40 mg/pkt | **Adults: Cap/Susp: Symptomatic GERD:** 20 mg qd x up to 4 wks. **Erosive Esophagitis: Healing:** 20 mg qd x 4-8 wks. May give up to additional 4 wks if no response after 8 wks or may consider 4-8 wk courses if there is recurrence. **Maint:** 20 mg qd. **Asian Population:** Consider dose reduction. | ●C ✿v H |

Laxatives
BOWEL EVACUANTS

| Bisacodyl/ Polyethylene Glycol 3350/ Sodium Chloride/ Sodium Bicarbonate/ Potassium Chloride (HalfLytely) | **Kit: Tab,Delay:** (Bisacodyl) 5 mg; **Pow for Sol:** (Polyethylene Glycol 3350-Potassium Chloride-Sodium Bicarbonate-Sodium Chloride) 210-0.74-2.86-5.6 gm/2 L | **Adults:** Consume only clear liquids on day of preparation. Take 1 bisacodyl tab w/ water. Do not crush or chew tab. After 1st bowel movement (or max of 6h) drink 2000 ml sol at a rate of 8 oz q10min. Drink all sol. Drink each portion at longer intervals or d/c temporarily if abdominal distension/discomfort occurs until symptoms improve. | ●C ✿> |
| Dibasic Sodium Phosphate/ Monobasic Sodium Phosphate (Visicol) | **Tab:** 1.102-0.398 gm | **Adults: Colonoscopy:** pm before exam, 3 tabs w/ 8 oz clear liq q15min for total of 20 tabs (last dose is 2 tabs). Repeat day of exam 3-5h before procedure. May retreat after 7d. | ●C ✿> W [109] |

NAME	FORM/STRENGTH	DOSAGE	COMMENTS
Monobasic Sodium Phosphate Monohydrate/ Dibasic Sodium Phosphate (Osmoprep)	**Tab:** (Sodium Phosphate Monobasic Monohydrate-Sodium Phosphate Dibasic Anhydrous) 1.102-0.398 gm	**Adults: ≥18 yo: Evening Before Colonoscopy Procedure:** 4 tabs w/ 8 oz of clear liq q15min for total of 20 tabs. **Day of Colonoscopy Procedure:** Take 4 tabs w/ 8 oz of clear liq q15min for total of 12 tabs starting 3-5h before procedure. Drink only clear liq. Adequately hydrate before, during, & after use. Do not use w/in 7d of previous administration. Do not take any additional enema or laxative.	▣C ❊> W [103]
Polyethylene Glycol 3350/ Potassium Chloride/ Sodium Sulfate/ Sodium Chloride/ Sodium Bicarbonate (GoLYTELY)	**Sol:** 236-2.97-22.74-5.86-6.74 gm/4 L; 227.1-2.82-21.5-5.53-6.36 gm/gallon	**Adults: PO:** 240 ml q10min until fecal discharge is clear or 4 L consumed. **NG-Tube:** 20-30 ml/min (1.2-1.8 L/h).	▣C ❊>
Polyethylene Glycol 3350/ Sodium Chloride/ Sodium Bicarbonate/ Potassium Chloride (NuLYTELY, Trilyte)	**Pow for Sol:** 420-1.48-5.72-11.2 gm/4 L	**Adults: GI Exam Prep: PO:** 240 ml q10min until fecal discharge is clear or 4 L consumed. **NG-Tube:** 20-30 ml/min (1.2-1.8 L/h). **Peds: ≥6 mths: PO/NG-Tube:** 25 ml/kg/h until fecal discharge is clear.	▣C ❊>
Polyethylene Glycol 3350/ Sodium Sulfate/ Ascorbic Acid/ Potassium Chloride/ Sodium Ascorbate/ Sodium Chloride (MoviPrep)	**Pow for Sol:** 100-7.5-4.7-1.015-5.9-2.691 gm/L	**Adults: ≥18 yo:** Split-Dose Regimen: 1 L over 1h (8 oz q15min) followed by 0.5 L of clear liq the pm prior to colonoscopy, then 1 L over 1h followed by 0.5 L of clear liq in the am, at least 1h prior to colonoscopy. **PM-Only Regimen:** Around 6 pm, take 1 L over 1h (8 oz q15min), after 1.5h, take 1 L over 1h. Additionally, take 1 L of clear liq during the pm prior to colonoscopy.	▣C ❊>

| Sodium Sulfate Sulfate/ Potassium Sulfate/ Magnesium Sulfate (Suprep) | Sol: 17.5 gm-3.13 gm-1.6 gm | Adults: Day prior to colonoscopy: May consume light breakfast or have only clear liq. Early in evening prior to colonoscopy, dilute one bottle w/ 16 oz of water & drink entire amt. Drink additional 32 oz of water over the next hr. Day of Colonoscopy: Have only clear liq until after colonoscopy. Morning of Colonoscopy (10-12h after pm dose): Repeat steps taken on day prior w/ second bottle. Complete all Suprep Bowel Prep Kit and required water at least 1h prior to colonoscopy. | ◐C ❄> |

OSMOTIC AGENTS

| Lactulose (Constilac, Constulose, Enulose, Generlac, Lactulose) | Sol: 10 gm/15 ml | Adults: 15-30 ml qd. Max: 60 ml/d. | ◐B ❄> |
| Polyethylene Glycol 3350 (MiraLax) | Pow: 17 gm/dose | Adults & Peds: ≥17 yo: Dissolve 17 gm in 4-8 oz of beverage & drink qd. Use no more than 7d. | ◐N ❄> |

STOOL SOFTENERS

| Docusate Sodium (Colace) | Cap: 50 mg, 100 mg; Syr: 60 mg/15 ml | Adults & Peds: ≥12 yo: Cap: (50 mg) 1-6 cap/d. (100 mg) 1-3 cap/d. Syr: 1-6 tbsp/d or ud. 2-<12 yo: Cap: (50 mg) 1-3 cap/d. (100 mg) 1 cap/d. Syr: 1-2.5 tbsp/d or ud. Give syr in 6-8 oz of milk or fruit juice. Doses may be taken qd or in divided doses. | ◐N ❄> |

NAME	FORM/STRENGTH	DOSAGE	COMMENTS
Mineral Oil (Fleet Mineral Oil Enema)	**Enema:** (Babylax) 2.3 gm, (Liquid Glycerin) 5.6 gm; **Sup:** 1 gm, 2 gm, 3 gm	**Adults & Peds:** ≥6 yo: 1 enema (5.6 gm) or 1 sup (2 gm or 3 gm) PR. **2-5 yo:** 1 enema (2.3 gm) or 1 sup (1 gm) PR.	⊕N ✿>

Ulcerative Colitis

ANTI-INFLAMMATORY/IMMUNOMODULATORY AGENT

Sulfasalazine (Azulfidine)	**Tab:** 500 mg	**Adults:** Individualize dose. **Initial:** 3-4 gm/d in evenly divided doses w/ intervals not >8h. May initiate at 1-2 gm/d to reduce GI intolerance. **Maint:** 2 gm/d. **Peds:** ≥6 yo: **Initial:** 40-60 mg/kg/24h divided into 3-6 doses. **Maint:** 30 mg/kg/24h divided into 4 doses. **Desensitization:** Refer to PI.	⊕B ✿>

SALICYLATES

Mesalamine (Asacol, Asacol HD)	**Tab, Delay:** (Asacol) 400 mg, (Asacol HD) 800 mg	**Adults: Asacol: Mildly-Moderately Active Ulcerative Colitis:** 800 mg tid x 6 wks. **Remission Maint:** 1.6 gm/d in divided doses. **Asacol HD: Moderately Active Ulcerative Colitis:** 1600 mg tid x 6 wks.	⊕C ✿> H R
Mesalamine (Lialda)	**Tab, Delay:** 1.2 gm	**Adults: Remission Induction, Active Mild-to-Moderate:** 2-4 tabs qd w/ meals. **Remission Maint:** 2 tabs qd w/ meals.	⊕B ✿> H R

| Mesalamine (Pentasa) | Cap,ER: 250 mg, 500 mg | **Mild-to-Moderately Active Ulcerative Colitis: Adults:** 1 gm qid x up to 8 wks. | ⊕B ❄v> |

Zollinger-Ellison Agents
H₂ ANTAGONISTS

Cimetidine (Tagamet)	**Sol:** 300 mg/5 ml; **Tab:** 200 mg, 300 mg, 400 mg, 800 mg	**Adults & Peds: ≥16 yo:** 300 mg qid. **Max:** 2400 mg/d.	⊕B ❄v R
Famotidine (Pepcid)	**Inj:** (Generic) 20 mg/ 50 ml, 10 mg/ml; **Susp:** (Pepcid) 40 mg/5 ml; **Tab:** 20 mg, 40 mg	**Adults: PO: Initial:** 20 mg q6h, then adjust as needed. **Max:** 160 mg q6h. IV: 20 mg q12h, then adjust as needed. Switch to PO when possible.	⊕B ❄v R
Ranitidine HCl (Zantac)	**Inj:** 1 mg/ml, 25 mg/ml; **Syr:** 15 mg/ml; **Tab:** 150 mg, 300 mg; **Tab,Eff:** 25 mg	**Adults: PO: Initial:** 150 mg bid, then adjust as needed. May give up to 6 gm/d w/ severe disease. **IM/IV (Intermittent):** 50 mg q6-8h. **IV (Continuous):** 1 mg/kg/h IV. **Titrate:** May increase after 4h by 0.5 mg/kg/h increments. **Max:** 2.5 mg/kg/h or 220 mg/h.	⊕B ❄> R

NAME	FORM/STRENGTH	DOSAGE	COMMENTS
PROTON PUMP INHIBITORS AND COMBINATIONS			
Esomeprazole Magnesium (Nexium)	**Cap,Delay:** 20 mg, 40 mg; **Susp,Delay:** 2.5 mg, 5 mg, 10 mg, 20 mg, 40 mg (granules/pkt)	**Adults: Initial:** 40 mg bid, then adjust as needed. **Max:** 240 mg/d.	⊞B ❄v H
Lansoprazole (Prevacid, Prevacid SoluTab)	**Cap,Delay:** 15 mg, 30 mg; **Tab,Delay,Dissolve:** (SoluTab) 15 mg, 30 mg.	**Adults: Initial:** 60 mg qd. **Titrate:** Individualize dose. **Max:** 90 mg bid. Divide dose if >120 mg/d.	⊞B ❄v H
Omeprazole (Prilosec)	**Cap,Delay:** 10 mg, 20 mg, 40 mg; **Sus,Delay:** 2.5 mg, 10 mg (granules/pkt)	**Adults: Initial:** 60 mg qd. **Titrate:** Adjust if needed. Divide dose if >80 mg/d. **Max:** 120 mg tid.	⊞C ❄v H
Pantoprazole Sodium (Protonix, Protonix IV)	**Inj:** 40 mg; **Susp,Delay:** 40 mg (granules/pkt); **Tab,Delay:** 20 mg, 40 mg	**Adults: PO: Initial:** 40 mg bid. **Titrate:** Individualize dose. **Max:** 240 mg/d. **IV: Usual:** 80 mg q12h. **Titrate:** Adjust frequency based on acid output. Switch to PO when possible. **Max:** 240 mg/d or 6d of treatment.	⊞B ❄v
Rabeprazole Sodium (Aciphex)	**Tab,Delay:** 20 mg	**Adults: Initial:** 60 mg bid. **Titrate:** Individualize dose. **Max:** 100 mg qd or 60 mg bid. Some have been treated up to 1 yr.	⊞B ❄v

Miscellaneous

Adalimumab (Humira)	**Inj:** 20 mg/0.4 ml, 40 mg/0.8 ml	**Crohn's Disease: Adults: Initial:** 160 mg SC (may be given as 4 inj on Day 1 or 2 inj/d x 2 consecutive days), then 80 mg in 2 wks (Day 15). **Maint:** 40 mg SC qow starting Wk 4 (Day 29).	B v W [86]
Alosetron HCl (Lotronex)	**Tab:** 0.5 mg, 1 mg	**Diarrhea-Predominant Irritable Bowel Syndrome (Women): Adults: Initial:** 1 mg qd x 4 wks. **Titrate:** May increase to 1 mg bid. D/C after 4 wks if symptoms uncontrolled on 1 mg bid.	B > W [43]
Certolizumab Pegol (Cimzia)	**Inj:** 200 mg/ml	**Adults: Crohn's Disease: Initial:** 400 mg SC, and at Wks 2 & 4. **Maint:** 400 mg SC q4wks.	B v W [86]
Infliximab (Remicade)	**Inj:** 100 mg	**Adults: Crohn's Disease: Induction:** 5 mg/kg IV at 0, 2, & 6 wks. **Maint:** 5 mg/kg q8wks. For patients who respond then lose response, may increase to 10 mg/kg. Consider d/c if no response by Wk 14. **Peds: ≥6 yo: Crohn's Disease: Induction:** 5 mg/kg IV at 0, 2 & 6 wks. **Maint:** 5 mg/kg q8wks.	B v Hepatosplenic T-cell lymphoma & other malignancies reported. W [86]
Lubiprostone (Amitiza)	**Cap:** 8 mcg, 24 mcg	**Adults: Chronic Idiopathic Constipation:** 24 mcg bid w/ food & water. **Women: ≥18 yo: Irritable Bowel Syndrome w/ Constipation:** 8 mcg bid w/ food & water.	C v H

NAME	FORM/STRENGTH	DOSAGE	COMMENTS
Methylnaltrexone Bromide (Relistor)	**Inj:** 12 mg/0.6 ml, 8 mg/ 0.4 ml	**Opioid-Induced Constipation: Adults:** Inject SC in upper arm, abdomen, or thigh. **Usual:** 1 dose qod prn. **Max:** 1 dose/24h. **Patient Wt:** 38-<62 kg (84-<136 lbs): 8 mg. 62-114 kg (136-251 lbs): 12 mg. **Patients Outside These Ranges:** 0.15 mg/kg. To calculate inj volume for these patients, multiply wt in lbs by 0.0034 or wt in kg by 0.0075 & round volume up to nearest 0.1 ml.	●B ✿> R
Metoclopramide HCl (Metozolv ODT)	**Tab,Dissolve:** 5 mg, 10 mg	**Diabetic Gastroparesis: Adults:** 10 mg up to qid on empty stomach ≥30 min ac and qhs. **Max:** 12 wks of therapy. If severe, begin with inj ≤10d.	●B ✿v May cause tardive dyskinesia. R
Natalizumab (Tysabri)	**Inj:** 300 mg/15 ml	**Crohn's Disease: Adults: Usual:** 300 mg IV infusion over 1h q4wks. D/C if benefit not seen by 12 wks, if cannot taper off corticosteroids w/in 6 mths, or if require additional steroid use that exceeds 3 mths w/in calendar yr.	●C ✿> W [85]
Pancrelipase (Zenpep)	**Cap,Delay:** (Amylase-Lipase-Protease) (Zenpep 3) 16,000 U-3000 U-10,000 U; (Zenpep 5) 27,000 U-5000 U-17,000 U; (Zenpep 10) 55,000 U-10,000 U-34,000 U; (Zenpep 15) 82,000	**Exocrine Pancreatic Insufficiency: Adults & Peds:** Individualize dose based on clinical symptoms, degree of steatorrhea & fat content of diet. **≥4 yo: Initial:** 500 lipase U/kg/meal. **Max:** 2500 lipase U/kg/meal (or ≤10,000 lipase U/kg/d) or <4000 lipase U/gm fat ingested/d. **12 mths-4 yo: Initial:** 1000 lipase U/kg/meal. **Max:** 2500 lipase U/kg/ meal. **≤12 mths:** 3000 lipase U/120 ml of formula or breastfeeding.	●C ✿> R

	U-15,000 U-51,000 U; (Zenpep 20) 109,000 U-20,000 U-68,000 U		
Rifaximin (Xifaxan)	**Tab:** 200 mg, 550 mg	**Hepatic Encephalopathy: Adults: ≥18 yo:** 550 mg bid.	⊞C ✿v

GYNECOLOGY

Anti-Infective Agents
ANTIBACTERIALS

Clindamycin Phosphate (Clindesse)	**Cre:** 2%	**Bacterial Vaginosis: Adults & Peds: Postmenarchal:** 1 applicatorful intravaginally any time of day.	⊞B ✿v
Metronidazole (Flagyl)	**Cap:** 375 mg; **Tab:** 250 mg, 500 mg	**Adults: Trichomoniasis:** 375 mg (cap) bid or 250 mg (tab) tid x 7d. **Alternate Regimen:** If nonpregnant, 2 gm (tab) as single or 2 divided doses in 1d.	⊞B ✿v CI in 1st trimester in trichomoniasis. **H W** [83]
Metronidazole (Flagyl ER)	**Tab,ER:** 750 mg	**Bacterial Vaginosis: Adults:** 750 mg qd x 7d. Take ≥1h ac or ≥2h pc.	⊞B ✿v CI in 1st trimester. **H W** [83]
Metronidazole (MetroGel-Vaginal)	**Gel:** 0.75%	**Bacterial Vaginosis: Adults:** Insert 1 applicatorful intravaginally qd-bid x 5d. For qd dosing, give hs.	⊞B ✿v

NAME	FORM/STRENGTH	DOSAGE	COMMENTS
Metronidazole (Vandazole)	Gel: 0.75%	**Bacterial Vaginosis: Adults & Peds: Postmenarchal:** Insert 1 applicatorful intravaginally qhs x 5d.	◉B ✿v W [83]
ANTIFUNGALS			
Fluconazole (Diflucan)	Tab: 150 mg	**Vaginal Candidiasis: Adults:** 150 mg single dose.	◉C ✿v
Terconazole (Terazol 3)	Cre: (Terazol 7) 0.4%, (Terazol 3) 0.8%; Sup: (Terazol 3) 80 mg	**Vulvovaginal Candidiasis: Adults:** 1 applicatorful of 0.8% or 80 mg sup intravaginally qhs x 3d.	◉C ✿>
QUINOLONES			
Ciprofloxacin HCl (Cipro Oral)	Susp: 250 mg/5 ml, 500 mg/5 ml; Tab: 250 mg, 500 mg	**Uncomplicated Urethral/Cervical Gonococcal Infections: Adults:** 250 mg PO single dose.	◉C ✿v R W [98]
Norfloxacin (Noroxin)	Tab: 400 mg	**Uncomplicated Gonorrhea: Adults:** 800 mg single dose.	◉C ✿v R W [98]
Ofloxacin	Tab: 200 mg, 300 mg, 400 mg	**Gonorrhea: Adults: ≥18 yo:** 400 mg single dose.	◉C ✿v H R W [98]

Contraceptives
PROGESTOGEN

Levonorgestrel (Mirena)	IUD: 52 mg	**Adults: Contraception/Heavy Menstrual Bleeding:** Insert into uterine cavity initially w/in 7d of menses onset or immediately after 1st trimester abortion. May replace any time in the cycle. Delay insertion until ≥6 wks postpartum or until uterine involution is complete. Re-examine/evaluate 4-12 wks after insertion.	ⓒN ❊v CI in pregnancy.
Medroxyprogesterone Acetate (Depo-Provera Contraceptive)	Inj: 150 mg/ml	**Adults & Peds: Postmenarchal Adolescents:** 150 mg IM q3mths. Give 1st inj during 1st 5d of menses; w/in 1st 5d postpartum if not nursing; or at 6th postpartum wk if nursing. If >13 wks between inj, determine that patient is not pregnant before administration.	ⓒN ❊>CI in pregnancy.

Dysmenorrhea
NSAIDs

Celecoxib (Celebrex)	Cap: 50 mg, 100 mg, 200 mg, 400 mg	**Adults: Day 1:** 400 mg, then 200 mg if needed. **Maint:** 200 mg bid prn. **Poor Metabolizers of CYP2C9 Substrates:** Half lowest recommended dose.	ⓒC ⓒD (≥30 wks gestation) ❊v H W [66, 67]
Naproxen (Anaprox, Anaprox DS, EC-Naprosyn, Naprosyn)	Tab: 275 mg, 550 mg	**Adults: Initial:** Anaprox/Anaprox DS: 550 mg, then 550 mg q12h or 275 mg q6-8h prn. **Max:** 1375 mg/d initially, then 1100 mg/d thereafter.	ⓒC ❊v H R W [66, 67]

NAME	FORM/STRENGTH	DOSAGE	COMMENTS

Hormone Therapy
ESTROGEN/PROGESTIN COMBINATION

NAME	FORM/STRENGTH	DOSAGE	COMMENTS
Drospirenone/Estradiol (Angeliq)	**Tab:** 0.25-0.5 mg; 0.5-1 mg	**Vasomotor Symptoms, Vulvar/Vaginal Atrophy: Adults:** 1 tab qd. Reevaluate periodically.	●N ✿> **H R W** [4, 28]
Estradiol/Levonorgestrel (Climara Pro)	**Patch:** 0.045-0.015 mg/d	**Adults: Vasomotor Symptoms:** Apply 1 patch qwk to lower abdomen (avoid breasts/waistline). Rotate application site; allow 1 wk between applications to same site.	●N ✿> CI in pregnancy. **H W** [4, 28]
Estradiol/Norgestimate (Prefest)	**Tab:** 1 mg-none, 1 mg-0.09 mg	**Vasomotor Symptoms, Vulvar/Vaginal Atrophy: Adults: Intact Uterus:** 1 mg estradiol x 3d alternating w/ 1-0.09 mg x 3d on continuous schedule.	●X ✿v **W** [28]
Medroxyprogesterone Acetate/Conjugated Estrogens (Premphase, Prempro)	**Tab:** (Premphase) 0.625 mg (conjugated estrogens), 5-0.625 mg; (Prempro) 1.5-0.3 mg, 1.5-0.45 mg, 2.5-0.625 mg, 5-0.625 mg	**Adults: Vasomotor Symptoms, Vulvar/Vaginal Atrophy: Premphase:** 0.625 mg tab qd on Days 1-14 & 5-0.625 mg tab qd on Days 15-28. **Prempro:** 1 tab qd. Reevaluate treatment need periodically.	●N ✿v CI in pregnancy. **H W** [4, 28]
Norethindrone Acetate/Estradiol (Activella)	**Tab:** 0.5-1 mg, 0.1-0.5 mg	**Vulval/Vaginal Atrophy, Vasomotor Symptoms: Adults: Intact Uterus:** 1 tab qd. Reevaluate treatment need periodically (eg, 3-6 mth intervals).	●N ✿>CI in pregnancy. **W** [28]
Norethindrone Acetate/Ethinyl Estradiol (femhrt)	**Tab:** 0.5 mg-2.5 mcg, 1 mg-5 mcg	**Vasomotor Symptoms: Adults:** 1 tab qd.	●N ✿> **H W** [4, 28]

ESTROGENS

Conjugated Estrogens (Cenestin)	**Tab:** 0.3 mg, 0.45 mg, 0.625 mg, 0.9 mg, 1.25 mg	**Adults: Vasomotor Symptoms: Initial:** 0.45 mg qd. Adjust dose based on response. **Vulvar/Vaginal Atrophy:** 0.3 mg qd.	⊕X ❀> W [4, 28]
Conjugated Estrogens (Enjuvia)	**Tab:** 0.3 mg, 0.45 mg, 0.625 mg, 0.9 mg, 1.25 mg	**Vasomotor Symptoms/Vulvar & Vaginal Atrophy/Vaginal Dryness & Pain w/ Intercourse: Adults: Initial:** 0.3 mg qd. Adjust dose based on response.	⊕N ❀>CI in pregnancy. **W** [4, 28]
Conjugated Estrogens (Premarin Tablets)	**Tab:** 0.3 mg, 0.45 mg, 0.625 mg, 0.9 mg, 1.25 mg	**Adults:** Individualize dose. **Vasomotor Symptoms/Vulvar & Vaginal Atrophy: Initial:** 0.3 mg qd continuous or cyclically (25d on, 5d off). **Female Hypogonadism:** 0.3 or 0.625 mg qd cyclically (3 wks on, 1 wk off). **Female Castration/ Primary Ovarian Failure:** 1.25 mg qd cyclically.	⊕N ❀v CI in pregnancy **W** [4, 28]
Conjugated Estrogens (Premarin Vaginal)	**Cre:** 0.625 mg/gm	**Adults: Atrophic Vaginitis/Kraurosis Vulvae: Initial:** 0.5 gm intravaginally qd cyclically (3 wks on, 1 wk off). **Titrate:** 0.5-2 gm based on individual response. **Moderate to Severe Dyspareunia:** 0.5 gm intravaginally biw (eg, Mon & Thurs) continuous regimen or cyclically (3 wks on, 1 wk off).	⊕N ❀v **W** [4, 28]
Estradiol Acetate (Femtrace)	**Tab:** 0.45 mg, 0.9 mg, 1.8 mg	**Vasomotor Symptoms: Adults:** 1 tab qd. Use lowest effective dose. Reevaluate need periodically.	⊕N ❀> CI in pregnancy. **H W** [4, 28]

NAME	FORM/STRENGTH	DOSAGE	COMMENTS
Estradiol (Climara)	**Patch:** 0.025 mg/d, 0.0375 mg/d, 0.05 mg/d, 0.06 mg/d, 0.075 mg/d, 0.1 mg/d	**Vasomotor Symptoms, Vulval/Vaginal Atrophy, Hypoestrogenism: Adults: Initial:** Apply 0.025 mg/d qwk. **Titrate:** Adjust dose prn. Wait 1 wk after withdrawal of PO therapy before initiating patch.	⊕X ❄> W [4, 28]
Estradiol (Divigel)	**Gel:** 0.1%	**Adults: Initial:** 0.25 gm gd applied on skin of right or left upper thigh. Adjust dose based on response.	⊕N ❄> W [4, 28]
Estradiol (Evamist)	**Spr:** 1.53 mg/spr	**Adults: Initial:** 1 spr qd on inner surface of forearm. Adjust dose based on response. **Usual:** 1-3 spr qam.	⊕N ❄>CI in pregnancy. W [4, 28]

Premenstrual Dysphoric Disorder

SSRIs & COMBINATIONS

NAME	FORM/STRENGTH	DOSAGE	COMMENTS
Fluoxetine (Sarafem)	**Cap:** 10 mg, 20 mg; **Tab:** 10 mg, 15 mg, 20 mg	**Adults: Continuous: Initial:** 20 mg qd. **Intermittent: Initial:** 20 mg qd; start 14d before menses onset through 1st full day of menses. At 20 mg/d, efficacy has been shown for up to 6 mths (continuous) and for up to 3 mths (intermittent). **Max:** 80 mg/d.	⊕C ❄v H W [29]
Paroxetine HCl (Paxil CR)	**Tab,CR:** 12.5 mg, 25 mg, 37.5 mg	**Adults: Initial:** 12.5 mg qam throughout menstrual cycle or limited to luteal phase. 25 mg/d also shown to be effective. **Titrate:** Changes should occur at intervals of ≥1 wk.	⊕D ❄> H R W [29]

| Sertraline HCl (Zoloft) | **Sol:** 20 mg/ml; **Tab:** 25 mg, 50 mg, 100 mg | **Adults: Initial:** 50 mg qd continuous or limited to luteal phase. **Titrate:** Increase by 50 mg/cycle up to 150 mg/d for continuous dosing or 100 mg/d for luteal phase dosing. If 100 mg/d is established for luteal phase dosing, then titrate by 50 mg/d x 3d at beginning of each luteal phase dosing period. | ⊛C
⊛> H W [29] |

Miscellaneous

| Hydroxyprogesterone Caproate (Makena) | **Inj:** 250 mg/ml | **Prevention of Preterm Birth: Adults & Peds: ≥16 yo:** 250 mg IM in upper outer quadrant of gluteus maximus q7d. Begin between 16 wks, 0d & 20 wks, 6d of gestation. Continue once wkly until wk 37 (through 36 wks, 6d) of gestation or delivery, whichever is 1st. | ⊛B
⊛v |
| Tranexamic Acid (Lysteda) | **Tab:** 650 mg | **Cyclic Heavy Menstrual Bleeding: Adults:** 2 tabs tid x ≤5d. Do not chew or break; swallow tab whole. | ⊛B
⊛> CI w/ active/ history of thromboembolic disease. **R** |

NAME	FORM/STRENGTH	DOSAGE	COMMENTS

HEMATOLOGY/IMMUNOLOGY

Anemia
IRON/VITAMINS

NAME	FORM/STRENGTH	DOSAGE	COMMENTS
Folic Acid	**Inj:** 5 mg/ml; **Tab:** 0.4 mg, 0.8 mg, 1 mg	**Adults & Peds:** Up to 1 mg/d. **Maint:** 0.1-0.8 mg qd.	●A ❀^
Iron Carbonyl (Feosol)	**Tab:** 200 mg (65 mg iron)	**Adults & Peds:** ≥12 yo: 1 tab qd w/ food.	●N ❀> W[22]
Iron Carbonyl (Feosol)	**Tab:** 50 mg (45 mg iron)	**Adults & Peds:** ≥12 yo: 1 tab qd w/ food.	●N ❀> W[22]
Iron Dextran (INFeD)	**Inj:** 50 mg/ml	**Iron-Deficiency Anemia: Adults & Peds:** ≥4 mths & >15 kg: Dose (ml) = 0.0442 (desired Hgb-observed Hgb) x LBW + (0.26 x LBW); LBW = lean body wt (kg). **Peds: 5-15 kg:** Use calculation above w/ wt in place of LBW.	●C ❀> W[33]
Iron Sucrose (Venofer)	**Sol:** 20 mg/ml	**Adults:** Usual Total Treatment Course: 1000 mg. May repeat therapy if iron deficiency reoccurs. **Hemodialysis-Dependent Chronic Kidney Disease:** 100 mg undiluted as slow IV inj over 2-5 min or 100 mg diluted in a max of 100 ml of 0.9% NaCl as infusion over a period of at least 15 min per consecutive hemodialysis session (administer early during dialysis). **Non-Dialysis-Dependent Chronic Kidney Disease:** 200 mg undiluted as slow IV inj over 2-5 min on 5 different occasions over a 14d period.	●B ❀>

		Receiving Peritoneal Dialysis: Administer in 3 divided doses and by slow IV infusion, w/in 28d. 2 infusions each of 300 mg over 1.5h 14d apart, then one 400 mg infusion over 2.5h 14d later (should be diluted in a max of 250 ml of 0.9% NaCl).	
Sodium Ferric Gluconate Complex (Ferrlecit)	Inj: 62.5 mg elemental iron/5 ml	Iron-Deficiency Anemia in Chronic Kidney Disease on Dialysis: Adults: 10 ml (125 mg) as IV infusion (diluted) or as slow IV inj (undiluted); see PI. Cumulative Dose: 1000 mg elemental iron over 8 dialysis sessions. Peds: ≥6 yo: 0.12 ml/kg (1.5 mg/kg) as IV infusion over 1h/ dialysis session. Max: 125 mg/dose.	⊕B ❀>

Hematopoietic Agents

| Darbepoetin Alfa (Aranesp) | Inj: (Syr) 25 mcg/ 0.42 ml, 40 mcg/0.4 ml, 60 mcg/0.3 ml, 100 mcg/ 0.5 ml, 150 mcg/0.3 ml, 200 mcg/0.4 ml, 300 mcg/0.6 ml, 500 mcg/ml; (Single-Dose Vial) 25 mcg/ml, 40 mg/ml, 60 mcg/ml, 100 mcg/ml, | CKD: Adults: On Dialysis: Initial: 0.45 mcg/kg IV/SC wkly or 0.75 mcg/kg IV/SC q2wks. Not on Dialysis: Initial: 0.45 mcg/kg IV/SC q4wks. Titrate: Adjust dose based on Hgb levels; see PI. Adults & Peds: >1 yo: Conversion from Epoetin Alfa: See PI. Malignancy: Adults: Initial: 2.25 mcg/kg SC wkly or 500 mcg SC q3wks until completion of chemotherapy. Titrate: Adjust dose based on Hgb levels; see PI. | ⊕C ❀> Initiate only if Hgb less than 10 gm/dl (see PI). W [75] |

Continued on Next Page

NAME	FORM/STRENGTH	DOSAGE	COMMENTS
Darbepoetin Alfa (Aranesp) *Continued*	150 mcg/0.75 ml, 200 mcg/ml, 300 mcg/ml, 500 mcg/ml		
Eltrombopag (Promacta)	**Tab:** 12.5 mg, 25 mg, 50 mg, 75 mg	**Thrombocytopenia: Adults: Initial:** 50 mg qd. **East Asian Ancestry: Initial:** 25 mg qd. **Titrate:** Maintain platelet count ≥50 x 10^9/l. **Max:** 75 mg/d. Refer to PI for dosing according to platelet count.	⊞C ✿v May cause hepatotoxicity. **H**
Epoetin Alfa (Epogen)	**Inj:** (Single-Dose Vial) 2000 U/ml, 3000 U/ml, 4000 U/ml, 10,000 U/ml, 40,000 U/ml; (Multi-Dose Vials) 10,000 U/ml, 20,000 U/ml	**CKD: Adults: On Dialysis/Not on Dialysis: Initial:** 50-100 U/kg IV/SC tiw. **Titrate:** Adjust based on Hgb levels; see PI. **Peds: On Dialysis:** 1 mth-16 yo: **Initial:** 50 U/kg IV/SC tiw. **Titrate:** Adjust based on Hgb levels; see PI. **Zidovudine-Treated HIV Patients: Adults: Initial:** 100 U/kg IV/SC tiw. **Titrate:** Adjust dose based on Hgb levels; see PI. **Malignancy: Adults: Initial:** 150 U/kg SC tiw or 40,000 U SC wkly until completion of chemotherapy. **Titrate:** Adjust based on Hgb; see PI. **Peds:** ≥5 yo: **Initial:** 600 U/kg IV wkly until completion of chemotherapy. **Titrate:** Adjust dose based on Hgb levels; see PI. **Max:** 60,000 U/wk. **Surgery Patients:** 300 U/kg/d SC x 10d prior to surgery, on day of, & 4d after surgery (14d total); or 600 U/kg SC, 21, 14, & 7d prior to surgery & a 4th dose on day of surgery.	⊞C ✿> (CKD & Malignancy) Initiate only if Hgb less than 10 gm/dl (see PI). **W** [75]

Epoetin Alfa (Procrit)	**Inj:** 2000 U/ml, 3000 U/ml, 4000 U/ml, 10,000 U/ml, 40,000 U/ml (Single-dose Vials); 10,000 U/ml, 20,000 U/ml (Multidose Vials)	**CKD: Adults: On Dialysis/Not on Dialysis: Initial:** 50-100 U/kg IV/SC tiw. **Titrate:** Adjust based on Hgb levels; see PI. **Peds: On Dialysis:** 1 mth-16 yo: **Initial:** 50 U/kg IV/SC tiw. **Titrate:** Adjust based on Hgb levels; see PI. **Zidovudine-Treated HIV Patients: Adults: Initial:** 100 U/kg IV/SC tiw. **Titrate:** Adjust dose based on Hgb levels; see PI. **Malignancy: Adults: Initial:** 150 U/kg SC tiw or 40,000 U SC wkly until completion of chemotherapy. **Titrate:** Adjust based on Hgb; see PI. **Peds: ≥5 yo: Initial:** 600 U/kg IV wkly until completion of chemotherapy. **Titrate:** Adjust dose based on Hgb levels; see PI. **Max:** 60,000 U. **Surgery Patients:** 300 U/kg/d SC x 10d prior to surgery, on day of, & 4d after surgery (14d total); or 600 U/kg SC, 21, 14, & 7d prior to surgery & a 4th dose on day of surgery.	◉C ✿> (CKD & Malignancy) Initiate only if Hgb less than 10 gm/dl (see PI). **W** [75]
Filgrastim (Neupogen)	**Inj:** 300 mcg/0.5 ml, 300 mcg/ml, 480 mcg/0.8 ml, 480 mcg/1.6 ml	**Adults:** Adjust dose based on ANC. **Myelosuppressive Chemo: Initial:** 5 mcg/kg/d IV/SC. **Bone Marrow Transplant: Initial:** 10 mcg/kg/d IV/SC. **Peripheral Blood Progenitor Cell Collection: Initial:** 10 mcg/kg/d SC x at least 4d before & x 6-7d w/ leukapheresis on Days 5, 6, & 7. **Congenital Neutropenia: Initial:** 6 mcg/kg SC bid. **Idiopathic/Cyclic Neutropenia: Initial:** 5 mcg/kg SC qd.	◉C ✿>
Oprelvekin (Neumega)	**Inj:** 5 mg	**Severe Thrombocytopenia Prevention: Adults:** 50 mcg/kg SC qd. Initiate 6-24h after chemo completion. Continue therapy until post-nadir platelets ≥50,000 cells/mcl. D/C at least 2d before next chemo cycle. **Max:** 21d of therapy.	◉C ✿v

NAME	FORM/STRENGTH	DOSAGE	COMMENTS
Pegfilgrastim (Neulasta)	Inj: 6 mg/0.6 ml	Infection/Febrile Neutropenia w/ Non-Myeloid Malignancies: Adults: 6 mg SC, once per chemo cycle. Do not administer in period 14d before & 24h after cytotoxic chemo.	▣C ✽>

Vaccines/Toxoids/Immunoglobulins

NAME	FORM/STRENGTH	DOSAGE	COMMENTS
Diphtheria Toxoid/ Pertussis Vaccine, Acellular/ Tetanus Toxoid (Infanrix)	Inj: 0.5 ml	Peds: 6 wks-7 yo: 3 doses of 0.5 ml given at 2, 4, & 6 mths IM at 4-8 wk intervals. Booster Doses: Give at 15-20 mths & at 4-6 yo.	▣C ✽>
Diphtheria Toxoid/ Tetanus Toxoid/ Pertussis Vaccine, Acellular (Tripedia)	Inj: 0.5 ml	Peds: ≥6 wks up to 7 yo: 3 doses of 0.5 ml IM at 4-8 wk intervals. Booster Doses: Give at 15-18 mths & at 4-6 yo.	▣C ✽>
Haemophilus b Conjugate Vaccine (ActHIB)	Inj: 10 mcg	Peds: 0.5 ml IM in the mid-thigh or deltoid at 2, 4, & 6 mths old (reconstituted w/ DTP or 0.4% NaCl); 4th dose at 15-18 mths old (reconstituted w/ DTP or Tripedia or 0.4% NaCl); 5th dose at 4-6 yo (DTP or Tripedia). Previously Unvaccinated: 7-11 mths: 2 doses at 8-wk intervals w/ a booster at 15-18 mths old. 12-14 mths: 1 dose followed by a booster 2 mths later.	▣C ✽>
Hepatitis A Vaccine (Inactivated) (Vaqta)	Inj: 25 U/0.5 ml, 50 U/ml	Adults: ≥19 yo: 1 ml IM. Booster: 1 ml IM 6-18 mths later. Peds: 1-18 yo: 0.5 ml IM. Booster: 1 ml IM 6-18 mths later.	▣C ✽>

Hepatitis A Vaccine/ Hepatitis B (Recombinant) (Twinrix)	Inj: 1 ml	**Adults: 3-Dose Schedule:** 1 ml IM at 0, 1, & 6 mths. **Alternative 4-Dose Schedule:** 1 ml IM on Days 0, 7, & 21-30 followed by booster dose at 12 mths. Inject into deltoid region.	⊛C ✿>
Hepatitis B (Recombinant) (Engerix-B)	Inj: 20 mcg/ml, 10 mcg/ 0.5 ml	**Adults: ≥20 yo:** 1 ml IM at 0, 1 & 6 mths. **Peds: ≤19 yo:** 0.5 ml IM at 0, 1, & 6 mths. **Booster: Adults & Peds: ≥11 yo:** 1 ml IM. **≤10 yo:** 0.5 ml IM.	⊛C ✿>
Hepatitis B (Recombinant)/ Haemophilus B Conjugate (Comvax)	Inj: 0.5 ml	**Peds: 6 wks-15 mths:** 0.5 ml IM at 2, 4, & 12-15 mths of age. If cannot follow schedule, wait at least 6 wks between 1st two doses. 2nd & 3rd dose should be close to 8-11 mths apart.	⊛C ✿>
Human Papillomavirus Recombinant Vaccine, Bivalent (Cervarix)	Inj: 0.5 ml	**Cervical Cancer Prevention: Adults and Peds: 9-25 yo:** Give 3 separate doses of 0.5 ml IM in deltoid region of the upper arm at 0, 1, & 6 mths.	⊛B ✿>
Human Papillomavirus Recombinant Vaccine, Quadrivalent (Gardasil)	Inj: 0.5 ml	**Genital Warts/Cervical/Vulvar/Vaginal/Anal Cancer Prevention: Adults & Peds: 9-26 yo:** Give 3 separate 0.5 ml IM doses in deltoid region of upper arm or in the higher anterolateral area of the thigh. 1st dose: at elected date; 2nd dose: 2 mths after 1st dose; 3rd dose: 6 mths after 1st dose.	⊛B ✿>

NAME	FORM/STRENGTH	DOSAGE	COMMENTS
Influenza Virus Vaccine (Fluvirin)	Inj: 45 mcg/0.5 ml	**Adults & Peds: >9 yo:** 0.5 ml IM as a single dose. **Peds: 4-8 yo: Previously Vaccinated w/ 2 Doses in the Previous Season or Received 1 Dose Year Prior to Previous Season:** 0.5 ml IM as a single dose. **Not Previously Vaccinated or Received Only 1 Dose in 1st Year of Vaccination in Previous Season:** 0.5 ml IM on Day 1. Repeat dose ≥4 wks later. Administer in deltoid (adults & peds) or anterolateral thigh (peds).	◐C ✿>
Influenza Virus Vaccine (Fluzone Intradermal)	Inj: 0.25 ml, 0.5 ml, 5 ml	**Adults & Peds: ≥9 yo:** 0.5 ml IM. **Peds: 3-8 yo:** 0.5 ml IM. **6-35 mths:** 0.25 ml IM. Children <9 yo who have not previously been vaccinated or were vaccinated for the 1st time last season w/ 1 dose should receive 2 doses of vaccine ≥1 mth apart. Administer in deltoid muscle for patients ≥12 mths & anterolateral aspect of thigh for infants 6-11 mths.	◐C ✿>
Influenza Virus Vaccine Live, Intranasal (FluMist)	Nasal Spr: 0.2 ml/spr	**Adults & Peds: 9-49 yo:** One 0.2 ml (0.1 ml/nostril) dose. **2-8 yo: Not Previously Vaccinated w/ Influenza Vaccine:** 0.2 ml (0.1 ml/nostril) x 2 doses at least 1 mth apart. **Previously Vaccinated w/ Influenza Vaccine:** One 0.2 ml (0.1 ml/nostril) dose.	◐C ✿>
Influenza Virus Vaccine (Afluria)	Inj: (Syringe) 0.5 ml, (MDV) 5 ml	**Adults & Peds: ≥9 yo:** 0.5 ml IM in deltoid muscle of upper arm. **Peds: 5-8 yo: Not Previously Vaccinated/Received Only 1 Dose for the 1st Time Last Season:** Two 0.5-ml IM doses, one on Day 1 followed by another approx. 4 wks later. **Previously Vaccinated w/ 2 Doses Last Season/1**	◐B ✿>

		Dose ≥2 yrs ago: One 0.5-ml IM dose. Preferred site is the deltoid muscle of the upper arm.	
Influenza Virus Vaccine (FluLaval)	Inj: 5 ml	**Adults: ≥18 yo:** 0.5 ml IM as a single dose, preferably in the deltoid muscle of the upper arm.	⬛B ❀>
Measles Vaccine Live/ Rubella Vaccine Live/ Mumps Vaccine Live (M-M-R II)	Inj: 0.5 ml/dose	**Adults & Peds: ≥12 mths:** 0.5 ml SC in upper arm. Recommended primary vaccination is at 12-15 mths; repeat before elementary school entry. If first vaccinated at <12 mths, repeat dose at 12-15 mths & before elementary school entry.	⬛C ❀>
Meningococcal (groups A, C, Y and W-135) Oligosaccharide Diphtheria CRM 197 Conjugate (Menveo)	Inj: 0.5 ml	**Adults & Peds: 2-55 yo:** 0.5 ml IM into deltoid muscle (upper arm). **2-5 yo (Continued High Risk):** May give 2nd dose 2 mths after 1st dose.	⬛B ❀>
Meningococcal Polysaccharide A/C/Y/W-135 (Menomune-A/C/Y/W-135)	Inj: 0.6 ml, 6 ml	**Adults & Peds: ≥2 yo:** 0.5 ml SC. **Revaccination (persons at high risk who were previously vaccinated):** 0.5 ml SC.	⬛C ❀>
Meningococcal Polysaccharide Diptheria Toxoid Conjugate Vaccine (Menactra)	Inj: 0.5 ml	**Adults & Peds: 2-55 yo:** 0.5 ml IM. **9-23 mths:** 0.5 ml IM and repeat after 3 mths.	⬛C ❀>
Pneumococcal Vaccine Polyvalent (Pneumovax 23)	Inj: 0.5 ml	**Adults & Peds: ≥2 yo:** Usual/Revaccination: 0.5 ml SC/IM into the deltoid muscle or lateral mid-thigh.	⬛C ❀>

NAME	FORM/STRENGTH	DOSAGE	COMMENTS
Pneumococcal Vaccine, Diphtheria Conjugate (Prevnar 13)	**Inj:** 0.5 ml	**Adults: ≥50 yo:** *S. pneumoniae*: 0.5 ml IM single dose. **Peds:** *S. pneumoniae*/Otitis Media: 0.5 ml IM. 1st dose at 6 wks-2 mths old, then q2mths x 2 more doses. 4th dose given at 12-15 mths. **Unvaccinated: ≥24 mths-5 yo:** 0.5 ml IM single dose. **12-23 mths:** 0.5 ml IM x 2 doses given at least 2 mths apart. **7-11 mths:** 0.5 ml IM. 1st 2 doses at least 4 wks apart, then 3rd dose after 1st birthday at least 2 mths after 2nd dose.	◐B ❄>
Tetanus Toxoid/ Pertussis Vaccine Acellular, Adsorbed/Diphtheria Toxoid, Reduced (Adacel)	**Inj:** 0.5 ml	**Adults & Peds: 11-64 yo:** 0.5 ml IM. Inject preferably into the deltoid muscle.	◐C ❄>
Varicella Virus Vaccine Live (Varivax)	**Inj:** 0.5 ml	**Adults & Peds: ≥13 yo:** 0.5 ml SC, repeat in 4-8 wks. **12 mth-12 yo:** 0.5 ml SC. Minimum 3 mths later if second dose given.	◐C ❄> CI in pregnancy.
Zoster Vaccine Live (Zostavax)	**Inj:** 0.65 ml	**Adults: ≥50 yo:** Single 0.65 ml SC in deltoid region of upper arm.	◐N ❄> CI in pregnancy.

ADHD/Narcolepsy Agents

ALPHA ADRENERGIC AGONIST

Clonidine HCl (Kapvay ER)	**Tab,ER:** 0.1 mg, 0.2 mg	**Peds: 6-17 yo: Initial:** 0.1 mg hs. **Titrate:** Adjust in increments of 0.1 mg/d at wkly intervals until desired response is achieved. **Max:** 0.4 mg/d. D/C in decrements of no more than 0.1 mg q3-7d. Refer to PI for further dosing information.	⊙C ✿> R

NOREPINEPHRINE REUPTAKE INHIBITOR

Atomoxetine HCl (Strattera)	**Cap:** 10 mg, 18 mg, 25 mg, 40 mg, 60 mg, 80 mg, 100 mg	**ADHD: Adults & Peds: ≥6 yo & >70 kg: Initial:** 40 mg/d given qam or evenly divided doses in am & late afternoon/early pm. **Titrate:** Increase after minimum of 3d to target dose of about 80 mg/d. After 2-4 wks, may increase to max of 100 mg/d. **Max:** 100 mg/d. **≥6 yo & ≤70 kg: Initial:** 0.5 mg/kg/d given qam or evenly divided doses in am & late afternoon/early pm. **Titrate:** Increase after minimum of 3d to target dose of about 1.2 mg/kg/d. **Max:** 1.4 mg/kg/d or 100 mg, whichever is less. Adjust w/ CYP2D6 inhibitors.	⊙C ✿> Increased risk of suicidal ideation in children or adolescents. **H**

NAME	FORM/STRENGTH	DOSAGE	COMMENTS

SYMPATHOMIMETICS

NAME	FORM/STRENGTH	DOSAGE	COMMENTS
Amphetamine Salt Combo CII (Adderall XR)	Cap,ER: 5 mg, 10 mg, 15 mg, 20 mg, 25 mg, 30 mg	**ADHD: Adults: Initial:** 20 mg qam. **Peds: 13-17 yo: Initial:** 10 mg qam. **Titrate:** May increase to 20 mg/d after 1 wk if symptoms not controlled. **6-12 yo: Initial:** 10 mg qam or 5 mg qam when lower initial dose is appropriate. **Titrate:** May increase qwk by 5-10 mg/d. **Max:** 30 mg/d. **Currently Using Adderall:** May switch to Adderall XR at same total daily dose taken qd. Titrate at wkly intervals prn.	◉C ✿v W [49]
Amphetamine Salt Combo CII (Adderall)	Tab: 5 mg, 7.5 mg, 10 mg, 12.5 mg, 15 mg, 20 mg, 30 mg	**Peds: ≥6 yo: ADHD:** 5 mg qd-bid. **Titrate:** May increase qwk by 5 mg. **Max:** 40 mg/d. **3-5 yo:** 2.5 mg qd. **Titrate:** May increase qwk by 2.5 mg until optimal response. **Adults & Peds: ≥12 yo: Narcolepsy: Initial:** 10 mg/d. **Titrate:** May increase by 10 mg qwk. **Usual:** 5-60 mg/d. **6-12 yo: Initial:** 5 mg/d. **Titrate:** May increase by 5 mg qwk. Give 1st dose upon awakening & additional doses q4-6h.	◉C ✿v W [49]
Dexmethylphenidate HCl CII (Focalin XR)	Cap,ER: 5 mg, 10 mg, 15 mg, 20 mg, 25 mg, 30 mg, 35 mg, 40 mg	**ADHD: Methylphenidate-Naive: Adults: Initial:** 10 mg/d. **Titrate:** May adjust wkly by 10 mg/d. **Max:** 40 mg/d. **Peds: ≥6 yo: Initial:** 5 mg/d. **Titrate:** May adjust wkly by 5 mg/d. **Max:** 30 mg/d. **Adults & Peds: ≥6 yo: Currently on Methylphenidate: Initial:** Take 1/2 methylphenidate daily dose. **Currently on Dexmethylphenidate IR:** Switch to same daily dose of XR. Take qam. Reduce or d/c if paradoxical aggravation of symptoms. D/C if no	◉C ✿> W [102]

		improvement after dose adjustments over 1 mth. Swallow whole or sprinkle on applesauce.	
Dexmethylphenidate HCl CII (Focalin)	**Tab:** 2.5 mg, 5 mg, 10 mg	**ADHD: Methylphenidate-Naive: Initial:** Adults & Peds: ≥6 yo: 2.5 mg bid at least 4h apart. **Titrate:** May adjust wkly by 2.5-5 mg/d. **Max:** 20 mg/d. **Currently on Methylphenidate: Initial:** Take 1/2 methylphenidate dose. **Max:** 20 mg/d. D/C if no improvement after 1 mth.	⊙C ❄> W [102]
Dextroamphetamine Sulfate CII (Procentra)	**Sol:** (Procentra) 5 mg/ml; **Tab:** 5 mg, 10 mg	**Peds: ≥6 yo:** Individualize dose. Administer at lowest effective dose. **ADHD: Initial:** 5 mg qd-bid. **Titrate:** Increase qwk by 5 mg. Only in rare cases will it be necessary to exceed a total of 40 mg/d. **3-5 yo: Initial:** 2.5 mg qd. **Titrate:** Increase qwk by 2.5 mg. **Adults & Peds: ≥12 yo:** Individualize dose. Administer at lowest effective dose. **Narcolepsy: Initial:** 10 mg qd. **Titrate:** Increase qwk by 10 mg/d. **Usual:** 5-60 mg/d in divided doses. **6-12 yo: Initial:** 5 mg/d. **Titrate:** Increase qwk by 5 mg.	⊙C ❄v W [49]
Dextroamphetamine Sulfate CII (Dexedrine Spansules)	**Cap:** (Spansules) 5 mg, 10 mg, 15 mg	**Narcolepsy: Adults & Peds: ≥12 yo: Initial:** 10 mg/d. **Titrate:** May increase by 10 mg/d at wkly intervals until optimal response obtained. **Usual:** 5-60 mg/d in divided doses. May give once daily. **6-12 yo: Initial:** 5 mg qd. **Titrate:** May increase wkly by 5 mg/d until optimal response obtained. **ADHD: ≥6 yo: Initial:** 5 mg qd-bid. **Titrate:** May	⊙C ❄v W [49]

Continued on Next Page

NAME	FORM/STRENGTH	DOSAGE	COMMENTS
Dextroamphetamine Sulfate CII (Dexedrine Spansules) *Continued*		increase 5 mg/d at wkly intervals until optimal response obtained. Only in rare cases will it be necessary to exceed a total of 40 mg/d. May give once daily.	
Lisdexamfetamine Dimesylate CII (Vyvanse)	**Cap:** 20 mg, 30 mg, 40 mg, 50 mg, 60 mg, 70 mg	**ADHD: Adults & Peds: ≥6 yo:** Individualize dose. **Initial:** 30 mg qam. **Titrate:** May increase by 10 or 20 mg/d at wkly intervals. **Max:** 70 mg/d.	⊞C ❋v W [49]
Methylphenidate CII (Daytrana)	**Patch:** 10 mg/9h, 15 mg/9h, 20 mg/9h, 30 mg/9h	**ADHD: Adults & Peds ≥6 yo:** Individualize dose. Apply to hip area 2h before effect needed & remove 9h after application. **Recommended Titration Schedule: Wk 1:** 10 mg/9h. **Wk 2:** 15 mg/9h. **Wk 3:** 20 mg/9h. **Wk 4:** 30 mg/9h.	⊞C ❋> W [102]
Methylphenidate HCl CII (Concerta)	**Tab,ER:** 18 mg, 27 mg, 36 mg, 54 mg	**Adults & Peds: Methylphenidate-Naive or Receiving Other Stimulant: Initial: 6-17 yo:** 18 mg qam. **18-65 yo:** 18 or 36 mg qam. **Titrate:** Adjust dose by 18 mg wkly. **Max: 6-12 yo:** 54 mg/d. **13-17 yo:** 72 mg/d not to exceed 2 mg/kg/d. **18-65 yo:** 72 mg/d. **Currently on Methylphenidate: Initial:** 18 mg qam if previous dose 10-15 mg/d; 36 mg qam if previous dose 20-30 mg/d; 54 mg qam if previous dose 30-45 mg/d; 72 mg qam if previous dose 40-60 mg/d. **Titrate:** Adjust dose by 18 mg wkly. **Max: Adults:** 72 mg/d. **Peds: 6-12 yo:** 54 mg/d; **13-17 yo:** 72 mg/d. Reduce dose or d/c if paradoxical aggravation of symptoms occurs. D/C if no improvement after appropriate dosage adjustments over 1 mth.	⊞C ❋> W [102]

Methylphenidate HCl CII (Metadate CD)	**Cap,ER:** 10 mg, 20 mg, 30 mg, 40 mg, 50 mg, 60 mg	**Peds: ≥6 yo: Usual:** 20 mg qam before breakfast. **Titrate:** Increase wkly by 10-20 mg depending on tolerability/ efficacy. **Max:** 60 mg/d. Reduce dose or d/c if paradoxical aggravation of symptoms occurs. D/C if no improvement after appropriate dose adjustments over 1 mth. Swallow whole w/ liq or open & sprinkle on 1 tbsp applesauce followed by water.	⊞C ❄> W [102]
Methylphenidate HCl CII (Metadate ER)	**Tab,ER:** 20 mg	**ADHD: Adults:** (IR-Methylphenidate) 10-60 mg/d given bid-tid 30-45 min ac. **Peds: ≥6 yo: Initial:** (IR-Methylphenidate) 5 mg bid before breakfast & lunch. **Titrate:** Increase gradually by 5-10 mg wkly. **Max:** 60 mg/d. (Tab,ER) May use in place of IR tabs when 8h dose corresponds to titrated 8h IR dose.	⊞C ❄> W [102]
Methylphenidate HCl CII (Methylin, Methylin ER)	**Sol:** (Methylin) 5 mg/ 5 ml, 10 mg/5 ml; **Tab:** (Methylin) 5 mg, 10 mg, 20 mg; **Tab,Chew:** (Methylin) 2.5 mg, 5 mg, 10 mg; **Tab,ER:** (Methylin ER) 10 mg, 20 mg	**ADHD: Adults:** Methylin: 10-60 mg/d divided bid-tid 30-45 min ac. **Peds: ≥6 yo:** Methylin: 5 mg bid. **Titrate:** May increase by 5-10 mg qwk. **Max:** 60 mg/d. May use Methylin ER when 8h ER dose corresponds to titrated 8h IR dose.	⊞C ❄> W [102]

NAME	FORM/STRENGTH	DOSAGE	COMMENTS
Methylphenidate HCl CII (Ritalin, Ritalin LA, Ritalin SR)	**Cap,ER:** (Ritalin LA) 10 mg, 20 mg, 30 mg, 40 mg; **Tab:** (Ritalin) 5 mg, 10 mg, 20 mg; **Tab,ER:** (Ritalin-SR) 20 mg	Individualize dose. **ADHD: Adults & Peds: ≥6 yo: Ritalin LA: Initial:** 10-20 mg qam. **Titrate:** May adjust wkly by 10 mg increments. **Max:** 60 mg/d. **ADHD & Narcolepsy: Adults: Ritalin:** 10-60 mg/d divided bid-tid 30-45 min ac. **Peds: ≥6 yo: Ritalin: Initial:** 5 mg bid before breakfast & lunch. **Titrate:** May increase by 5-10 mg qwk. **Max:** 60 mg/d. May use Ritalin-SR when 8h ER dose corresponds to titrated 8h IR dose.	⊙C ❄️> W [102]

MISCELLANEOUS

NAME	FORM/STRENGTH	DOSAGE	COMMENTS
Armodafinil CIV (Nuvigil)	**Tab:** 50 mg, 150 mg, 250 mg	**Adults & Peds: ≥17 yo: Narcolepsy/Obstructive Sleep Apnea:** 150 mg or 250 mg qam. **Shift Work Disorder:** 150 mg qd 1h prior to work shift. **Elderly:** Consider dose reduction.	⊙C ❄️> H
Guanfacine (Intuniv)	**Tab,ER:** 1 mg, 2 mg, 3 mg, 4 mg	**ADHD: Peds: 6-17 yo: Monotherapy/Adjunctive Therapy: Initial:** 1 mg qd. **Titrate:** Adjust dose by increments of ≤1 mg/wk. **Maint:** 1-4 mg qd. **Monotherapy:** 0.05-0.08 mg/kg/d based on clinical response and tolerability; if well tolerated, doses up to 0.12 mg/kg/d may provide additional benefit. **Max:** 4 mg/d. **Adjunctive Therapy:** 0.05-0.12 mg/kg/d. **D/C:** Taper in decrements of ≤1 mg every 3-7d. See PI for dosage reinitiation and adjustment.	⊙B ❄️> H R

| Modafinil CIV (Provigil) | Tab: 100 mg, 200 mg | Adults & Peds: ≥17 yo: 200 mg qd. Max: 400 mg/d as single dose (no evidence of additional benefit). Narcolepsy/Obstructive Sleep Apnea: Take as single dose in am. Shift Work Disorder: Take 1h prior to start of work shift. | ⬤C ❄️> H |

Alzheimer's Therapy
CHOLINESTERASE INHIBITORS

| Donepezil HCl (Aricept) | Tab: 5 mg, 10 mg, 23 mg; Tab,Dissolve: 5 mg, 10 mg | Adults: Mild-to-Moderate: Initial: 5 mg qhs. Titrate: May increase to 10 mg qhs after 4-6 wks. Usual: 5-10 mg qhs. Moderate-to-Severe: Initial: 5 mg qhs. Titrate: May increase to 10 mg qhs after 4-6 wks, then to 23 mg qhs after ≥3 mths. Usual: 10-23 mg qhs. | ⬤C ❄️> |
| Galantamine HBr (Razadyne, Razadyne ER) | Sol: 4 mg/ml; Tab: 4 mg, 8 mg, 12 mg; Cap,ER: 8 mg, 16 mg, 24 mg | Adults: Sol/Tab: Initial: 4 mg bid w/ am & pm meals. Titrate: Increase to 8 mg bid after 4 wks if tolerated, then 12 mg bid after 4 wks if tolerated. Usual: 16-24 mg/d. Max: 24 mg/d. Cap,ER: Initial: 8 mg qd w/ am meal. Titrate: Increase to 16 mg qd after 4 wks, then 24 mg/d after 4 wks if tolerated. Usual: 16-24 mg/d. Max: 24 mg/d. | ⬤B ❄️v H R |

NAME	FORM/STRENGTH	DOSAGE	COMMENTS
Rivastigmine Tartrate (Exelon)	**Cap:** 1.5 mg, 3 mg, 4.5 mg, 6 mg; **Sol:** 2 mg/ml; **Patch:** 4.6 mg/24h, 9.5 mg/24h	**Alzheimer's Dementia: Adults: PO: Initial:** 1.5 mg bid. **Titrate:** May increase by 1.5 mg bid q2wks. **Usual:** 6-12 mg/d. **Max:** 12 mg/d. If not tolerated, suspend therapy for several doses & restart at same or next lower dose. If interruption is longer than several days, reinitiate w/ lowest daily dose & titrate as before. **Patch: Initial:** 4.6 mg/24h qd. **Maint:** May increase dose after 4 wks. **Max:** 9.5 mg/24h if well tolerated. **Switching from PO: Total PO Daily Dose <6 mg:** Switch to 4.6 mg/24h patch. **Total PO Daily Dose 6-12 mg:** Switch to 9.5 mg/24h patch. Apply 1st patch on the day following last PO dose.	●B ❄v

NMDA-RECEPTOR ANTAGONISTS

NAME	FORM/STRENGTH	DOSAGE	COMMENTS
Memantine HCl (Namenda XR)	**Sol:** 2 mg/ml; **Tab:** 5 mg, 10 mg	**Adults: Initial:** 5 mg qd. **Maint:** 10 mg bid. **Titrate:** Increase at intervals ≥1 wk in 5 mg increments to 10 mg/d (5 mg bid), 15 mg/d (5 mg & 10 mg as separate doses), then 20 mg/d (10 mg bid).	●B ❄> R
Memantine HCl (Namenda XR)	**Cap,ER:** 7 mg, 14 mg, 21 mg, 28 mg	**Adults: Initial:** 7 mg qd. **Maint:** 28 mg qd. **Titrate:** Increase at intervals ≥1 wk in 7 mg increments. **Max:** 28 mg qd. **Switching from Tabs to Caps,ER:** Switch from 10 mg bid tabs to 28 mg qd ER caps the day following the last dose of 10-mg tab. Swallow caps intact or may be opened, sprinkled on applesauce. Do not divide, chew, or crush.	●B ❄> R

Antianxiety/Hypnotic Agents
BENZODIAZEPINES

Drug	Form	Dosing	Ratings
Alprazolam CIV (Niravam)	**Tab, Dissolve:** 0.25 mg, 0.5 mg, 1 mg, 2 mg	**Adults: Anxiety: Initial:** 0.25-0.5 mg tid. **Titrate:** May increase q3-4d. **Max:** 4 mg/d. **Panic Disorder: Initial:** 0.5 mg tid. **Titrate:** Increase by no more than 1 mg/d q3-4d; slower titration if >4 mg/d. **Usual:** 1-10 mg/d. Decrease dose slowly (no more than 0.5 mg/d q3d). **Elderly/Debilitated: Initial:** 0.25 mg bid-tid. **Titrate:** Increase gradually as tolerated.	⊕D ❀v H
Alprazolam CIV (Xanax XR)	**Tab, ER:** 0.5 mg, 1 mg, 2 mg, 3 mg	**Panic Disorder: Adults: Initial:** 0.5-1 mg qd, preferably in am. **Titrate:** Increase by no more than 1 mg/d q3-4d. **Maint:** 1-10 mg/d. **Usual:** 3-6 mg/d. Decrease dose slowly (no more than 0.5 mg q3d). **Elderly/Debilitated: Initial:** 0.5 mg qd.	⊕D ❀v H
Alprazolam CIV (Xanax)	**Tab:** 0.25 mg, 0.5 mg, 1 mg, 2 mg	**Adults: Anxiety: Initial:** 0.25-0.5 mg tid. **Titrate:** May increase q3-4d. **Max:** 4 mg/d. **Panic Disorder: Initial:** 0.5 mg tid. **Titrate:** Increase by no more than 1 mg/d q3-4d; slower titration if ≥4 mg/d. **Usual:** 1-10 mg/d. Decrease dose slowly (no more than 0.5 mg q3d). **Elderly/Debilitated: Initial:** 0.25 mg bid-tid. **Titrate:** Increase gradually as tolerated.	⊕D ❀v H
Clorazepate Dipotassium CIV (Tranxene T-Tab)	**Tab:** 3.75 mg, 7.5 mg, 15 mg	**Anxiety: Adults: Initial:** 15 mg qhs. **Usual:** 30 mg/d in divided doses. **Max:** 60 mg/d.	⊕N ❀v

NAME	FORM/STRENGTH	DOSAGE	COMMENTS
Diazepam CIV (Valium)	**Tab:** 2 mg, 5 mg, 10 mg	**Adults: Anxiety:** 2-10 mg bid-qid. **Acute Alcohol Withdrawal:** 10 mg tid-qid for 24h. Reduce to 5 mg tid-qid prn. **Elderly/Debilitated:** 2-2.5mg qd-bid. **Titrate:** May increase gradually prn and tolerated. **Peds: ≥6 mths: Initial:** 1-2.5 mg tid-qid. **Titrate:** May increase gradually prn and tolerated.	●D ❄v
Lorazepam CIV (Ativan)	**Tab:** 0.5 mg, 1 mg, 2 mg	**Adults & Peds: ≥12 yo: Anxiety: Initial:** 2-3 mg/d given bid-tid. **Usual:** 2-6 mg/d. **Insomnia:** 2-4 mg qhs.	●N ❄v
Midazolam HCl CIV	**Syr:** 2 mg/ml	**Sedation, Anxiolysis & Amnesia: Peds: ≥6 mths:** Individualize dose. **Usual:** 0.25-0.5 mg/kg single dose. **Max:** 20 mg. **6-<16 yo/Cooperative Patients: Usual:** 0.25 mg/kg. **6 mths-<6 yo/Less Cooperative Patients:** May require higher than usual dose, up to 1 mg/kg. **W/ Cardiac or Respiratory Compromise/Higher Risk Surgical Patients/Concomitant Narcotics or Other CNS Depressants:** Consider 0.25 mg/kg. **Obese Patients:** Calculate dose based on ideal body wt.	●D ❄> Associated w/ respiratory depression & respiratory arrest.
Temazepam CIV (Restoril)	**Cap:** 7.5 mg, 15 mg, 22.5 mg, 30 mg	**Adults: Insomnia: Usual:** 15 mg qhs. **Range:** 7.5-30 mg qhs. **Transient Insomnia:** 7.5 mg qhs.	●X ❄> H R

SEROTONIN/NOREPINEPHRINE REUPTAKE INHIBITORS

Duloxetine HCl (Cymbalta)	Cap, Delay: 20 mg, 30 mg, 60 mg	**Generalized Anxiety Disorder: Adults: Initial:** 60 mg qd or 30 mg qd x 1 wk before increasing to 60 mg qd. **Titrate:** Increase in increments of 30 mg qd. **Maint:** 60-120 mg qd. **Max:** 120 mg/d.	⊞C ❋v H R W [29]
Venlafaxine HCl (Effexor XR)	Cap, ER: 37.5 mg, 75 mg, 150 mg	**Adults: Generalized Anxiety Disorder: Initial:** 75 mg/d or 37.5 mg/d x 4-7d and then increase to 75 mg/d. **Titrate:** Increase by increments of up to 75 mg/d at intervals of ≥4d. **Max:** 225 mg/d. **Panic Disorder: Initial:** 37.5 mg/d x 7d. **Titrate:** Increase by increments of up to 75 mg/d at intervals of ≥7d. **Max:** 225 mg/d. **Social Anxiety Disorder:** 75 mg/d.	⊞C ❋v H R W [29]

SSRIs & COMBINATIONS

Escitalopram Oxalate (Lexapro)	Sol: 5 mg/5 ml; Tab: 5 mg, 10 mg, 20 mg	**Generalized Anxiety Disorder: Adults: Initial:** 10 mg qd. **Titrate:** May increase to 20 mg after ≥1 wk.	⊞C ❋> H W [29]
Fluoxetine HCl (Prozac)	Cap: 10 mg, 20 mg, 40 mg	**Panic Disorder: Adults: Initial:** 10 mg/d. May increase to 20 mg/d after 1 wk. May increase further after several wks if no improvement observed. **Max:** 60 mg/d.	⊞C ❋v H W [29]
Paroxetine HCl (Paxil CR)	Tab, CR: 12.5 mg, 25 mg, 37.5 mg	**Adults: Panic Disorder: Initial:** 12.5 mg qam. **Titrate:** May increase by 12.5 mg/d at intervals of ≥1 wk. **Max:** 75 mg/d. **Social Anxiety Disorder: Initial:** 12.5 mg qam. **Titrate:** May increase by 12.5 mg/d at intervals of ≥1 wk. **Max:** 37.5 mg/d.	⊞D ❋> H R W [29]

NAME	FORM/STRENGTH	DOSAGE	COMMENTS
Paroxetine HCl (Paxil)	**Susp:** 10 mg/5 ml; **Tab:** 10 mg, 20 mg, 30 mg, 40 mg	**Adults: Panic Disorder: Initial:** 10 mg qam. **Titrate:** May increase by 10 mg/d at intervals ≥1 wk. **Usual:** 40 mg/d. **Max:** 60 mg/d. **Social Anxiety Disorder: Initial/Usual:** 20 mg qam. **Generalized Anxiety Disorder/PTSD: Initial/Usual:** 20 mg qam. **Titrate:** If indicated may increase by 10 mg/d at intervals of ≥1 wk. **Range:** 20-50 mg/d.	●D ❄> H R W [29]
Paroxetine Mesylate (Pexeva)	**Tab:** 10 mg, 20 mg, 30 mg, 40 mg	**Panic Disorder: Adults: Initial:** 10 mg/d. **Titrate:** 10 mg/d wkly. **Max:** 40 mg/d.	●C ❄> H R W [29]
Sertraline HCl (Zoloft)	**Sol:** 20 mg/ml; **Tab:** 25 mg, 50 mg, 100 mg	**Panic Disorder/Social Anxiety Disorder/PTSD: Adults: Initial:** 25 mg qd. **Titrate:** Increase to 50 mg qd after 1 wk. Adjust wkly. **Max:** 200 mg/d.	●C ❄> H W [29]

MISCELLANEOUS

NAME	FORM/STRENGTH	DOSAGE	COMMENTS
Buspirone	**Tab:** 5 mg, 7.5 mg, 10 mg, 15 mg, 30 mg	**Anxiety: Adults: Initial:** 7.5 mg bid. **Titrate:** Increase by 5 mg/d q2-3d. **Usual:** 20-30 mg/d. **Max:** 60 mg/d.	●B ❄v
Doxepin (Silenor)	**Tab:** 3 mg, 6 mg	**Adults: Insomnia: Usual:** 6 mg qd w/in 30 min of hs. May decrease to 3 mg. **Max:** 6 mg/d. **Elderly:** 3 mg qd w/in 30 min of hs. May increase to 6 mg. **Max:** 6 mg/d. Do not take w/ in 3h of a meal.	●C ❄v H
Eszopiclone CIV (Lunesta)	**Tab:** 1 mg, 2 mg, 3 mg	**Insomnia: Adults 18-64 yo: Initial:** 2 mg qhs **Max:** 3 mg qhs. **≥65 yo: Difficulty Falling Asleep: Initial:** 1 mg qhs. **Max:** 2 mg qhs. **Difficulty Staying Asleep:** 2 mg qhs.	●C ❄> H

Ramelteon (Rozerem)	Tab: 8 mg	**Insomnia: Adults:** 8 mg w/in 30 min of hs. **Max:** 8 mg/d. Do not take w/ or after high-fat meal.	⊞C ❄>H
Zaleplon CIV (Sonata)	Cap: 5 mg, 10 mg	**Insomnia: Adults:** 10 mg qhs. **Max:** 20 mg qhs. **Low-Wt Patients:** 5 mg qhs. **Max:** 20 mg qhs. **Elderly/Debilitated Patients:** 5 mg qhs. **Max:** 10 mg qhs. **Concomitant Cimetidine: Initial:** 5 mg qhs.	⊞C ❄v H
Zolpidem Tartrate CIV (Ambien CR)	Tab,ER 6.25 mg, 12.5 mg	**Insomnia: Adults:** ≥18 yo: 12.5 mg qhs. **Elderly/Debilitated:** 6.25 mg qhs.	⊞C ❄v H
Zolpidem Tartrate CIV (Ambien)	Tab: 5 mg, 10 mg	**Insomnia: Adults:** 10 mg qhs. **Elderly/Debilitated:** 5 mg qhs. Adjust dose w/ other CNS depressants.	⊞B ❄>H
Zolpidem Tartrate CIV (Intermezzo)	Tab,SL: 1.75 mg, 3.5 mg	**Adults: Usual/Max:** (Women) 1.75 mg, (Men) 3.5 mg once per night prn if a middle-of-the-night awakening is followed by difficulty returning to sleep. **Concomitant CNS Depressants/Elderly (>65 yrs):** Use the 1.75 mg dose.	⊞C ❄>H

Anticonvulsants
BENZODIAZEPINES

| Diazepam CIV (Valium) | Tab: 2 mg, 5 mg, 10 mg | **Adults:** 2-10 mg bid-qid. **Elderly/Debilitated:** 2-2.5 mg qd-bid. **Titrate:** May increase gradually prn and tolerated. **Peds:** ≥6 mths: **Initial:** 1-2.5 mg tid-qid. **Titrate:** May increase gradually prn and tolerated. | ⊞D ❄v |
| Lorazepam CIV (Ativan Injection) | Inj: 2 mg/ml, 4 mg/ml | **Status Epilepticus: Adults:** ≥18 yo: 2 mg/min IV x 2 min, may repeat x 1 dose after 10-15 min. **Max:** 8 mg. | ⊞D ❄v |

NAME	FORM/STRENGTH	DOSAGE	COMMENTS

CARBOXYLIC ACID DERIVATIVES

NAME	FORM/STRENGTH	DOSAGE	COMMENTS
Valproate Sodium (Depacon)	Inj: 100 mg/ml	**Adults & Peds: ≥10 yo: IV: Complex Partial Seizures: Initial:** 10-15 mg/kg/d. **Titrate:** Increase by 5-10 mg/kg/wk. **Max:** 60 mg/kg/d. **≥2 yo: Simple/Complex Absence Seizures: Initial:** 15 mg/kg/d. **Titrate:** Increase wkly by 5-10 mg/kg/d. **Max:** 60 mg/kg/d. Divide doses >250 mg/d into multiple doses.	▣D ❄v H W [101]
Valproic Acid (Depakene)	Cap: 250 mg; Syr: 250 mg/5 ml	**Adults & Peds: ≥10 yo: Complex Partial Seizures: Initial:** 10-15 mg/kg/d. **Titrate:** Increase wkly by 5-10 mg/kg/wk. **Max:** 60 mg/kg/d. **Adults: Simple/Complex Absence Seizures: Initial:** 15 mg/kg/d. **Titrate:** Increase wkly by 5-10 mg/kg/d. **Max:** 60 mg/kg/d.	▣D ❄v H W [101]
Valproic Acid (Stavzor)	Cap, Delay: 125 mg, 250 mg, 500 mg	**Adults & Peds: ≥10 yo: Complex Partial Seizures: Initial:** 10-15 mg/kg/d. **Titrate:** Increase by 5-10 mg/kg/wk until optimal response (50-100 mcg/ml). **Max:** 60 mg/kg/d. **Conversion to Monotherapy:** Reduce concomitant antiepileptic drug (AED) dosage by 25% q2wks; withdrawal of AED highly variable, monitor closely for seizure frequency. **Simple/Complex Absence Seizures: Initial:** 15 mg/kg/d. **Titrate:** Increase at 1-wk interval by 5-10 mg/kg/d until optimal response (50-100 mcg/ml). **Max:** 60 mg/kg/d. If dose >250 mg/d, give in divided doses. **Elderly:** Reduce starting dose & increase slowly.	▣D ❄v W [101]

HYDANTOIN DERIVATIVES

Phenytoin (Dilantin Infatabs, Dilantin-125)	**Cap,ER:** 30 mg, 100 mg	**Tonic-Clonic & Complex Partial Seizures/Seizure Treatment or Prevention w/ Neurosurgery: Adults: Cap,ER: Initial:** 100 mg tid. **Titrate:** Increase q7-10d. **Maint:** 100 mg tid-qid. **Max:** 200 mg tid if necessary. May give ER qd if controlled on 300 mg/d. **LD:** 1 gm in 3 divided doses (400 mg, 300 mg, 300 mg) given 2h apart. Start maint 24h later. **Peds: Initial:** 5 mg/kg/d given in 2 or 3 equally divided doses. **Titrate:** Increase q7-10d. **Maint:** 4-8 mg/kg/d. **Max:** 300 mg/d. **>6 yo:** May require minimum adult dose (300 mg/d).	⊞D ✿v

SODIUM CHANNEL INACTIVATOR

Lacosamide CV (Vimpat)	**Inj:** 200 mg/20 ml; **Tab:** 50 mg, 100 mg, 150 mg, 200 mg; **Sol:** 10 mg/ml	**Partial Onset Seizures: Adults & Peds: ≥17 yo: PO/IV: Initial:** 50 mg bid. **Titrate:** May increase at wkly intervals by 100 mg/d given bid. **Maint:** 200-400 mg/d based on response & tolerability. **Switching from PO to IV; IV to PO:** See PI.	⊞C ✿v H R

SUCCINIMIDES

Ethosuximide (Zarontin)	**Cap:** 250 mg; **Syr:** 250 mg/5 ml	**Adults & Peds: Absence Seizures: Initial: ≥6 yo:** 500 mg qd. **3-6 yo: Initial:** 250 mg qd. **Titrate:** Increase daily dose by 250 mg q4-7d. Optimal dose for peds is 20 mg/kg/d. Caution w/ doses >1.5 gm/d.	⊞N ✿>

NAME	FORM/STRENGTH	DOSAGE	COMMENTS
Methsuximide (Celontin)	**Cap:** 150 mg, 300 mg	**Absence Seizures: Adults & Peds:** Individualize dose. **Initial:** 300 mg qd for the 1st wk. **Titrate:** Increase wkly by 300 mg/d x 3 wks. **Max:** 1.2 gm/d.	⊞N ❄>

SULFONAMIDE

NAME	FORM/STRENGTH	DOSAGE	COMMENTS
Zonisamide (Zonegran)	**Cap:** 25 mg, 100 mg	**Partial Seizures: Adults & Peds:** ≥16 yo: **Initial:** 100 mg/d. **Titrate:** Increase by 100 mg q2wks, given qd-bid. **Max:** 400 mg/d.	⊞C ❄v H R

TRIAZOLE DERIVATIVE

NAME	FORM/STRENGTH	DOSAGE	COMMENTS
Rufinamide (Banzel)	**Susp:** 40 mg/ml; **Tab:** 200 mg, 400 mg	**Adults: Initial:** 400-800 mg/d in 2 equally divided doses. **Titrate:** May increase by 400-800 mg/d qod until max is reached. **Max:** 3200 mg/d. **Peds:** ≥4 yo: **Initial:** 10 mg/kg/d in 2 equally divided doses. **Titrate:** May increase by 10 mg/kg increments qod to target dose of 45 mg/kg/d or 3200 mg/d, whichever is less, given in 2 equally divided doses. Take w/ food.	⊞C ❄v H

MISCELLANEOUS

NAME	FORM/STRENGTH	DOSAGE	COMMENTS
Carbamazepine (Tegretol, Tegretol-XR)	**Chewtab:** 100 mg; **Susp:** 100 mg/5 ml; **Tab:** 200 mg; **Tab,ER:** 100 mg, 200 mg, 400 mg	**Partial/Tonic-Clonic/Mixed Seizures: Adults & Peds:** >12 yo: **Initial: Chewtab/Tab/Tab,ER:** 200 mg bid. **Susp:** 100 mg qid. **Titrate:** May increase wkly by 200 mg/d given tid-qid (Chewtab/Susp/Tab) or bid (Tab,ER). **Maint:** 800-1200 mg/d. **Max:** 1200 mg/d (>15 yo) or 1000 mg/d	⊞D ❄v H W [87]

		(12-15 yo). **6-12 yo: Chewtab/Tab/Tab,ER: Initial:** 100 mg bid. **Susp:** 50 mg qid. **Titrate:** May increase wkly by 100 mg/d given tid-qid (Chewtab/Susp/Tab) or bid (Tab,ER). **Maint:** 400-800 mg/d. **Max:** 1000 mg/d. **6 mths-6 yo: Chewtab/Tab: Initial:** 10-20 mg/kg/d given bid-tid. **Susp:** 10-20 mg/kg/d given qid. **Titrate:** (Chewtab/ Susp/Tab) May increase wkly tid-qid. **Max:** 35 mg/kg/d.	
Divalproex Sodium (Depakote)	**Cap,Delay:** (Sprinkle) 125 mg; **Tab,Delay:** 125 mg, 250 mg, 500 mg	**Adults & Peds: >10 yo: Complex Partial Seizures: Initial:** 10-15 mg/kg/d. **Titrate:** Increase by 5-10 mg/kg/ wk. **Max:** 60 mg/kg/d. **Adults: Absence Seizures: Initial:** 15 mg/kg/d. **Titrate:** Increase by 5-10 mg/kg/wk. **Max:** 60 mg/kg/d.	⊛D ❁v H W [101]
Divalproex Sodium (Depakote ER)	**Tab,ER:** 250 mg, 500 mg	**Adults & Peds: ≥10 yo: Complex Partial Seizures: Monotherapy/Conversion to Monotherapy/Adjunctive Therapy: Initial:** 10-15 mg/kg qd. **Titrate:** Increase by 5-10 mg/kg/wk. **Max:** 60 mg/kg/d. **Absence Seizures: Initial:** 15 mg/kg qd. **Titrate:** Increase by 5-10 mg/kg/wk. **Max:** 60 mg/kg/d.	⊛D ❁v W [101]
Ezogabine CV (Potiga)	**Tab:** 50 mg, 200 mg, 300 mg, 400 mg	**Partial Seizures: Adults:** Increase dose gradually at wkly intervals no more than 50 mg tid. **Initial:** 100 mg tid. **Maint:** 200-400 mg tid. **Max:** 400 mg tid. **Elderly: >65 yo: Initial:** 50 mg tid. **Max:** 250 mg tid.	⊛C ❁v H R

NAME	FORM/STRENGTH	DOSAGE	COMMENTS
Gabapentin (Neurontin)	**Cap:** 100 mg, 300 mg, 400 mg; **Sol:** 250 mg/ 5 ml; **Tab:** 600 mg, 800 mg	**Partial Seizures: Adults & Peds: >12 yo: Initial:** 300 mg tid. Titrate: Increase up to 1800 mg/d. **Max:** 3600 mg/d. **3-12 yo: Initial:** 10-15 mg/kg/d given tid. **Titrate:** Increase over 3d. **Usual: ≥5 yo:** 25-35 mg/kg/d given tid. **3-4 yo:** 40 mg/kg/d given tid. **Max:** 50 mg/kg/d.	⊕C ❄️> R
Lamotrigine (Lamictal, Lamictal ODT)	**Chewtab:** 2 mg, 5 mg, 25 mg; **Tab:** 25 mg, 100 mg, 150 mg, 200 mg; **Tab, Dissolve:** 25 mg, 50 mg, 100 mg, 200 mg	**Partial/Primary Generalized Tonic-Clonic/Generalized Seizures of Lennox-Gastaut Syndrome: Adults & Peds: >12 yo: Concomitant Valproate (VPA): Wks 1 & 2:** 25 mg qod. **Wks 3 & 4:** 25 mg qd. **Wk 5 Onward:** Increase by 25-50 mg/d q1-2wks. **Maint:** 100-200mg/d if VPA alone or 100-400 mg/d if VPA w/ other drugs inducing glucuronidation (1-2 divided doses). **Not Taking Carbamazepine, Phenytoin, Phenobarbital, Primidone, or VPA: Wks 1 & 2:** 25 mg qd. **Wks 3 & 4:** 50 mg/d. **Wk 5 Onward:** Increase by 50 mg/d q1-2wks. **Maint:** 225-375 mg/d (2 divided doses). **Concomitant Carbamazepine, Phenytoin, Phenobarbital, Primidone w/o VPA: Wks 1 & 2:** 50 mg qd. **Wks 3 & 4:** 100 mg/d (2 divided doses). **Wk 5 Onward:** Increase by 100 mg/d q1-2wks. **Maint:** 300-500 mg/d (2 divided doses). **2-12 yo:** Round dose down to nearest whole tab and give in 1-2 divided daily doses. **Concomitant VPA: Wks 1 & 2:** 0.15 mg/kg/d. **Wks 3 & 4:** 0.3 mg/kg/d. **Wk 5 Onward:** Increase q1-2wks by 0.3 mg/kg/d. **Maint:** 1-3 mg/kg/d if VPA alone or 1-5 mg/kg/d. **Max:** 200 mg/d. **Initial**	⊕C ❄️> Serious rashes, Stevens-Johnson syndrome reported. **H R**

		Wt-Based Dosing Guide (Wks 1-4): See PI. Not Taking Carbamazepine, Phenytoin, Phenobarbital, Primidone, or VPA: Wks 1 & 2: 0.3 mg/kg/d. Wks 3 & 4: 0.6 mg/kg/d. Wk 5 Onward: Increase q1-2wks by 0.6 mg/kg/d. Maint: 4.5-7.5 mg/kg/d. Max: 300 mg/d. Concomitant Carbamazepine, Phenytoin, Phenobarbital, Primidone w/o VPA: Wks 1 & 2: 0.6 mg/kg/d. Wks 3 & 4: 1.2 mg/kg/d. Wk 5 Onward: Increase q1-2wks by 1.2 mg/kg/d. Maint: 5-15 mg/kg/d. Max: 400 mg/d. <30 kg: May increase maint dose by up to 50%. ≥16 yo: Conversion to Monotherapy: See PI.	
Lamotrigine (Lamictal XR)	Tab, ER: 25 mg, 50 mg, 100 mg, 200 mg, 250mg, 300 mg	Primary Generalized Tonic-Clonic/Partial Onset Seizure: Adults & Peds ≥13 yo: Concomitant Valproate (VPA): Wks 1 & 2: 25 mg qod. Wks 3 & 4: 25 mg qd. Wk 5: 50 mg qd. Wk 6: 100 mg qd. Wk 7: 150 mg qd. Maint (Wk 8 & Onward): 200-250 mg qd. Patients Not Taking Carbamazepine, Phenytoin, Phenobarbital, Primidone, or VPA: Wks 1 & 2: 25 mg qd. Wks 3 & 4: 50 mg qd. Wk 5: 100 mg qd. Wk 6: 150 mg qd. Wk 7: 200 mg qd. Maint (Wk 8 & Onward): 300-400 mg qd. Patients Taking Carbamazepine, Phenytoin, Phenobarbital, Primidone w/o VPA: Wks 1 & 2: 50 mg qd. Wks 3 & 4: 100 mg qd. Wk 5: 200 mg qd. Wk 6: 300 mg qd. Wk 7: 400 mg qd. Maint (Wk 8 & Onward): 400-600 mg qd. Dose increases	◎C ❁> Serious rashes, including Stevens-Johnson syndrome reported. H R

Continued on Next Page

NAME	FORM/STRENGTH	DOSAGE	COMMENTS
Lamotrigine (Lamictal XR) *Continued*		at Wk 8 or later should not exceed 100 mg qd at wkly intervals. **Conversion to Monotherapy:** See PI.	
Levetiracetam (Keppra XR)	**Tab,ER:** 500 mg, 750 mg	**Partial Onset Seizures: Adults & Peds: ≥16 yo:** Initial: 1000 mg qd. **Titrate:** Adjust dose in increments of 1000 mg q2wks. **Max:** 3000 mg/d.	●C ❄v R
Levetiracetam (Keppra)	**Inj:** 500 mg/ml; **Sol:** 100 mg/ml; **Tab:** 250 mg, 500 mg, 750 mg, 1000 mg	**Adults: ≥16 yo: PO/IV: Partial Onset Seizures/Juvenile Myoclonic Epilepsy (JME)/Primary Generalized Tonic-Clonic Seizures (PGTC):** Initial: 500 mg bid. **Titrate:** Increase q2wks by 1000 mg/d. **Max:** 3 gm/d. **Replacement Therapy:** IV: Initial total daily dosage & frequency should equal total daily dosage & frequency of PO therapy. **Peds:** PO: JME: Initial: 500 mg bid. **Titrate:** Increase q2wks by 1000 mg/d. **Max:** 3 gm/d. **Partial Onset Seizures (4-<16 yo) or PGTC (6-<16 yo):** PO: Initial: 10 mg/kg bid. **Titrate:** Increase q2wks by 20 mg/kg/d. **Max:** 30 mg/kg bid. **Partial Onset Seizures: <4 yo:** Refer to PI.	●C ❄v R
Oxcarbazepine (Trileptal)	**Susp:** 300 mg/5 ml; **Tab:** 150 mg, 300 mg, 600 mg	**Partial Seizures: Monotherapy: Adults:** Initial: 300 mg bid. **Titrate:** Increase by 300 mg/d q3d. **Maint:** 1200 mg/d. **4-16 yo:** Initial: 4-5 mg/kg/d bid. **Titrate:** Increase by 5 mg/kg/d q3d. **Maint:** Refer to PI. **Adjunct Therapy: Adults:** Initial: 300 mg bid. **Titrate:** Increase wkly by max of 600 mg/d. **Maint:** 600 mg bid. **4-16 yo:** Initial: 4-5 mg/kg bid. **Max:** 600 mg/d. **Titrate:** Increase over 2 wks. **Maint:** 20-29 kg: 900 mg/d. **29.1-39 kg:**	●C ❄v R

		1200 mg/d. **>39 kg:** 1800 mg/d. **2-<4 yo: Initial:** 4-5 mg/kg bid. **Max:** 600 mg/d. **<20 kg: Initial:** 8-10 mg/kg bid. **Max:** 60 mg/kg/d. **Conversion to Monotherapy: Adults: Initial:** 300 mg bid while reducing other AEDs. **Titrate:** Increase wkly by 600 mg/d. **Maint:** 2400 mg/d. **4-16 yo: Initial:** 4-5 mg/kg bid while reducing other AEDs. **Titrate:** Increase wkly by max of 10 mg/kg/d to target dose. Withdraw other AEDs over 3-6 wks.	
Pregabalin CV (Lyrica)	**Cap:** 25 mg, 50 mg, 75 mg, 100 mg, 150 mg, 200 mg, 225 mg, 300 mg; **Sol:** 20 mg/ml	**Partial Onset Seizures: Adults: Initial:** 150 mg/d divided bid-tid. **Titrate:** May increase based on response & tolerability up to 600 mg/d. **Max:** 600 mg/d. **D/C:** Taper over a minimum of 1 wk.	⊛C ❄v R
Primidone (Mysoline)	**Tab:** 50 mg, 250 mg	**Grand Mal/Psychomotor/Focal Seizures: Adults & Peds: ≥8 yo: No Prior Antiepileptic Therapy: Initial/Titrate: Days 1-3:** 100-125 mg qhs. **Days 4-6:** 100-125 mg bid. **Days 7-9:** 100-125 mg tid. **Day 10/Maint:** 250 mg tid. **Max:** 500 mg qid. **Prior Antiepileptic Therapy: Initial:** 100-125 mg qhs. **Titrate:** Increase gradually to maint as other drug is d/c over ≥2 wks. **Max:** 2 gm/d. **<8 yo: Initial/Titrate: Days 1-3:** 50 mg qhs. **Days 4-6:** 50 mg bid. **Days 7-9:** 100 mg bid. **Day 10/Maint:** 125-250 mg tid or 10-25 mg/kg/d in divided doses.	⊛N ❄v

NAME	FORM/STRENGTH	DOSAGE	COMMENTS
Topiramate (Topamax, Topamax Sprinkle Capsules)	**Cap:** 15 mg, 25 mg; **Tab:** 25 mg, 50 mg, 100 mg, 200 mg	**Partial Onset/Tonic-Clonic Seizures: Monotherapy: Adults & Peds: ≥10 yo: Initial:** 25 mg qam & qpm x 1 wk. **Titrate:** Refer to PI. **Usual:** 200 mg bid. **2-<10 yo:** Based on wt. **Initial:** 25mg/day qpm x 1 wk. **Titrate:** Refer to PI. **Max Maint Dose:** 25-50mg/day weekly increments. **Partial Onset/Tonic-Clonic/Lennox-Gastaut Seizures: Adjunctive Therapy: Adults & Peds: ≥17 yo: Initial:** 25-50 mg/d. **Titrate:** Increase by 25-50 mg/wk. **Usual:** 100-200 mg bid (partial seizures) or 200 mg bid (tonic-clonic seizures). **Max:** 1600 mg/d. **Peds: 2-16 yo: Initial:** 25 mg or 1-3 mg/kg/d qpm x 1 wk. **Titrate:** Increase by 1-3 mg/kg/d q1-2wks. **Usual:** 5-9 mg/kg/d given bid.	▣D ✵> R
Vigabatrin (Sabril)	**Pow:** 500 mg/pkt; **Tab:** 500 mg	**Refractory Complex Partial Seizures: Adults: Tab: Initial:** 500 mg bid (1 gm/d). **Titrate:** Increase by 500 mg wkly depending on response. **Maint:** 1.5 gm bid (3 gm/d). **Infantile Spasms: Peds: 1 mth-2 yo: Pow: Initial:** 50 mg/kg/d in 2 divided doses. **Titrate:** Increase by 25-50 mg/kg/d q3d. **Max:** 150 mg/kg/d in 2 divided doses. Gradually taper to d/c.	▣C ✵v R W [106]

Antidepressant Agents

5-HT, AGONIST & COMBINATION

| Vilazodone HCl (Viibryd) | **Tab:** 10 mg, 20 mg, 40 mg | **Adults: Initial:** 10 mg qd x 7d. **Titrate:** Increase to 20 mg qd x 7d, then increase to 40 mg qd. **Usual:** 40 mg qd. Reassess periodically. **D/C of Therapy:** Reduce dose gradually. Take w/ food. | ⒸC ❄> W [29] |

DIBENZAPINE DERIVATIVES

| Olanzapine (Zyprexa, Zyprexa Zydis) | **Tab:** 2.5 mg, 5 mg, 7.5 mg, 10 mg, 15 mg, 20 mg; **Tab,Dissolve:** (Zydis) 5 mg, 10 mg, 15 mg, 20 mg | **Combination Therapy w/ Fluoxetine for Treatment-Resistant Depression: Adults: PO: Initial:** 5 mg qd olanzapine and 20 mg qd fluoxetine given in pm. **Range:** 5-20 mg olanzapine and 20-50 mg fluoxetine. **Max:** 18 mg olanzapine and 75 mg fluoxetine. **Predisposition to Hypotension/Hepatic Impairment/Slow Metabolizers:** See PI. | ⒸC ❄v H W [30] |
| Quetiapine Fumarate (Seroquel XR) | **Tab,ER:** 50 mg, 150 mg, 200 mg, 300 mg, 400 mg | **Adults: Adjunct for MDD:** Give qd in pm. **Initial:** 50 mg/d. **Titrate:** May increase to 150 mg/d on Day 3. **Max:** 300 mg/d. | ⒸC ❄v H W [29, 30] |

NAME	FORM/STRENGTH	DOSAGE	COMMENTS
DOPAMINE/NOREPINEPHRINE REUPTAKE INHIBITORS			
Bupropion HCl (Budeprion SR, Wellbutrin, Wellbutrin SR)	**Tab:** 75 mg, 100 mg; (Wellbutrin SR) **Tab,ER:** 100 mg, 150 mg, 200 mg; (Budeprion SR) **Tab,ER:** 100 mg, 150 mg	**Adults: Tab: Initial:** 100 mg bid. **Usual:** 100 mg tid. **Max:** 450 mg/d. **Tab,ER: Initial:** 150 mg qam. **Usual:** 150 mg bid. **Max:** 200 mg bid.	▣C ❋v H R W [29]
Bupropion HCl (Budeprion XL, Wellbutrin XL)	(Budeprion XL) **Tab,ER:** 150 mg; (Wellbutrin XL) **Tab,ER:** 150 mg, 300 mg	**Adults: Initial:** 150 mg qam, may increase to 300 mg qam on Day 4. **Usual:** 300 mg qam. **Max:** 450 mg/d.	▣C ❋v H R W [29]
Bupropion Hydrobromide (Aplenzin)	**Tab,ER:** 174 mg, 348 mg, 522 mg	**Adults:** Give in am. Swallow whole. **Initial:** 174 mg qd. **Titrate:** May increase to 348 mg qd as early as Day 4 if tolerated. There should be an interval of ≥24h between successive doses. **Usual:** 348 mg qd. **Max:** 522 mg/d given as single dose if no clinical improvement after several wks. **Maint:** Reassess periodically for need of maint treatment and dose. **Switching from Wellbutrin, Wellbutrin SR, or Wellbutrin XL:** See PI.	▣C ❋v H R W [29]

PARTIAL D₂/5-HT₁ₐ AGONIST/5-HT₂ₐ ANTAGONIST

Aripiprazole (Abilify, Abilify Discmelt)	**Sol:** 1 mg/ml; **Tab:** 2 mg, 5 mg, 10 mg, 15 mg, 20 mg, 30 mg; **Tab,Dissolve:** (Discmelt) 10 mg, 15 mg	**Adjunctive Treatment for Major Depressive Disorder:** **Adults: PO: Initial:** 2-5 mg/d. **Titrate:** Dose adjustments of up to 5 mg/d should occur gradually at intervals of no less than 1 wk. **Usual:** 2-15 mg/d. **Oral Sol:** Can be substituted for tabs on mg-per-mg basis up to 25 mg. Patients receiving 30-mg tabs should receive 25 mg of sol. Adjust dose w/ CYP3A4/CYP2D6 inhibitors, CYP3A4 inducers, & in poor CYP2D6 metabolizers.	⊞C ❀v W [29, 30]

SEROTONIN/NOREPINEPHRINE REUPTAKE INHIBITORS

Desvenlafaxine (Pristiq)	**Tab,ER:** 50 mg, 100 mg	**Adults: Usual:** 50 mg qd.	⊞C ❀v H R W [29]
Duloxetine HCl (Cymbalta)	**Cap,Delay:** 20 mg, 30 mg, 60 mg	**Adults: Initial:** 20 mg bid-60 mg/d (given qd or 30 mg bid) or 30 mg qd x 1 wk before increasing to 60 mg qd. **Maint:** 60 mg qd. **Max:** 120 mg/d.	⊞C ❀v H R W [29]
Venlafaxine HCl (Effexor XR)	**Cap,ER:** 37.5 mg, 75 mg, 150 mg	**Adults: Initial:** 75 mg/d or 37.5 mg/d x 4-7d and then increase to 75 mg/d. **Titrate:** Increase by increments of up to 75 mg/d at intervals ≥4d. **Max:** 225 mg/d.	⊞C ❀v H R W [29]
Venlafaxine HCl (Effexor)	**Tab:** 25 mg, 37.5 mg, 50 mg, 75 mg, 100 mg	**Adults: Initial:** 75 mg/d given bid-tid w/ food. **Titrate:** May increase to 150 mg/d. If needed, increase up to 225 mg/d. Increase by ≤75 mg/d q4d. **Max:** 375 mg/d given tid.	⊞C ❀v H R W [29]

NAME	FORM/STRENGTH	DOSAGE	COMMENTS
SSRIs & COMBINATIONS			
Citalopram HBr (Celexa)	**Sol:** 10 mg/5 ml; **Tab:** 10 mg, 20 mg, 40 mg	**Adults: Initial:** 20 mg qd. **Titrate:** Increase dose to 40 mg at an interval ≥1 wk. **Max:** 40 mg/d. **≥60 yo/Hepatic Impairment/CYP2C19 Poor Metabolizers/CYP2C19 Inhibitors: Max:** 20 mg/d.	⊙C ❄v H W [29]
Escitalopram Oxalate (Lexapro)	**Sol:** 5 mg/5 ml; **Tab:** 5 mg, 10 mg, 20 mg	**Adults & Peds: ≥12 yo: Initial:** 10 mg qd. **Titrate:** May increase to 20 mg after ≥1 wk (adults) or ≥3 wks (peds).	⊙C ❄> H W [29]
Fluoxetine HCl (Prozac)	**Cap:** 10 mg, 20 mg, 40 mg	**Adults: Initial:** 20 mg qam. **Titrate:** Increase dose after several wks if clinical improvement is insufficient. Give doses >20 mg/d qam or bid (am & noon). **Max:** 80 mg/d. **Peds: ≥8 yo & Higher Wt Peds: Initial:** 10 or 20 mg/d. After 1 wk at 10 mg/d, may increase to 20 mg/d. **Lower Wt Peds: Initial:** 10 mg/d. **Titrate:** May increase to 20 mg/d after several wks if clinical improvement not observed.	⊙C ❄v H W [29]
Olanzapine/Fluoxetine HCl (Symbyax)	**Cap:** 3-25 mg, 6-25 mg, 6-50 mg, 12-25 mg, 12-50 mg	**Depressive Episodes Associated w/Bipolar I Disorder/ Treatment-Resistant Depression: Adults: Initial:** 6-25 mg qpm. **Titrate:** Adjust dose based on efficacy and tolerability. **Max:** 18-75 mg/d. **Hypotension Risk/Slow Metabolizers/ Olanzapine-Sensitive/Pregnant:** Adjust dose.	⊙C ❄v H W [29, 30]
Paroxetine HCl (Paxil CR)	**Tab,CR:** 12.5 mg, 25 mg, 37.5 mg	**Adults: Initial:** 25 mg qam. **Titrate:** May increase by 12.5 mg/d at intervals of ≥1 wk. **Max:** 62.5 mg/d.	⊙D ❄> H R W [29]

Paroxetine HCl (Paxil)	**Susp:** 10 mg/5 ml; **Tab:** 10 mg, 20 mg, 30 mg, 40 mg	**Adults: Initial:** 20 mg qam. **Titrate:** May increase by 10 mg/d at intervals of ≥1 wk. **Max:** 50 mg/d.	⊙D ❀> **H R W** [29]
Paroxetine Mesylate (Pexeva)	**Tab:** 10 mg, 20 mg, 30 mg, 40 mg	**Adults: Initial:** 20 mg/d. **Max:** 50 mg/d.	⊙C ❀> **H R W** [29]
Sertraline HCl (Zoloft)	**Sol:** 20 mg/ml; **Tab:** 25 mg, 50 mg, 100 mg	**Adults: Initial:** 50 mg qd. **Titrate:** Adjust wkly. **Max:** 200 mg/d.	⊙C ❀> **H W** [29]

TETRACYCLICS

Mirtazapine (Remeron, Remeron SolTab)	**Tab,Dissolve:** (SolTab) 15 mg, 30 mg, 45 mg; **Tab:** 15 mg, 30 mg, 45 mg	**Adults: Initial:** 15 mg qhs. **Titrate:** Increase q1-2wks. **Max:** 45 mg qd.	⊙C ❀> **W** [29]

TRICYCLIC ANTIDEPRESSANTS

Amitriptyline	**Tab:** 10 mg, 25 mg, 50 mg, 75 mg, 100 mg, 150 mg	**Adults: Initial:** (Outpatient) 75 mg/d in divided doses or 50-100 mg qhs. (Inpatient) 100 mg/d. **Titrate:** (Outpatient) Increase by 25-50 mg qhs. (Inpatient) Increase to 200 mg/d. **Maint:** 50-100 mg qhs. **Max:** 150 mg/d (3 mg/kg/d for a 50 kg patient). **Peds:** ≥**12 yo & Elderly:** 10 mg tid & 20 mg qhs.	⊙C ❀v **W** [29]
Desipramine (Norpramin)	**Tab:** 10 mg, 25 mg, 50 mg, 75 mg, 100 mg, 150 mg	**Adults: Usual:** 100-200 mg qd. **Max:** 300 mg/d. **Adolescents/Elderly: Usual:** 25-100 mg qd. **Max:** 150 mg/d.	⊙N ❀> **W** [29]

249 KEY: ⊙ PREGNANCY RATING; ❀ BREASTFEEDING SAFETY; H HEPATIC ADJUSTMENT; R RENAL ADJUSTMENT

NAME	FORM/STRENGTH	DOSAGE	COMMENTS
Imipramine HCl (Tofranil)	Tab: 10 mg, 25 mg, 50 mg	**Adults: Inpatient: Initial:** 100 mg/d in divided doses. **Titrate:** May increase to 200 mg/d, then to 250-300 mg/d after 2 wks if needed. **Outpatient: Initial:** 75 mg/d. **Titrate:** Increase to 150 mg/d. **Maint:** 50-150 mg/d. **Max:** 200 mg/d. **Adolescents/Elderly: Initial:** 30-40 mg/d. **Max:** 100 mg/d.	◐N ❋v **H R W** [29]
Nortriptyline HCl (Pamelor)	Cap: 10 mg, 25 mg, 50 mg, 75 mg; Sol: 10 mg/5 ml	**Adults: Usual:** 25 mg tid-qid. **Max:** 150 mg/d. **Adolescents:** 30-50 mg/d.	◐N ❋> **W** [29]

MISCELLANEOUS

NAME	FORM/STRENGTH	DOSAGE	COMMENTS
Trazodone HCl (Oleptro)	Tab, ER: 150 mg, 300 mg	**Adults: Initial:** 150 mg hs. **Titrate:** May increase by 75 mg/d q3d. **Max:** 375 mg/d. Take on an empty stomach.	◐C ❋> **W** [29]

Antiparkinson's Agents
ANTICHOLINERGIC AGENT

NAME	FORM/STRENGTH	DOSAGE	COMMENTS
Benztropine Mesylate (Cogentin)	Inj: 1 mg/mL; Tab: 0.5 mg, 1 mg, 2 mg	**Adults:** Individualize dose. **Titrate:** May increase by 0.5 mg/d q5-6d. **Idiopathic Parkinsonism: Initial:** 0.5-1 mg qhs. **Postencephalitic Parkinsonism:** 2 mg/d given in ≥1 doses. **Extrapyramidal Disorders:** 1-4 mg/d given qd-bid. D/C and reevaluate necessity after 1-2 wks; may reinstitute if disorders recur. **Acute Dystonic Reactions: (Inj)** 1-2 mg IM/IV.	◐N ❋>

CHOLINESTERASE INHIBITOR

Rivastigmine Tartrate (Exelon)	**Cap:** 1.5 mg, 3 mg, 4.5 mg, 6 mg; **Patch:** 4.6 mg/24h, 9.5 mg/24h; **Sol:** 2 mg/ml	**Dementia Associated w/ Parkinson's Disease: Adults: PO: Initial:** 1.5 mg bid. **Titrate:** May increase by 1.5 mg q4wks. **Usual:** 3-12 mg/d. **Patch: Initial:** 4.6 mg/24h qd. **Maint:** May increase dose after 4 wks. **Max:** 9.5 mg/24h if well tolerated. **Switching from PO:** See PI.	⊙B ❈v

COMT INHIBITOR

Entacapone (Comtan)	**Tab:** 200 mg	**Adults:** 200 mg w/ each levodopa/carbidopa dose. **Max:** 1600 mg/d.	⊙C ❈> H

DOPAMINE AGONISTS

Bromocriptine Mesylate (Parlodel)	**Cap:** 5 mg; **Tab:** 2.5 mg	**Adults: Initial:** 1.25 mg bid. **Titrate:** Increase by 2.5 mg/d q2-4wks. **Max:** 100 mg/d.	⊙B ❈v
Pramipexole Dihydrochloride (Mirapex ER)	**Tab,ER:** 0.375 mg, 0.75 mg, 1.5 mg, 2.25 mg, 3 mg, 3.75 mg, 4.5 mg	**Adults: Initial:** 0.375 mg qd. **Titrate:** May increase q5-7d, first to 0.75 mg/d and then by 0.75 mg increments based on efficacy and tolerability. **Max:** 4.5 mg/d. **D/C:** Taper dose gradually over 1 wk. **Dose Adjustment:** No more frequently than at weekly intervals. **Switching from Immediate-Release Dosing (IR):** See PI.	⊙C ❈v R
Pramipexole Dihydrochloride (Mirapex)	**Tab:** 0.125 mg, 0.25 mg, 0.5 mg, 0.75 mg, 1 mg, 1.5 mg	**Adults: Initial:** 0.125 mg tid. **Titrate:** Increase q5-7d (eg, **Wk 2:** 0.25 mg tid; **Wk 3:** 0.5 mg tid; **Wk 4:** 0.75 mg tid; **Wk 5:** 1 mg tid; **Wk 6:** 1.25 mg tid; **Wk 7:** 1.5 mg tid). **Maint:** 0.5-1.5 mg tid. **Max:** 1.5 mg tid.	⊙C ❈v R

NAME	FORM/STRENGTH	DOSAGE	COMMENTS
Ropinirole HCl (Requip XL)	**Tab:** 0.25 mg, 0.5 mg, 1 mg, 2 mg, 3 mg, 4 mg, 5 mg	**Adults: Initial:** 0.25 mg tid. **Titrate/Maint:** Increase wkly by 0.25 mg tid x 4 wks. After wk 4, increase wkly by 1.5 mg/d up to 9 mg/d, then by 3 mg/d wkly to 24 mg/d. **Max:** 24 mg/d. **Withdrawal:** Decrease dose to bid x 4d, then qd x 3d.	●C ☀v
Ropinirole HCl (Requip XL)	**Tab,ER:** 2 mg, 4 mg, 8 mg, 12 mg	**Adults: Initial:** 2 mg qd x 1-2 wks. **Titrate:** May increase by 2 mg/d at ≥1-wk interval, depending on response & tolerability. **Max:** 24 mg/d. Swallow whole. **Switching from Immediate-Release (IR) to XL:** Initial dose should match total daily dose of IR formulation. See PI for more info.	●C ☀v

DOPAMINE PRECURSOR/DOPA-DECARBOXYLASE INHIBITOR

NAME	FORM/STRENGTH	DOSAGE	COMMENTS
Carbidopa/Levodopa (Sinemet, Sinemet CR)	**Tab:** 10-100 mg, 25-100 mg, 25-250 mg; **Tab,ER:** (CR) 25-100 mg, 50-200 mg	**Adults: ≥18 yo: Tab: Initial:** 10-100 mg tab tid-qid or 25-100 mg tab tid. **Titrate:** May increase by 1 tab qd or qod until 8 tabs/d. **Maint:** 70-100 mg/d carbidopa required. **Max:** 200 mg/d carbidopa. **Conversion from Levodopa:** See PI. **Tab,ER: No Prior Levodopa Use: Initial:** 50-200 mg tab bid at intervals ≥6h. **Titrate:** May increase/decrease dose or interval accordingly. Adjust dose at interval ≥3d. **Usual:** 400-1600 mg/d levodopa, given in 4-8h intervals w/a. **Conversion to Tab,ER/Addition of Other Antiparkinson Medication/Interruption of Therapy:** See PI.	●C ☀>

DOPAMINE PRECURSOR/DOPA-DECARBOXYLASE INHIBITOR/COMT INHIBITOR

Carbidopa/Entacapone/ Levodopa (Stalevo)	**Tab:** 12.5/200/50 mg, 18.75/200/75 mg, 25/200/100 mg, 31.25/200/125 mg, 37.5/200/150 mg, 50/200/200 mg	**Adults:** ≤75 yo: Individualize dose. **Titrate:** Adjust according to desired therapeutic response. **Currently Taking Carbidopa/Levodopa & Entacapone:** May switch directly to corresponding strength of levodopa/ carbidopa/entacapone. **Currently Taking Carbidopa/Levodopa but not Entacapone:** 1st titrate individually w/ carbidopa/ levodopa product & entacapone product, then transfer to corresponding dose. **Max:** 8 tabs/d (Stalevo 50/Stalevo 75/Stalevo 100/Stalevo 125/Stalevo 150) or 6 tabs/d (Stalevo 200).	⊞C ✿>

MAOIs

Rasagiline (Azilect)	**Tab:** 0.5 mg, 1 mg	**Adults:** Monotherapy: 1 mg qd. **Adjunctive Therapy: Initial:** 0.5 mg qd. **Titrate:** May increase to 1 mg qd. Adjust dose of levodopa w/ concomitant use. **Concomitant Ciprofloxacin or Other CYP1A2 Inhibitors:** 0.5 mg qd.	⊞C ✿> H
Selegiline HCl (Eldepryl)	**Cap:** 5 mg; **Tab:** 5 mg	**Adults:** 5 mg bid, at breakfast & lunch. **Max:** 10 mg/d.	⊞C ✿v

NAME	FORM/STRENGTH	DOSAGE	COMMENTS

Antipsychotic Agents
BENZISOXAZOLE DERIVATIVE

NAME	FORM/STRENGTH	DOSAGE	COMMENTS
Iloperidone (Fanapt)	**Tab:** 1 mg, 2 mg, 4 mg, 6 mg, 8 mg, 10 mg, 12 mg	**Adults: Initial:** 1 mg bid. **Titrate: Day 2:** 2 mg bid. **Day 3:** 4 mg bid. **Day 4:** 6 mg bid. **Day 5:** 8 mg bid. **Day 6:** 10 mg bid. **Day 7:** 12 mg bid. **Range:** 6-12 mg bid. **Max:** 12 mg bid (24 mg/d). **Concomitant Strong CYP2D6 or CYP3A4 Inhibitors/Poor CYP2D6 Metabolizers:** Reduce dose by 50%. **Maint:** Responding patients may continue beyond acute response; periodically reassess need for maintenance treatment. **Reinitiation of Treatment:** Follow initial titration schedule if have had an interval off for >3d. **Switching From Other Antipsychotics:** Minimize overlapping period of antipsychotics.	●C ❄v H W [30]
Paliperidone Palmitate (Invega Sustenna)	**Inj,ER:** 39 mg, 78 mg, 117 mg, 156 mg, 234 mg	**Schizophrenia: Adults: Initial:** 234 mg IM on Day 1, then 156 mg 1 wk later (in deltoid muscle). **Maint:** 117 mg/mth (in deltoid or gluteal muscle). **Range:** 39-234 mg based on tolerability and/or efficacy. Switching from other antipsychotics: See PI.	●C ❄v R W [30]
Paliperidone (Invega)	**Tab,ER:** 1.5 mg, 3 mg, 6 mg, 9 mg	**Adults: Schizophrenia:** 6 mg qd. **Titrate:** If indicated may increase by 3mg/d; dose increases >6mg/d should be made at intervals of >5d. **Usual:** 3-12 mg/d. **Max:** 12mg/d. **Schizoaffective Disorder:** 6 mg qd. **Titrate:** If indicated may increase by 3 mg/d at intervals of >4d. **Usual:** 3-12 mg/d. **Max:** 12 mg/d. **Peds: 12-17 yo: Schizophrenia:**	●C ❄v R W [30]

		3 mg qd. **Titrate:** If indicated may increase by 3 mg/d at intervals of >5d. **Max:** **<51 kg:** 6 mg/d. **≥51 kg:** 12 mg/d.	
Risperidone (Risperdal Consta)	**Inj:** 12.5 mg, 25 mg, 37.5 mg, 50 mg	**Adults: Schizophrenia:** In risperidone-naive patients, establish tolerability w/ PO risperidone prior to treatment. Give 1st inj w/ PO risperidone or other antipsychotic, continue x 3 wks, then d/c PO. **Usual:** 25 mg IM q2wks. **Titrate:** May increase to 37.5 mg or 50 mg. Increase at intervals of no more than q4wks. **Max:** 50 mg q2wks. **Elderly:** 25 mg IM q2wks. **Poor Tolerability: Initial:** 12.5 mg IM. **Switching from Other Antipsychotics/ Concomitant Use w/ Enzyme Inducers/Fluoxetine/ Paroxetine:** See PI.	⊚C ❋v **H R W** [30]
Risperidone (Risperdal, Risperdal M-Tab)	**Sol:** 1 mg/ml; **Tab:** 0.25 mg, 0.5 mg, 1 mg, 2 mg, 3 mg, 4 mg; **Tab,Dissolve:** 0.5 mg, 1 mg, 2 mg, 3 mg, 4 mg	**Schizophrenia: Adults: Initial:** 2 mg/d given qd or bid. **Titrate:** Adjust dose at intervals not <24h, in increments of 1-2 mg/d to recommended dose of 4-8 mg/d. **Range:** 4-16 mg/d. **Max:** 16 mg/d. **Maint Therapy:** 2-8 mg/d. **Peds: 13-17 yo: Initial:** 0.5 mg qd in am or pm. **Titrate:** Adjust dose in increments of 0.5 or 1 mg/d & at intervals not <24h as tolerated to a recommended dose of 3 mg/d. **Max:** 6 mg/d. **Elderly/Debilitated/Hypotension/Severe Renal or Hepatic Impairment: Initial:** 0.5 mg bid. **Titration:** See PI. **Coadministration w/ Enzyme Inducers/ Fluoxetine/Paroxetine:** May affect plasma concentrations; titrate accordingly.	⊚C ❋v **H R W** [30]

NAME	FORM/STRENGTH	DOSAGE	COMMENTS
Ziprasidone (Geodon)	**Cap:** 20 mg, 40 mg, 60 mg, 80 mg; **Inj:** 20 mg/ml	**Adults: Schizophrenia: PO: Initial:** 20 mg bid w/ food. **Titrate:** Adjust dose at intervals not <2d. **Max:** 80 mg bid. **Acute Agitation in Schizophrenia: IM:** 10 mg q2h or 20 mg q4h. **Max:** 40 mg/d x 3d.	⊛C ❈v W [30]

BENZOISOTHIAZOL DERIVATIVE

NAME	FORM/STRENGTH	DOSAGE	COMMENTS
Lurasidone HCl (Latuda)	**Tab:** 20 mg, 40 mg, 80 mg, 120 mg	**Adults: Initial:** 40 mg qd. **Max:** 160 mg/d. **Concomitant Use w/Potential CYP3A4 Inhibitors/Inducers: Initial:** 20 mg/d. **Concomitant Use w/ Moderate CYP3A4 Inhibitors (eg, diltiazem): Max:** 80 mg/d. Take w/ food (at least 350 calories).	⊛B ❈v H R W [30]

DIBENZAPINE DERIVATIVES

NAME	FORM/STRENGTH	DOSAGE	COMMENTS
Asenapine (Saphris)	**Tab,SL:** 5 mg, 10 mg	**Adults: Schizophrenia: Acute Treatment: Initial/Usual:** 5 mg bid. **Titrate:** May increase up to 10 mg bid after 1 wk based on tolerability. **Max:** 10 mg bid.	⊛C ❈v H W [30]
Clozapine (Clozaril)	**Tab:** (Generic) 25 mg, 50 mg, 100 mg; (Clozaril) 25 mg, 100 mg	**Schizophrenia/Suicidal Behavior Risk Reduction: Adults: Initial:** 12.5 mg qd-bid. **Titrate:** Increase by 25-50 mg/d, up to 300-450 mg/d by end of 2 wks, then increase once or twice wkly in increments ≤100 mg. **Usual:** 300-600 mg/d on a divided basis. **Titrate:** May increase to 600-900 mg/d. **Max:** 900 mg/d. To d/c, gradually reduce dose over 1-2 wks.	⊛B ❈v W [26, 30]

Clozapine (Fazaclo)	**Tab,Dissolve:** 12.5 mg, 25 mg, 100 mg, 150 mg, 200 mg	**Schizophrenia/Suicidal Behavior Risk Reduction: Adults: Initial:** 12.5 mg qd-bid. **Titrate:** Increase by 25-50 mg/d, up to 300-450 mg/d by end of 2 wks, then increase once or twice wkly by increments ≤100 mg. **Usual:** 300-600 mg/d given on a divided basis. **Titrate:** May increase to 600-900 mg/d. **Max:** 900 mg/d. To d/c, gradually reduce dose over 1-2 wks.	⊞B ❄v W [26]
Olanzapine (Zyprexa, Zyprexa Zydis)	**Inj:** 10 mg; **Tab:** 2.5 mg, 5 mg, 7.5 mg, 10 mg, 15 mg, 20 mg; **Tab,Dissolve:** (Zydis) 5 mg, 10 mg, 15 mg, 20 mg	**Schizophrenia: Adults: PO: Initial/Usual:** 5-10 mg qd. **Titrate:** Adjust wkly by 5 mg/d. **Max:** 20 mg/d. **Peds: 13-17 yo: PO: Initial/ Usual:** 2.5-5 mg qd. **Titrate:** Adjust by 2.5-5 mg qd. **Max:** 20 mg/d. Periodically reassess to determine the need for maint treatment. Use lowest dose to maintain remission. **Debilitated/Predisposition to Hypotension/Slow Metabolizers: PO: Initial:** 5 mg qd. **Titrate:** Caution w/ dose escalation. **Agitation Associated w/ Schizophrenia: IM: Initial:** 10 mg. May initiate PO therapy when clinically appropriate. **Range:** 2.5-10 mg. **Max:** 3 doses of 10 mg q2-4h. **Geriatric Patients: IM:** 5 mg. **Debilitated/Predisposed to Hypotension: IM:** 2.5 mg.	⊞C ❄v H W [30]

NAME	FORM/STRENGTH	DOSAGE	COMMENTS
Olanzapine (Zyprexa Relprevv)	**Inj,ER:** 210 mg, 300 mg, 405 mg	**Schizophrenia: Adults: IM: Usual:** 150-300 mg q2wks or 405 mg q4wks. Refer to PI for recommended dosing based on corresponding oral olanzapine doses. **Max:** 405 mg q4wks or 300 mg q2wks. **Debilitated/Predisposition to Hypotension/Slow Metabolizers/Pharmacodynamic Sensitivity:** See PI.	▣C ☼v W [30]
Quetiapine Fumarate (Seroquel XR)	**Tab,ER:** 50 mg, 150 mg, 200 mg, 300 mg, 400 mg	**Adults: Schizophrenia:** Give qd, preferably in pm. **Initial:** 300 mg/d. **Titrate:** May increase to 400-800 mg/d depending on response & tolerance. Dose increases may be made at intervals ≥1 day and in increments up to 300 mg/d. Reevaluate periodically. **Max:** 800 mg/d.	▣C ☼v H W [29, 30]
Quetiapine Fumarate (Seroquel)	**Tab:** 25 mg, 50 mg, 100 mg, 200 mg, 300 mg, 400 mg	**Schizophrenia: Adults: Initial:** 25 mg bid. **Titrate:** Increase by 25-50 mg divided bid-tid on Days 2 & 3, up to target dose of 300-400 mg/d by Day 4. May adjust by 25-50 mg divided bid at ≥2-d intervals. **Max:** 800 mg/d. **Peds: 13-17 yo:** Give bid-tid. **Day 1:** 50 mg/d. **Day 2:** 100 mg/d. **Day 3:** 200 mg/d. **Day 4:** 300 mg/d. **Day 5:** 400 mg/d. **Titrate:** Increase by increments ≤100 mg/d. **Max:** 800 mg/d.	▣C ☼v H W [29, 30]

PARTIAL D₂/5-HT₁ₐ AGONIST/5-HT₂ₐ ANTAGONIST

Aripiprazole (Abilify, Abilify Discmelt)	**Inj:** 7.5 mg/ml; **Sol:** 1 mg/ml; **Tab:** 2 mg, 5 mg, 10 mg, 15 mg, 20 mg, 30 mg; **Tab,Dissolve:** (Discmelt) 10 mg, 15 mg	**Schizophrenia: PO: Adults: Initial/Target:** 10 or 15 mg qd. **Titrate:** Should not increase before 2 wks. **Usual:** 10-30 mg/d. **Peds: 13-17 yo: Initial:** 2 mg/d. **Titrate:** May increase to 5 mg/d after 2d, then to target of 10 mg/d after 2 add'l days. May increase in 5 mg increments thereafter. **Usual:** 10-30 mg/d. **Oral Sol:** Can be substituted for tabs on mg-per-mg basis up to 25 mg. Patients receiving 30-mg tabs should receive 25 mg of sol. **Agitation Associated w/ Schizophrenia: Adults: IM:** 9.75 mg. **Usual:** 5.25-15 mg. **Max:** 30 mg/d. Not more frequently than q2h. If clinically indicated, may replace w/ PO at 10-30 mg/d ASAP. Adjust dose w/ CYP3A4/CYP2D6 inhibitors, CYP3A4 inducers, & in poor CYP2D6 metabolizers.	⊞C ❄v W [29, 30]

PHENOTHIAZINES

Chlorpromazine HCl	**Inj:** 25 mg/ml; **Tab:** 10 mg, 25 mg, 50 mg, 100 mg, 200 mg	**Adults: Inpatient: Acute Schizophrenic/Manic State: IM:** 25 mg, then 25-50 mg in 1h if needed. **Titrate:** Increase up to 400 mg q4-6h until controlled then switch to PO. **PO: Usual:** 500 mg/d. Gradual increases to ≥2000 mg/d may be needed. **Less Acutely Disturbed: PO:** 25 mg tid. **Titrate:** Gradually increase to 400 mg/d. **Outpatient: PO:** 10 mg tid-qid or 25 mg bid-tid. **More Severe Cases: PO:** 25 mg	⊞N ❄v H R W [30]

Continued on Next Page

NAME	FORM/STRENGTH	DOSAGE	COMMENTS
Chlorpromazine HCl *Continued*		tid. **Titrate:** After 1-2d, increase by 20-50 mg semiwkly until calm. **Prompt Control of Severe Symptoms: Initial:** IM: 25 mg, may repeat in 1h. **Subsequent Doses:** PO: 25-50 mg tid.	
Fluphenazine	**Cnt:** 5 mg/ml; **Inj:** 2.5 mg/ml; **Eli:** 2.5 mg/5 ml, **Tab:** 1 mg, 2.5 mg, 5 mg, 10 mg	**Adults: PO: Initial:** 2.5-10 mg/d given q6-8h. **Max:** 40 mg/d. **Maint:** 1-5 mg qd. **Inj: Initial:** 2.5-10 mg/d IM divided q6-8h. Caution w/ >10 mg/d.	⊕N ❋> W [30]
Perphenazine	**Tab:** 2 mg, 4 mg, 8 mg, 16 mg	**Adults & Peds: ≥12 yo: Outpatients: Initial:** 4-8 mg tid. **Maint:** Reduce to min effective dose. **Inpatients:** 8-16 mg bid-qid. **Max:** 64 mg/d.	⊕N ❋> R W [30]
Thioridazine	**Tab:** 10 mg, 15 mg, 25 mg, 50 mg, 100 mg, 150 mg, 200 mg	**Adults: Initial:** 50-100 mg tid. **Maint:** 200-800 mg/d given bid-qid. **Max:** 800 mg/d. **Peds: Initial:** 0.6 mg/kg/d in divided doses. **Max:** 3 mg/kg/d.	⊕N ❋> QTc prolongation.
Trifluoperazine HCl	**Tab:** 1 mg, 2 mg, 5 mg, 10 mg	**Adults: Initial:** 2-5 mg tid. **Usual:** 15-20 mg/d. **Max:** 40 mg/d or more if needed. **Peds: 6-12 yo: Initial:** 1 mg qd-bid. **Titrate:** Increase gradually until symptoms controlled. **Usual Max:** 15 mg/d.	⊕N ❋v W [30]
THIOXANTHENE DERIVATIVES			
Thiothixene (Navane)	**Cap:** 1 mg, 2 mg, 5 mg, 10 mg	**Adults & Peds: ≥12 yo: Mild Condition: Initial:** 2 mg tid. **Titrate:** May increase to 15 mg/d. **Severe Condition: Initial:** 5 mg bid. **Usual:** 20-30 mg/d. **Max:** 60 mg/d.	⊕N ❋v W [30]

Bipolar Agents

Drug	Forms	Dosing	
Aripiprazole (Abilify, Abilify Discmelt)	**Inj:** 7.5 mg/ml; **Sol:** 1 mg/ml; **Tab:** 2 mg, 5 mg, 10 mg, 15 mg, 20 mg, 30 mg; **Tab,Dissolve:** (Discmelt) 10 mg, 15 mg	**Bipolar I Disorder: Acute Manic & Mixed Episodes: PO: Adults: Initial: Monotherapy:** 15 mg qd. **Adjunct:** 10-15 mg qd. **Target:** 15 mg qd. **Titrate:** May increase to 30 mg/d. **Max:** 30 mg/d. **Peds: 10-17 yo: Initial:** 2 mg/d. **Titrate:** May increase to 5 mg/d after 2d, then to target of 10 mg/d after 2 add'l days. May increase in 5 mg increments thereafter. **Oral Sol:** Can be substituted for tabs on mg-per-mg basis up to 25 mg. Patients receiving 30-mg tabs should receive 25 mg of sol. **Agitation Associated w/ Manic or Mixed Episodes: IM: Adults:** 9.75 mg. **Usual:** 5.25-15 mg. **Max:** 30 mg/d. Not more frequently than q2h. If clinically indicated, may replace w/ PO at 10-30 mg/d ASAP. Adjust dose w/ CYP3A4/CYP2D6 inhibitors, CYP3A4 inducers, & in poor CYP2D6 metabolizers.	⊕C ❅v W [29, 30]
Carbamazepine (Equetro)	**Cap,ER:** 100 mg, 200 mg, 300 mg	**Bipolar I Disorder: Acute Manic & Mixed Episodes: Adults: Initial:** 400 mg/d, given bid. **Titrate:** Adjust in increments of 200 mg/d. **Max:** 1600 mg/d.	⊕D ❅v W [87]
Divalproex Sodium (Depakote)	**Tab,Delay:** 125 mg, 250 mg, 500 mg	**Mania: Adults: Initial:** 750 mg/d in divided doses. **Titrate:** May increase rapidly to clinical effect. **Max:** 60 mg/kg/d.	⊕D ❅v H W [101]
Divalproex Sodium (Depakote ER)	**Tab,ER:** 250 mg, 500 mg	**Mania: Adults: Initial:** 25 mg/kg/d. **Titrate:** May increase rapidly to clinical effect. **Max:** 60 mg/kg/d.	⊕D ❅v W [101]

NAME	FORM/STRENGTH	DOSAGE	COMMENTS
Lamotrigine (Lamictal, Lamictal ODT)	**Chewtab:** 2 mg, 5 mg, 25 mg; **Tab:** 25 mg, 100 mg, 150 mg, 200 mg; **Tab, Dissolve:** 25 mg, 50 mg, 100 mg, 200 mg	**Adults: Patients Not Taking Carbamazepine, Phenytoin, Phenobarbital, Primidone, or VPA: Wks 1 & 2:** 25 mg/d. **Wks 3 & 4:** 50 mg/d. **Wk 5:** 100 mg/d. **Wks 6 & 7:** 200 mg/d. **Concomitant VPA: Wks 1 & 2:** 25 mg qod. **Wks 3 & 4:** 25 mg/d. **Wk 5:** 50 mg/d. **Wks 6 & 7:** 100 mg/d. **Concomitant Carbamazepine, Phenytoin, Phenobarbital, Primidone w/o VPA: Wks 1 & 2:** 50 mg/d. **Wks 3 & 4:** 100 mg/d (divided doses). **Wk 5:** 200 mg/d (divided doses). **Wk 6:** 300 mg/d (divided doses). **Wk 7:** Up to 400 mg/d (divided doses). **After D/C of Psychotropic Drugs Excluding Carbamazepine, Phenytoin, Phenobarbital, Primidone, or VPA:** Maintain current dose. **After D/C of VPA & Current Lamotrigine Dose of 100 mg/d: Wk 1:** 150 mg/d. **Wk 2 & Onward:** 200 mg/d. **After D/C of Carbamazepine, Phenytoin, Phenobarbital, Primidone & Current Lamotrigine Dose of 400 mg/d: Wk 1:** 400 mg/d. **Wk 2:** 300 mg/d. **Wk 3 & Onward:** 200 mg/d.	●C ❄> Serious rashes, Stevens-Johnson syndrome reported. **H R**
Lithium Carbonate	**Cap:** 150 mg, 300 mg, 600 mg; **Tab:** 300 mg; **Sol:** 8 mEq/5 ml	**Adults & Peds: ≥12 yo: Acute Mania:** 600 mg or 10 ml tid. Effective serum levels range 1-1.5 mEq/L; monitor levels twice wkly until stabilized. **Maint:** 300 mg or 5 ml tid-qid to maintain serum levels of 0.6-1.2 mEq/L; monitor levels q2mths.	●D ❄v Lithium toxicity related to serum levels.

Drug	Forms	Dosage	Rating
Lithium Carbonate (Lithobid)	**Tab,ER:** 300 mg, 450 mg; (Lithobid) 300 mg	**Adults & Peds:** ≥12 yo: 900 mg bid or 600 mg tid to achieve effective serum levels of 1-1.5 mEq/L; monitor levels twice wkly until stabilized. **Maint:** 900-1200 mg/d, given bid-tid to maintain serum levels of 0.6-1.2 mEq/L; monitor levels q2mths.	⊕D ❁v Lithium toxicity related to serum levels.
Olanzapine (Zyprexa, Zyprexa Zydis)	**Inj:** 10 mg; **Tab:** 2.5 mg, 5 mg, 7.5 mg, 10 mg, 15 mg, 20 mg; **Tab,Dissolve:** (Zydis) 5 mg, 10 mg, 15 mg, 20 mg	**Adults: Bipolar I Disorder: Acute Manic & Mixed Episodes: Monotherapy: PO: Initial:** 10-15 mg qd. **Range:** 5-20 mg/d. **Titrate:** May adjust by 5 mg/d at intervals of not <24h. **Max:** 20 mg/d. **Maint Monotherapy: PO:** 5-20 mg qd. **Combination Therapy w/ Lithium or Valproate: PO: Initial:** 10 mg qd. **Range:** 5-20 mg/d. **Max:** 20 mg/d. **Peds: 13-17 yo: PO: Initial:** 2.5-5 mg qd. **Titrate:** Adjust by 2.5-5 mg. **Max:** 20 mg/d. **Agitation Associated w/ Bipolar Mania: IM: Initial:** 10 mg. May initiate PO therapy when clinically appropriate. **Range:** 2.5-10 mg. **Max:** 3 doses of 10 mg q2-4h. **Geriatric Patients: IM:** 5 mg. **Debilitated/Predisposed to Hypotension:** See PI. **Combination Therapy w/ Fluoxetine for Depressive Episodes Associated w/ Bipolar I Disorder: PO: Initial:** 5 mg qd olanzapine and 20 mg qd fluoxetine given in the pm. **Range:** 5-12.5 mg olanzapine and 20-50 mg fluoxetine. **Max:** 18 mg olanzapine & 75 mg fluoxetine. **Predisposition to Hypotension/Slow Metabolizers/ Hepatic Impairment:** See PI.	⊕C ❁v H W [30]

NAME	FORM/STRENGTH	DOSAGE	COMMENTS
Quetiapine Fumarate (Seroquel XR)	Tab,ER: 50 mg, 150 mg, 200 mg, 300 mg, 400 mg	**Adults: Bipolar Depressive Episodes:** Give qd in pm. **Day 1:** 50 mg/d. **Day 2:** 100 mg/d. **Day 3:** 200 mg/d. **Day 4:** 300 mg/d. **Bipolar Mania: Monotherapy/Adjunct Therapy w/ Lithium or Divalproex:** Give qd in pm. **Day 1:** 300 mg/d. **Day 2:** 600 mg/d. **Titrate:** May adjust dose between 400-800 mg/d beginning on Day 3 depending on response and tolerance. **Maint of Bipolar I Disorder:** 400-800 mg/d given bid as adjunct to lithium or divalproex. Reevaluate periodically.	☢ⓒ ✿ v H W 29, 30
Quetiapine Fumarate (Seroquel)	Tab: 25 mg, 50 mg, 100 mg, 200 mg, 300 mg, 400 mg	**Bipolar I Disorder: Acute Manic Episodes: Monotherapy or Adjunct Therapy w/ Lithium or Divalproex: Adults: Initial:** 100 mg/d given bid on Day 1. **Titrate:** Increase to 400 mg/d given bid on Day 4 in increments of up to 100 mg/d divided bid. Adjust doses up to 800 mg/d by Day 6 in increments ≤200 mg/d. **Max:** 800 mg/d. **Peds: 10-17 yo:** Give bid-tid. **Day 1:** 50 mg/d. **Day 2:** 100 mg/d. **Day 3:** 200 mg/d. **Day 4:** 300 mg/d. **Day 5:** 400 mg/d. **Titrate:** Increase by increments ≤100 mg/d. **Range:** 400-600 mg/d. **Max:** 600 mg/d. **Bipolar I Disorder Maint: Adults:** 400-800 mg/d given bid as adjunct to lithium or divalproex. **Bipolar Depressive Episodes: Adults:** Give once daily hs. **Day 1:** 50 mg/d. **Day 2:** 100 mg/d. **Day 3:** 200 mg/d. **Day 4:** 300 mg/d. **Max:** 600 mg/d.	☢ⓒ ✿ v H W 29, 30

| **Risperidone**
(Risperdal Consta) | **Inj:** 12.5 mg, 25 mg,
37.5 mg, 50 mg | **Adults: Biopolar I Disorder:** In risperidone-naive patients, establish tolerability w/ PO risperidone prior to treatment. Give 1st inj w/ PO risperidone or other antipsychotic, continue x 3 wks, then d/c PO. **Usual:** 25 mg IM q2wks. **Titrate:** May increase to 37.5 mg or 50 mg. Increase at intervals of no more than q4wks. **Max:** 50 mg q2wks. **Elderly:** 25 mg IM q2wks. **Poor Tolerability:** Initial: 12.5 mg IM. **Switching from Other Antipsychotics/ Coadministration w/ Enzyme Inducers/Fluoxetine/ Paroxetine:** See PI. | ⊙C
❖v H R W [30] |
| **Risperidone**
(Risperdal, Risperdal M-Tab) | **Sol:** 1 mg/ml; **Tab:** 0.25 mg, 0.5 mg, 1 mg, 2 mg, 3 mg, 4 mg; **Tab, Dissolve:** 0.5 mg, 1 mg, 2 mg, 3 mg, 4 mg | **Bipolar I Disorder: Acute Manic & Mixed Episodes: Adults: Monotherapy or Adjunct Therapy w/ Lithium or Valproate:** Initial: 2-3 mg qd. **Titrate:** Adjust dose at intervals not <24h and in increments/decrements of 1 mg/d. **Range:** 1-6 mg/d. **Max:** 6 mg/d. **Peds: 10-17 yo: Monotherapy:** Initial: 0.5 mg qd in am or pm. **Titrate:** Adjust dose, in increments of 0.5 or 1 mg/d & at intervals not <24h as tolerated to recommended dose of 2.5 mg/d. **Range:** 0.5-6mg/d. **Max:** 6 mg/d. **Elderly/Debilitated/ Hypotension/Severe Renal or Hepatic Impairment:** Initial: 0.5 mg bid. **Titrate:** See PI. **Coadministration w/ Enzyme Inducers/Fluoxetine/Paroxetine:** May affect plasma concentrations; titrate accordingly. | ⊙C
❖v H R W [30] |

NAME	FORM/STRENGTH	DOSAGE	COMMENTS
Valproic Acid (Stavzor)	Cap, Delay: 125 mg, 250 mg, 500 mg	**Adults: Mania: Initial:** 750 mg qd in divided doses. **Titrate:** Increase rapidly to produce desired clinical effect or plasma level (50-125 mcg/ml). **Max:** 60 mg/kg/d. **Elderly:** Reduce starting dose & increase slowly.	⊕D ✿v W [101]
Ziprasidone (Geodon)	Cap: 20 mg, 40 mg, 60 mg, 80 mg	**Adults: Bipolar Disorder: Acute Manic & Mixed Episodes: Initial:** 40 mg bid w/ food. **Titrate:** May increase to 60-80 mg bid on Day 2 and thereafter based on tolerance and efficacy. **Range:** 40-80 mg bid. **Maint as Adjunct to Lithium or Valproate:** 40-80 mg bid.	⊕C ✿v W [30]

Migraine Therapy
5-HT, AGONISTS & COMBINATIONS

NAME	FORM/STRENGTH	DOSAGE	COMMENTS
Almotriptan Malate (Axert)	Tab: 6.25 mg, 12.5 mg	**Acute Therapy: Adults & Peds: 12-17 yo: Initial:** 6.25 mg or 12.5 mg; may repeat after 2h. **Max:** 2 doses/24h.	⊕C ✿> H R
Eletriptan HBr (Relpax)	Tab: 20 mg, 40 mg	**Acute Therapy: Adults: ≥18 yo: Initial:** 20 mg or 40 mg; may repeat after 2h. **Max:** 40 mg/dose or 80 mg/d.	⊕C ✿> H
Frovatriptan Succinate (Frova)	Tab: 2.5 mg	**Acute Therapy: Adults: ≥18 yo: Initial:** 2.5 mg; may repeat after 2h. **Max:** 7.5 mg/d.	⊕C ✿>
Naproxen Sodium/ Sumatriptan Succinate (Treximet)	Tab: 500 mg/85 mg	**Acute Therapy: Adults: Initial:** 1 tab; may repeat after 2h. **Max:** 2 tabs/24h. Do not split, crush, or chew.	⊕C ✿v H R W [66, 67]
Naratriptan HCl (Amerge)	Tab: 1 mg, 2.5 mg	**Acute Therapy: Adults: Initial:** 1 mg or 2.5 mg; may repeat once after 4h. **Max:** 5 mg/24h.	⊕C ✿> H R

Rizatriptan Benzoate (Maxalt, Maxalt-MLT)	Tab: 5 mg, 10 mg; Tab, Dissolve (ODT): (MLT) 5 mg, 10 mg	Acute Therapy: Adults: Initial: 5 or 10 mg; may repeat q2h. Max: 30 mg/24h. Place ODT on tongue.	⊕C ❄> Adjust dose w/ propranolol.
Sumatriptan Succinate (Imitrex)	Inj: 4mg/0.5 ml, 6 mg/0.5 ml; Nasal Spr: 5 mg/spr, 20 mg/spr; Tab: 25 mg, 50 mg, 100 mg	Acute Therapy: Adults: ≥18 yo: Initial: Inj: Max Single Dose: 6 mg SC. Max Dose/24h: Two 6 mg inj separated by at least 1h. Tab: Initial: 25 mg, 50 mg, or 100 mg single dose; may repeat in 2h. If headache returns after initial treatment w/ inj dose, may give additional single tabs (up to 100 mg/d), w/ an interval of at least 2h between tab doses. Max: 200 mg/24h. Nasal Spr: 5 mg, 10 mg, or 20 mg; may repeat once in 2h. Max: 40 mg/24h.	⊕C ❄> Avoid breastfeeding 12h after dose. (Tab) H
Sumatriptan (Alsuma)	Inj: 6 mg/0.5 ml	Acute Therapy & Cluster Headache: Adults: ≥18 yo: 6 mg SC. Max: 2 doses/24h separated by ≥1h.	⊕C ❄>
Zolmitriptan (Zomig, Zomig Nasal Spray, Zomig-ZMT)	Tab: 2.5 mg, 5 mg; Tab,Dissolve: 2.5 mg, 5 mg; Nasal Spr: 5 mg/spr	Acute Therapy: Adults: ≥18 yo: Initial: PO: 2.5 mg or lower; may repeat after 2h. Max: 10 mg/24h. Nasal Spr: 5 mg; may repeat after 2h. Max: 10 mg/24h.	⊕C ❄> H

MISCELLANEOUS

Divalproex Sodium (Depakote)	Tab,Delay: 125 mg, 250 mg, 500 mg	Prophylaxis: Adults & Peds: ≥16 yo: Initial: 250 mg bid. Max: 1000 mg/d.	⊕D ❄v H W [101]
Divalproex Sodium (Depakote ER)	Tab,ER: 250 mg, 500 mg	Prophylaxis: Adults: Initial: 500 mg qd x 1 wk. Titrate: Increase to 1000 mg/d. Max: 1000 mg/d.	⊕D ❄v W [101]

NAME	FORM/STRENGTH	DOSAGE	COMMENTS
Topiramate (Topamax, Topamax Sprinkle Capsules)	**Cap:** 15 mg, 25 mg; **Tab:** 25 mg, 50 mg, 100 mg, 200 mg	**Prophylaxis: Adults: Titrate: Wk 1:** 25 mg qpm. **Wk 2:** 25 mg bid. **Wk 3:** 25 mg qam & 50 mg qpm. **Wk 4:** 50 mg bid. **Usual:** 50 mg bid.	⊙D ❄>R
Valproic Acid (Stavzor)	**Cap, Delay:** 125 mg, 250 mg, 500 mg	**Prophylaxis: Adults: Initial:** 250 mg bid. **Max:** 1000 mg/d. **Elderly:** Reduce starting dose & increase slowly.	⊙D ❄v W [101]

Muscle Relaxants

NAME	FORM/STRENGTH	DOSAGE	COMMENTS
Cyclobenzaprine HCl (Amrix)	**Cap, ER:** 15 mg, 30 mg	**Adults: Usual:** 15 mg qd. **Titrate:** May increase to 30 mg qd if needed. Use for longer than 2-3 wks not recommended.	⊙B ❄>H
Cyclobenzaprine HCl (Flexeril)	**Tab:** 5 mg, 10 mg	**Adults & Peds: ≥15 yo: Usual:** 5 mg tid. **Titrate:** May increase to 10 mg tid. Do not exceed 2-3 wks of therapy.	⊙B ❄>H
Metaxalone (Skelaxin)	**Tab:** 800 mg	**Adults & Peds: >12 yo:** 800 mg tid-qid.	⊙N ❄v
Tizanidine HCl (Zanaflex)	**Cap:** 2 mg, 4 mg, 6 mg; **Tab:** 2 mg, 4 mg	**Adults: Initial:** 4 mg q6-8h. **Titrate:** Increase by 2-4 mg. **Usual:** 8 mg q6-8h. **Max:** 3 doses/24h or 36 mg/d.	⊙C ❄>

Obsessive-Compulsive Disorder

SSRIs & COMBINATIONS

Fluoxetine HCl (Prozac)	**Cap:** 10 mg, 20 mg, 40 mg	**Adults: Initial:** 20 mg qam. **Maint:** 20-60 mg/d given qd or bid (am & noon). **Max:** 80 mg/d. **Peds: ≥7 yo: Adolescents & Higher-Wt Peds: Initial:** 10 mg/d. **Titrate:** Increase to 20 mg/d after 2 wks. Consider additional dose increases after several more wks if clinical improvement not observed. **Usual:** 20-60 mg/d. **Lower-Wt Peds: Initial:** 10 mg/d. **Titrate:** Consider additional dose increases after several wks if clinical improvement not observed. **Usual:** 20-30 mg/d. **Max:** 60 mg/d.	⊕C ❅v H W [29]
Fluvoxamine Maleate (Luvox CR)	**Cap,ER:** 100 mg, 150 mg	**Adults: Initial:** 100 mg qhs. **Titrate:** May increase by 50 mg qwk. **Maint:** 100-300 mg/d. **Max:** 300 mg/d.	⊕C ❅v W [29]
Fluvoxamine	**Tab:** 25 mg, 50 mg, 100 mg	**Adults: Initial:** 50 mg qhs. **Titrate:** Increase by 50 mg q4-7d. **Maint:** 100-300 mg/d. **Max:** 300 mg/d. **Peds: 8-17 yo: Initial:** 25 mg qhs. **Titrate:** Increase by 25 mg q4-7d. **Maint:** 50-200 mg/d. **Max: 8-11 yo:** 200 mg/d. **Adolescents:** 300 mg/d.	⊕C ❅v H W [29]
Paroxetine HCl (Paxil)	**Susp:** 10 mg/5 ml; **Tab:** 10 mg, 20 mg, 30 mg, 40 mg	**Adults: Initial:** 20 mg qam. **Titrate:** May increase by 10 mg/d at intervals of ≥1 wk. **Usual:** 40 mg/d. **Max:** 60 mg/d.	⊕D ❅> H R W [29]
Paroxetine Mesylate (Pexeva)	**Tab:** 10 mg, 20 mg, 30 mg, 40 mg	**Adults: Initial:** 40 mg/d. **Max:** 60 mg/d.	⊕C ❅> H R W [29]

NAME	FORM/STRENGTH	DOSAGE	COMMENTS
Sertraline HCl (Zoloft)	Sol: 20 mg/ml; Tab: 25 mg, 50 mg, 100 mg	Adults & Peds: Initial: ≥13 yo: 50 mg qd. 6-12 yo: 25 mg qd. Titrate: Adjust wkly. Max: 200 mg/d.	⊕C ❋> H W [29]

Miscellaneous

NAME	FORM/STRENGTH	DOSAGE	COMMENTS
Aripiprazole (Abilify, Abilify Discmelt)	Sol: 1 mg/ml; Tab: 2 mg, 5 mg, 10 mg, 15 mg, 20 mg, 30 mg; Tab, Dissolve: (Discmelt) 10 mg, 15 mg	Irritability Associated w/ Autistic Disorder: Peds: 6-17 yo: Individualize dose. Initial: 2 mg/d. Titrate: Increase to 5mg/d. May increase to 10 or 15 mg/d if necessary. Dose adjustments of up to 5 mg/d should occur gradually at intervals of no less than 1 wk. Usual: 5-15 mg/d. Oral Sol: Can be substituted for tabs on mg-per-mg-basis up to 25 mg. Patients receiving 30-mg tabs should receive 25 mg of sol. Adjust dose w/ CYP3A4/CYP2D6 inhibitors, CYP3A4 inducers, & in poor CYP2D6 metabolizers.	⊕C ❋v W [29, 30]
Dextromethorphan Hydrobromide/Quinidine Sulfate (Nuedexta)	Cap: 20 mg-10 mg	Pseudobulbar Affect: Adults: Initial: 1 cap qd PO for 7d then 1 cap q12h.	⊕C ❋>
Pramipexole Dihydrochloride (Mirapex)	Tab: 0.125 mg, 0.25 mg, 0.5 mg, 0.75 mg, 1 mg, 1.5 mg	Moderate-to-Severe Primary Restless Legs Syndrome: Adults: Initial: 0.125 mg qd, 2-3h before hs. Titrate: May double dose q4-7d up to 0.5 mg/d.	⊕C ❋v R

| Risperidone (Risperdal, Risperdal M-Tab) | Sol: 1 mg/ml; Tab: 0.25 mg, 0.5 mg, 1 mg, 2 mg, 3 mg, 4 mg; Tab,Dissolve: 0.5 mg, 1 mg, 2 mg, 3 mg, 4 mg | Irritability Associated w/ Autistic Disorder: Peds: 5-16 yo: Individualize dose. Initial: <20 kg: 0.25 mg/d, given qd or bid; ≥20 kg: 0.5 mg/d, given qd or bid. Titrate: After at least 4d: <20 kg: Increase to 0.5 mg/d; ≥20 kg: 1 mg/d. Maint: For minimum of 14d. Inadequate Response: Increase at ≥2-wk intervals: <20 kg: Increase by 0.25 mg/d; ≥20 kg: Increase by 0.5 mg/d. Caution in patients <15 kg. Max: <20 kg: 1 mg/d; ≥20 kg: 2.5 mg/d; >45 kg: 3 mg/d. Coadministration w/ Enzyme Inducers/Fluoxetine/ Paroxetine: May affect plasma concentrations; titrate accordingly. | ●C ❀v H R W [30] |
| Ropinirole HCl (Requip XL) | Tab: 0.25 mg, 0.5 mg, 1 mg, 2 mg, 3 mg, 4 mg, 5 mg | Moderate-to-Severe Primary Restless Legs Syndrome: Adults: Initial: 0.25 mg qd, 1-3h before hs. Titrate: 0.5 mg qd on Days 3-7, then 1 mg qd during Wk 2, then increase by 0.5 mg wkly. Max: 4 mg/d. | ●C ❀v |

PULMONARY/RESPIRATORY

Asthma/COPD Preparations
ANTICHOLINERGICS

| Ipratropium Bromide (Atrovent HFA) | MDI: 17 mcg/inh | COPD: Adults: Initial: 2 inh qid. Max: 12 inh/24h. | ●B ❀> |
| Tiotropium Bromide (Spiriva) | Cap,Inh: 18 mcg | Adults: COPD: 2 inh of the powder contents of 1 cap qd w/ HandiHaler device. | ●C ❀> |

NAME	FORM/STRENGTH	DOSAGE	COMMENTS
BRONCHODILATOR (BETA AGONIST/ANTICHOLINERGIC)			
Albuterol Sulfate/ Ipratropium Bromide (Combivent)	**MDI:** 0.103-0.018 mg/inh	**COPD: Adults:** 2 inh qid. **Max:** 12 inh/24h.	⊕C ✲v
BRONCHODILATOR COMBINATIONS			
Albuterol Sulfate/ Ipratropium Bromide (Duoneb)	**Sol,Neb:** 3-0.5 mg/3 ml	**Adults: COPD:** 3 ml qid via neb. May give 2 additional doses/d if needed.	⊕C ✲v
Fluticasone Propionate/ Salmeterol (Advair HFA)	**MDI:** 45-21 mcg/inh, 115-21 mcg/inh, 230-21 mcg/inh	**Asthma: Adults & Peds: ≥12 yo: Usual:** 2 inh q12h. If inadequate response within 2 wks, may increase to higher strength. **Max:** 2 inh of 230-21 bid.	⊕C ✲v Asthma-related deaths reported.
Fluticasone Propionate/ Salmeterol (Advair)	**MDI:** (Diskus) 100-50 mcg/inh, 250-50 mcg/inh, 500-50 mcg/inh	**Asthma: Adults & Peds: ≥12 yo:** 1 inh q12h. If no response w/in 2 wks, may increase to higher strength. **Max:** 500-50 bid. **Symptomatic on Inhaled CS: 4-11 yo:** (100-50 only) 1 inh q12h. **COPD: Adults:** (250-50 only) 1 inh q12h. Rinse mouth after use.	⊕C ✲v Asthma-related deaths reported.
Formoterol Fumarate Dihydrate/Budesonide (Symbicort)	**MDI:** 80-4.5 mcg/inh, 160-4.5 mcg/inh	**Asthma: Adults & Peds: ≥12 yo: Initial:** Individualize dose. 2 inh bid of 80-4.5 or 160-4.5. **Maint:** 2 inh bid of 80-4.5 or 160-4.5. **No Current Inhaled Corticosteroid:** 2 inh bid of 80-4.5 or 160-4.5 depending on asthma severity. **Max:** 160-4.5 bid. Patients not responding to starting dose after	✲v ⊕C Asthma-related deaths reported.

		1-2 wks of therapy w/ 80-4.5, may replace w/ 160-4.5 for better asthma control. **COPD: Adults:** 2 inh bid of 160-4.5. If asthma or shortness of breath occurs in period between doses, use short-acting beta₂-agonist for immediate relief. Rinse mouth after use.	
Formoterol Fumarate Dihydrate/Mometasone Furoate (Dulera)	**MDI:** 100-5 mcg/inh, 200-5 mcg/inh	**Asthma: Adults & Peds:** ≥12 yo: 2 inh bid (am/pm). **Max:** 2 inh of 200/5 bid. **W/ Prior Medium-Dose Corticosteroid (CS): Initial:** 2 inh of 100/5 bid. **Max:** 400/20/d. **W/ Prior High-Dose CS: Initial:** 2 inh of 200/5 bid. **Max:** 800/20/d. Do not use >2 inh bid of prescribed strength. If no response after 2 wks, may increase to higher strength. Rinse mouth after use.	⊕C ❀> Asthma-related deaths reported.

BRONCHODILATORS (BETA AGONISTS)

Albuterol Sulfate (AccuNeb)	**Sol,Neb:** 0.63 mg/3 ml, 1.25 mg/3 ml	**Bronchospasm/Asthma: Peds:** 6-12 yo w/ Severe Asthma or >40 kg or 11-12 yo: **Initial:** 1.25 mg tid-qid. **2-12 yo:** 0.63 mg or 1.25 mg tid-qid prn via nebulizer over 5-15 min.	⊕C ❀v
Albuterol Sulfate (ProAir HFA)	**MDI:** 90 mcg/inh	**Adults & Peds:** ≥4 yo: Treatment/Prevention of Bronchospasm: 2 inh q4-6h or 1 inh q4h. **Exercise-Induced Bronchospasm Prevention:** 2 inh 15 min before exercise.	⊕C ❀v

NAME	FORM/STRENGTH	DOSAGE	COMMENTS
Albuterol Sulfate (Proventil HFA)	**MDI:** 0.09 mg/inh	**Adults & Peds: ≥4 yo: Bronchospasm:** 2 inh q4-6h or 1 inh q4h. **Exercise-Induced Bronchospasm:** 2 inh 15-30 min before exercise.	▣C ❁v
Albuterol Sulfate (Ventolin HFA)	**MDI:** 0.09 mg/inh	**Adults & Peds: ≥4 yo: Bronchospasm:** 2 inh q4-6h or 1 inh q4h. **Exercise-Induced Bronchospasm:** 2 inh 15-30 min before exercise.	▣C ❁v
Albuterol Sulfate (VoSpire ER)	**Tab,ER:** 4 mg, 8 mg	**Bronchospasm: Adults/Peds: >12 yo: Usual:** 4-8 mg q12h. **Low Body Wt: Initial:** 4 mg q12h. **Titrate:** May increase to 8 mg q12h. **Max:** 32 mg/d in divided doses. **6-12 yo: Usual:** 4 mg q12h. **Max:** 24 mg/d in divided doses. Swallow whole w/ liquids.	▣C ❁v
Arformoterol Tartrate (Brovana)	**Sol,Neb:** 15 mcg/2 ml	**COPD-Associated Bronchoconstriction: Adults: Usual:** 15 mcg bid (am & pm) via nebulizer. **Max:** 30 mcg/d.	▣C ❁> Asthma-related deaths reported.
Formoterol Fumarate (Foradil)	**MDI:** 12 mcg/inh	**Adults & Peds: ≥5 yo: Asthma:** 12 mcg q12h. **Max:** 24 mcg/d. **Exercise-Induced Bronchospasm Prevention:** 12 mcg 15 min prior to exercise (do not give preventive doses if already on bid dosing). **Adults: COPD:** 12 mcg q12h. **Max:** 24 mcg/d. Give only by inhalation w/ aerolizer inhaler.	▣C ❁> Asthma-related deaths reported.

Formoterol Fumarate (Perforomist)	Sol,Neb: 20 mcg/2 ml	COPD: Adults: 20 mcg bid (am & pm). Max: 40 mcg/d. Administer by nebulizer.	⊕C ✿> Asthma-related deaths reported.
Indacaterol (Arcapta Neohaler)	Cap,Inh: 75 mcg	COPD: Adults: 1 inh qd of contents of 1 cap (75mcg) w/ Neohaler device.	⊕C ✿>
Levalbuterol Tartrate (Xopenex HFA)	MDI: 45 mcg/inh	Adults & Peds: ≥4 yo: Bronchospasm: 2 inh (90 mcg) q4-6h or 1 inh (45 mcg) q4h may be sufficient.	⊕C ✿v
Salmeterol Xinafoate (Serevent)	Diskus: 50 mcg/inh	Adults & Peds: ≥4 yo: Asthma: 1 inh q12h. Exercise-Induced Bronchospasm Prevention: 1 inh ≥30 min before exercise (do not give preventive doses if already on bid dose). Adults: COPD: 1 inh q12h.	⊕C ✿v Asthma-related deaths reported.

INHALED CORTICOSTEROIDS

Beclomethasone Dipropionate (Qvar)	MDI: 40 mcg/inh, 80 mcg/inh	Adults: ≥12 yo: Previous Bronchodilator Only: 40-80 mcg bid. Max: 320 mcg bid. Previous Inhaled Corticosteroid Therapy: 40-160 mcg bid. Max: 320 mcg bid. 5-11 yo: Previous Bronchodilator Only or Inhaled Corticosteroid: 40 mcg bid. Max: 80 mcg bid. Adults & Peds: ≥5 yo: Maint w/ Oral Corticosteroids: May attempt gradual reduction of oral dose after 1 wk on inhaled therapy.	⊕C ✿v

NAME	FORM/STRENGTH	DOSAGE	COMMENTS
Budesonide (Pulmicort Flexhaler, Pulmicort Respules)	**Pow,Inh:** (Flexhaler) 90 mcg/dose, 180 mcg/dose; **Susp,Inh:** (Respules) 0.25 mg/2 ml, 0.5 mg/2 ml, 1 mg/2 ml	**Adults & Peds: Flexhaler: ≥6 yo:** Individualize dose. **Initial:** 180-360 mcg bid. **Max:** 720 mcg (adults) or 360 mcg (peds) bid. **Respules: 1-8 yo:** Individualize dose. Administer via jet neb. **Previous Bronchodilator Only: Initial:** 0.5 mg qd or 0.25 mg bid. **Max:** 0.5 mg/d. **Previous Inhaled Corticosteroid:** 0.5 mg qd or 0.25 mg bid. **Max:** 1 mg/d. **Previous Oral Corticosteroid:** 1 mg qd or 0.5 mg bid. **Max:** 1 mg/d. Gradually reduce PO corticosteroid after 1 wk of budesonide.	⬤B ❄>
Ciclesonide (Alvesco)	**MDI:** 80 mcg/inh, 160 mcg/inh	**Adults: Previous Bronchodilator Only: Initial:** 80 mcg bid. **Max:** 160 mcg bid. **Previous Inhaled Corticosteroids: Initial:** 80 mcg bid. **Max:** 320 mcg bid. **Previous Oral Corticosteroids: Initial:** 320 mcg bid. **Max:** 320 mcg bid.	⬤C ❄>
Fluticasone Propionate (Flovent HFA)	**MDI:** 44 mcg/inh, 110 mcg/inh, 220 mcg/ inh	**Adults & Peds: ≥12 yo: Previous Bronchodilator Only: Initial:** 88 mcg bid. **Max:** 440 mcg bid. **Previous Inhaled Corticosteroids: Initial:** 88-220 mcg bid. **Max:** 440 mcg bid. **Previous Oral Corticosteroids: Initial:** 440 mcg bid. **Max:** 880 mcg bid. **4-11 yo: Initial/Max:** 88 mcg bid. Reduce PO prednisone no faster than 2.5-5 mg/d wkly; begin ≥1 wk after start fluticasone. **Titrate:** Lowest effective dose. If inadequate response after 2 wks, may increase to higher strength.	⬤C ❄>

| Mometasone Furoate (Asmanex) | Twisthaler: 110 mcg/inh, 220 mcg/inh | Adults & Peds: ≥12 yo: Previous Therapy w/ Bronchodilators Alone or Inhaled Corticosteroids (CS): Initial: 220 mcg qpm. Max: 440 mcg qpm or 220 mcg bid. Previous Therapy w/ Oral CS: Initial: 440 mcg bid. Max: 880 mcg/d. Titrate to higher dose if inadequate response after 2 wks. Peds: 4-11 yo: 110 mcg qpm regardless of prior therapy. Adjust to lowest effective dose once asthma stability achieved. | ⊙C ❁> |
| Triamcinolone Acetonide (Azmacort) | MDI: 100 mcg/inh | Adults & Peds: >12 yo: 2 inh tid-qid or 4 inh bid. Severe Asthma: Initial: 12-16 inh/d. Max: 16 inh/d. 6-12 yo: 1-2 inh tid-qid or 2-4 inh bid. Max: 12 inh/d. | ⊙C ❁> |

LEUKOTRIENE MODIFIERS

| Montelukast Sodium (Singulair) | Chewtab: 4 mg, 5 mg; Granules: 4 mg/pkt; Tab: 10 mg | Asthma: Adults & Peds: ≥15 yo: 10 mg qpm. 6-14 yo: Chewtab: 5 mg qpm. 2-5 yo: Chewtab/Granules: 4 mg qpm. 12-23 mths: Granules: 4 mg qpm. Both Asthma and Allergic Rhinitis: 1 dose qpm. Exercise-Induced Bronchoconstriction: Adults & Peds: ≥15 yo: 10 mg ≥2h before exercise. Do not take additional dose w/in 24h of previous dose. | ⊙B ❁> |
| Zafirlukast (Accolate) | Tab: 10 mg, 20 mg | Adults & Peds: ≥12 yo: 20 mg bid. 5-11 yo: 10 mg bid. Administer ≥1h ac or 2h pc. | ⊙B ❁v H |

NAME	FORM/STRENGTH	DOSAGE	COMMENTS
MAST CELL STABILIZER			
Cromolyn Sodium	Sol: 10 mg/ml	**Asthma: Adults & Peds:** ≥5 yo: Sol: ≥2 yo: 20 mg qid via neb. **Acute Bronchospasm Prevention: Sol:** ≥2 yo: 20 mg via neb shortly before precipitant exposure.	●B ❋> H R
XANTHINE DERIVATIVE			
Theophylline (Theo-24)	Cap,ER: 100 mg, 200 mg, 300 mg, 400 mg	**Adults & Peds:** ≥12 yo & >45 kg: **Initial:** 300-400 mg/d. **Titrate:** Increase to 400-600 mg/d after 3d if tolerated, then to >600 mg/d if needed & tolerated after 3 more days. **Elderly/CHF: Max:** 400 mg/d. **Fast Metabolizers:** May give in divided doses q12h. ≥12 yo & <45 kg: **Initial:** 12-14 mg/kg/d (**Max:** 300 mg/d). After 3d, may increase to 16 mg/kg/d (**Max:** 400 mg/d). After 3 more days, may increase to 20 mg/kg/d (**Max:** 600 mg/d) if tolerated & needed.	●C ❋> H R
MISCELLANEOUS			
Roflumilast (Daliresp)	Tab: 500 mcg	**COPD: Adults:** 500 mcg/d.	●C ❋v H

Miscellaneous

BRONCHODILATORS (ALPHA/BETA AGONISTS)

Epinephrine (EpiPen, EpiPen Jr.)	Inj: (Epipen Jr) 0.15 mg/ 0.3ml, (Epipen) 0.3 mg/ 0.3ml	Allergic Reactions/Anaphylaxis: Adults & Peds: 15-30 kg: 0.15 mg. ≥30 kg: 0.3mg. Inject IM/SQ into anterolateral aspect of the thigh. May repeat w/ severe anaphylaxis.	●C ❀>
Epinephrine (Twinject)	Inj: 1 mg/ml (1:1000)	Allergic Reactions/Anaphylaxis: Adults/Peds: Inject IM or SC into thigh. 15-30 kg: (Twinject 0.15 mg) 0.15 mg. ≥30 kg: (Twinject 0.3 mg) 0.3 mg. May repeat if needed.	●C ❀>

LEUKOTRIENE MODIFIER

Montelukast Sodium (Singulair)	Chewtab: 4 mg, 5 mg; Granules: 4 mg/pkt; Tab: 10 mg	Seasonal/Perennial Allergic Rhinitis: Adults & Peds: ≥15 yo: 10 mg qd. 6-14 yo: Chewtab: 5 mg qd. 2-5 yo: Chewtab/Granules: 4 mg qd. Perennial Allergic Rhinitis: 6-23 mths: Granules: 4 mg qd.	●B ❀>

UROLOGY

Benign Prostatic Hypertrophy

ALPHA₁ RECEPTOR BLOCKERS

Alfuzosin HCl (Uroxatral)	Tab,ER: 10 mg	Adults: 10 mg w/ same meal qd. Swallow whole.	●B ❀> H
Doxazosin Mesylate (Cardura XL)	Tab,ER: 4 mg, 8 mg	Adults: Initial: 4 mg qd w/ breakfast. Titrate: May increase to 8 mg after 3-4 wks. Max: 8 mg. Swallow whole.	●C ❀v

NAME	FORM/STRENGTH	DOSAGE	COMMENTS
Doxazosin Mesylate (Cardura)	Tab: 1 mg, 2 mg, 4 mg, 8 mg	Adults: Initial: 1 mg qd (am or pm). Titrate: Based on response may increase to 2 mg, then 4 mg, 8 mg, and 16 mg. Allow titration interval of 1-2 wks. Max: 8 mg/d.	◕C ❄> Syncope w/ 1st dose.
Silodosin (Rapaflo)	Cap: 4 mg, 8 mg	Adults: 8 mg qd. Take w/ meal. CrCl 30-50 ml/min: 4 mg qd.	◕B ❄v H R W [24]
Tamsulosin HCl (Flomax)	Cap: 0.4 mg	Adults: Initial: 0.4 mg qd, 1/2 h after same meal qd. Titrate: If inadequate response after 2-4 wks, may increase to 0.8 mg qd.	◕B ❄v
Terazosin HCl	Cap: 1 mg, 2 mg, 5 mg, 10 mg	Adults: Initial: 1 mg qhs. Titrate: Increase stepwise to 10 mg qd. Usual: 10 mg/d. Assess clinical response after 4-6 wks. Max: 20 mg/d. If d/c for several days, restart at initial dose.	◕C ❄> Syncope w/ 1st dose.
ALPHA-REDUCTASE INHIBITORS			
Dutasteride (Avodart)	Cap: 0.5 mg	Adults: Monotherapy/Concomitant Tamsulosin: 0.5 mg qd. Swallow whole.	◕X ❄v
Finasteride (Proscar)	Tab: 5 mg	Adults: Monotherapy/Concomitant Doxazosin: 5 mg qd.	◕X ❄v
PHOSPHODIESTERASE TYPE 5 INHIBITOR			
Tadalafil (Cialis)	Tab: 2.5 mg, 5 mg, 10 mg, 20 mg	BPH and ED/BPH: Adults: 5 mg qd at the same time everyday. Concomitant Potent CYP3A4 Inhibitors: See PI.	◕B ❄v CI w/ nitrates. H R

| Tamsulosin HCl/Dutasteride (Jalyn) | Cap: 0.4 mg-0.5 mg | Adults: Initial: 1 cap qd, approx. 30 min after the same qd day. Swallow cap whole, do not chew or open. | ⊕X ❖v CI during pregnancy, in peds, and in women of childbearing potential. |

Erectile Dysfunction
PHOSPHODIESTERASE TYPE 5 INHIBITORS

| Avanafil (Stendra) | Tab: 50 mg, 100 mg, 200 mg | Adults: Initial: 100 mg prn 30 min before sexual activity. Titrate: May decrease to 50 mg or increase to max dose of 200 mg. Max Frequency: Dose qd. Concomitant α-Blockers or Moderate CYP3A4 Inhibitors: See PI. | ⊕C ❖> CI w/ nitrates. H R |
| Sildenafil Citrate (Viagra) | Tab: 25 mg, 50 mg, 100 mg | Adults: Usual: 50 mg prn 1h (range 0.5-4h) before sexual activity up to once daily. Titrate: May decrease to 25 mg qd or increase to 100 mg qd. Max: 100 mg qd. Elderly/ Concomitant Potent CYP3A4 Inhibitors, Ritonavir, or α-Blockers: See PI. | ⊕B ❖v CI w/ nitrates. H R |

NAME	FORM/STRENGTH	DOSAGE	COMMENTS
Tadalafil (Cialis)	**Tab:** 2.5 mg, 5 mg, 10 mg, 20 mg	**Adults: PRN Use: ED: Initial:** 10 mg prior to sexual activity. **Titrate:** May increase to 20 mg or decrease to 5 mg based on efficacy & tolerability. **Max Dosing Frequency:** qd. **Once-Daily Use: ED: Initial:** 2.5 mg qd. **Titrate:** May increase to 5 mg qd based on individual response. **BPH and ED:** 5 mg qd. Take at the same time every day. **Concomitant Alpha Blockers/Potent CYP3A4 Inhibitors:** See PI.	●B ❋v CI w/ nitrates. **H R**
Vardenafil HCl (Levitra)	**Tab:** 2.5 mg, 5 mg, 10 mg, 20 mg	**Adults: Initial:** 10 mg 60 min prior to sexual activity. **Titrate:** May decrease to 5 mg or increase to max of 20 mg based on response. **Max:** 1 tab/d. **Elderly:** ≥65 yo: **Initial:** 5 mg. **Concomitant Ritonavir/Indinavir/Saquinavir/ Atazanavir/Ketoconazole/Itraconazole/Erythromycin/α- Blocker:** See PI.	●B ❋v CI w/ nitrates or nitric oxide donors. **H**
Vardenafil HCl (Staxyn)	**Tab, Dissolve:** 10 mg	**Adults:** 10 mg prn. Take 1h before sexual activity. Place tab on tongue to disintegrate. Take w/o liquid. **Max:** 1 tab/d.	●B ❋> CI w/ nitrates and nitric oxide donors. **H R**

Urinary Tract Antispasmodics
PARASYMPATHOLYTICS

NAME	FORM/STRENGTH	DOSAGE	COMMENTS
Darifenacin (Enablex)	**Tab, ER:** 7.5 mg, 15 mg	**Adults: OAB: Initial:** 7.5 mg qd. **Titrate:** May increase to 15 mg qd after 2 wks. **Concomitant Potent CYP3A4 Inhibitors:** Do not exceed 7.5 mg/d.	●C ❋> **H**

Fesoterodine Fumarate (Toviaz)	Tab,ER: 4 mg, 8 mg	**OAB: Adults: Initial:** 4 mg qd. **Titrate:** May increase to 8 mg based on response & tolerability. **Potent CYP3A4 Inhibitors (eg, Ketoconazole, Itraconazole, Clarithromycin): Max:** 4 mg/d.	⊕C ✿> H R
Oxybutynin Chloride (Ditropan)	Syr: (Generic) 5 mg/5 ml; Tab: 5 mg	**OAB: Adults:** 5 mg bid-tid. **Max:** 5 mg qid. **Frail Elderly:** 2.5 mg bid-tid. **Peds: ≥5 yo:** 5 mg bid. **Max:** 5 mg tid.	⊕B ✿>
Oxybutynin Chloride (Gelnique)	Gel: 10%	**OAB: Adults:** Apply qd to dry, intact skin on abdomen, upper arms/shoulders, or thighs. Rotate sites.	⊕B ✿>
Oxybutynin (Oxytrol)	Patch: 3.9 mg/d	**OAB: Adults:** One 3.9 mg/d system applied 2X wkly (q3-4d) to dry, intact skin on the abdomen, hip, or buttock. Avoid reapplication to same site w/in 7d.	⊕B ✿>
Solifenacin Succinate (VESIcare)	Tab: 5 mg, 10 mg	**OAB: Adults: Usual:** 5 mg qd. **Titrate:** May increase to 10 mg qd if 5 mg dose is well tolerated. **Potent CYP3A4 Inhibitors: Max:** 5 mg qd.	⊕C ✿v H R
Tolterodine Tartrate (Detrol, Detrol LA)	Cap,ER: 2 mg, 4 mg; Tab: 1 mg, 2 mg	**OAB: Adults: Cap,ER: Usual:** 4 mg qd. May decrease to 2 mg qd depending on response & tolerability. **Tab: Initial:** 2 mg bid. May decrease to 1 mg bid depending on response & tolerability. See PI for dosing w/ potent CYP3A4 inhibitors.	⊕C ✿v H R
Trospium Chloride (Sanctura, Sanctura XR)	Cap,ER: 60 mg; Tab: 20 mg	**OAB: Adults:** (Tab) 20 mg bid ≥1h before meals or on empty stomach. **(Cap,ER)** 60 mg qd in am w/ water on an empty stomach, ≥1h before meals. **Elderly ≥75 yo:** (Tab) May titrate to 20 mg qd based on tolerability.	⊕C ✿> R

ANTIHISTAMINES

DRUG	RX/OTC	FORM/STRENGTH	DOSAGE	COMMENTS
Azelastine (Astelin)	RX	**Spr:** 137 mcg/spr	**Adults & Peds: ≥12 yo: Seasonal Allergic Rhinitis:** 1-2 spr per nostril bid. **5-11 yo:** 1 spr per nostril bid. **Adults & Peds: ≥12 yo: Vasomotor Rhinitis:** 2 spr per nostril bid.	⊞C ❄>
Azelastine (Astepro)	RX	**Spr:** 0.1% (137 mcg/spr), 0.15% (205.5 mcg/spr)	**Adults & Peds: ≥12 yo: Seasonal Allergic Rhinitis:** 1-2 spr per nostril bid. **0.15%:** May be given as 2 spr per nostril qd. **Perennial Allergic Rhinitis: 0.15%:** 2 spr/nostril bid.	⊞C ❄>
Brompheniramine Maleate-Pseudoephedrine HCl (Lodrane D)	OTC	**Cap:** 4-60 mg	**Adults & Peds: >12 yo:** 1 cap q4-6h. **Max:** 4 caps/d.	⊞N ❄>
Carbinoxamine Maleate	RX	**Sol:** 4 mg/5 ml; **Tab:** 4 mg	**Adults: Tab:** 4-8 mg tid-qid. **Peds: Tab: 6-11 yo:** 2-4 mg tid-qid. **Sol: Usual:** 0.2-0.4 mg/kg/d. **>6 yo:** 5-7.5 ml (4-6 mg) tid-qid. **3-6 yo:** 2.5-5 ml (2-4 mg) tid-qid. **2-3 yo:** 2.5 ml (2 mg) tid-qid.	⊞C ❄v
Cetirizine HCl (Zyrtec)	OTC	**Cap:** 10 mg; **Syr:** 1 mg/ml; **Tab:** 10 mg	**Adults: ≥65 yo: Syr:** 5 mg qd. **Max:** 5 mg/d. **Adults & Peds: ≥6 yo: Cap/Syr/Tab:** 5-10 mg qd. **Max:** 10 mg/d. **2-5 yo: Syr:** 2.5 mg qd. **Max:** 5 mg/d.	⊞N ❄v H R
Cetirizine HCl-Pseudoephedrine HCl (Zyrtec-D)	OTC	**Tab,ER:** 5-120 mg	**Adults & Peds: ≥12 yo:** 1 tab q12h. **Max:** 2 tabs/d.	⊞N ❄v H R

Chlorpheniramine Maleate (Chlor-Trimeton)	OTC	Tab: 4 mg; Tab,ER: 12 mg	Adults & Peds: ≥12 yo: Tab: 4 mg q4-6h. Max: 24 mg/d. Tab,ER: 12 mg q12h. Max: 24 mg/d. 6-<12 yo: Tab: 2 mg (1/2 tab) q4-6h. Max: 12 mg (3 tabs)/d.	⊞N ❊>
Chlorpheniramine Maleate-Phenylephrine HCl (Sudafed PE Sinus and Allergy)	OTC	Tab: 4-10 mg	Adults & Peds: ≥12 yo: 1 tab q4h. Max: 6 tabs/24h.	⊞N ❊>
Clemastine Fumarate	OTC (Tab 1.34 mg); RX (Tab 2.68 mg, Syr 0.5 mg/5 ml)	Syr: 0.5 mg/5 ml; Tab: 1.34 mg, 2.68 mg	Adults & Peds: ≥12 yo: Tab: 1.34 mg bid. Max: 8.04 mg/d. Syr: 1-2 mg bid. Max: 6 mg/d. 6-12 yo: Syr: 0.5-1 mg bid. Max: 3 mg/d.	⊞(Syr) B ⊞(Tab) N ❊v
Cyproheptadine HCl	RX	Syr: 2 mg/5 ml; Tab: 4 mg	Adults: Initial: 4 mg tid. Usual: 4-20 mg/d. Max: 0.5 mg/kg/d. 7-14 yo: 4 mg bid-tid. Max: 16 mg/d. 2-6 yo: 2 mg bid-tid. Max: 12 mg/d.	⊞B ❊v
Desloratadine (Clarinex)	RX	Syr: 0.5 mg/ml; Tab,Dissolve: (Reditab) 2.5 mg, 5 mg; Tab: 5 mg	Adults & Peds: ≥12 yo: Perennial Allergic Rhinitis/Urticaria: Tab: 5 mg qd. 6-11 yo: 2.5 mg qd. Syr: ≥12 yo: 10 ml (5 mg) qd. 6-11 yo: 5 ml (2.5 mg) qd. 12 mths-5 yo: 2.5 ml (1.25 mg) qd. 6-11 mths: 2 ml (1 mg) qd. Adults & Peds: ≥12 yo: Seasonal Allergic Rhinitis: Tab: 5 mg qd. 6-11 yo: 2.5 mg qd. Syr: ≥12 yo: 10 ml (5 mg) qd. 6-11 yo: 5 ml (2.5 mg) qd. 2-5 yo: 2.5 ml (1.25 mg) qd.	⊞C ❊v H R
Desloratadine-Pseudoephedrine Sulfate (Clarinex-D)	RX	Tab,ER: (12 Hr) 2.5 mg-120 mg, (24 Hr) 5 mg-240 mg	Seasonal Allergic Rhinitis: Adults & Peds: ≥12 yo: (12 Hr) 1 tab bid or (24 Hr) 1 tab qd w/ or w/o food.	⊞C ❊v H R

DRUG	RX/OTC	FORM/STRENGTH	DOSAGE	COMMENTS
Diphenhydramine HCl (Benadryl)	OTC (PO), RX (50 mg cap)	**Cap:** 25 mg, 50 mg; **Chewtab:** 12.5 mg; **Film:** 25 mg; **Inj:** 50 mg/ml; **Syr:** 12.5 mg/5 ml; **Tab:** 25 mg	**Adults: PO:** 25-50 mg q4-6h. **Max:** 6 doses/24h. **Inj:** 10-50 mg IV or up to 100 mg deep IM. **Max:** 400 mg/d. **≥12 yo:** 25-50 mg q4-6h. **Max:** 6 doses/24h. **6-11 yo: PO:** 12.5-25 mg q4-6h. **Max:** 6 doses/24h. **Peds: Inj:** 5 mg/kg/24h or 150 mg/m²/24h IV/IM in 4 divided doses. **Max:** 300 mg/d.	⊞ (RX) B ⊞ (OTC) N ❀v
Diphenhydramine HCl-Phenylephrine HCl (Benadryl-D Allergy and Sinus)	OTC	**Sol:** 12.5 mg-5 mg/5 ml; **Tab:** 25 mg-10 mg	**Adults & Peds: ≥12 yo: Sol/Tab:** 1 tab or 2 tsp q4h. **Max:** 6 doses/24h. **6-11 yo: Sol:** 1 tsp q4h. **Max:** 6 doses/24h.	⊞N ❀>
Fexofenadine HCl (Allegra)	OTC	**Susp:** 30 mg/5 ml; **Tab:** 30 mg, (12-Hr) 60 mg, (24-Hr) 180 mg; **Tab, Dissolve:** 30 mg	**Adults & Peds: ≥12 yo: 24 Hr Tab:** 180 mg qd. **Max:** 180 mg/24h. **Susp/12 Hr Tab/Tab, Dissolve:** 60 mg q12h. **Max:** 120 mg/24h. **6-11 yo: Tab/Tab, Dissolve:** 30 mg q12h. **Max:** 60 mg/24h. **2-11 yo: Susp:** 30 mg q12h. **Max:** 60 mg/24h.	⊞N ❀> R
Fexofenadine HCl-Pseudoephedrine HCl (Allegra-D)	OTC	**Tab, ER:** (12-Hr) 60 mg-120 mg, (24-Hr) 180 mg-240 mg	**Adults & Peds: ≥12 yo:** (12-Hr) 1 tab q12h or (24-Hr) 1 tab qd. **Max:** (12-Hr) 2 tab/24h or (24-Hr) 1 tab/24h.	⊞N ❀> R
Hydroxyzine HCl	RX	**Syr:** 10 mg/5 ml; **Tab:** 10 mg, 25 mg, 50 mg	**Adults:** 25 mg tid-qid. **Peds: ≥6 yo:** 50-100 mg/d in divided doses. **<6 yo:** 50 mg/d in divided doses.	⊞N ❀v CI in early pregnancy.
Hydroxyzine Pamoate (Vistaril)	RX	(Vistaril) **Cap:** 25 mg, 50 mg; (Generic) **Cap:** 25 mg, 50 mg	**Adults:** 25 mg tid-qid. **Peds: ≥6 yo:** 50-100 mg/d in divided doses. **<6 yo:** 50 mg/d in divided doses.	⊞N ❀v CI in early pregnancy.

Drug				
Levocetirizine Dihydrochloride (Xyzal)	RX	**Sol:** 2.5 mg/5 ml **Tab:** 5 mg	**Seasonal/Perennial Allergic Rhinitis/Urticaria: Tab: Adults & Peds: ≥12 yo:** 5 mg qd in pm. **6-11 yo:** 2.5 mg qd in pm. **Peds: 6 mths-5 yo: Sol:** 1.25 mg (2.5 ml) qd in pm.	◉B ✿v R
Loratadine (Alavert, Claritin, Claritin Reditabs)	OTC	**Tab, Dissolve:** (Alavert, Claritin Reditabs) 10 mg; **Syr:** 1 mg/ml; **Tab:** (Alavert, Claritin) 10 mg	**Adults & Peds: ≥6 yo:** 10 mg qd. **Max:** 10 mg/d. **2-<6 yo: Syr:** 5 mg qd. **Max:** 5 mg/d.	◉N ✿> H R
Loratadine-Pseudoephedrine Sulfate (Claritin-D)	OTC	**Tab, ER:** (12-Hr) 5 mg-120 mg, (24-Hr) 10 mg-240 mg	**Adults & Peds: ≥12 yo:** (12 Hr) 1 tab bid or (24 Hr) 1 tab qd. **Max:** (12 Hr) 2 tab/24h or (24 Hr) 1 tab/24h.	◉N ✿> H R
Olopatadine HCl (Pataday, Patanol)	RX	**Sol:** (Pataday) 0.2%, (Patanol) 0.1%	(Pataday) **Adults & Peds: ≥2 yo:** 1 gtt qd. (Patanol) **Adults & Peds: ≥3 yo:** 1 gtt bid (q6-8h).	◉C ✿>
Promethazine HCl	RX	**Inj:** 25 mg/ml, 50 mg/ml; **Sup:** 12.5 mg, 25 mg; **Syr:** 6.25 mg/5 ml	**Adults:** 25 mg PO/PR qhs or 12.5 mg before meals & hs. **Peds: ≥2 yo:** 25 mg or 0.5 mg/lb PO/PR qhs. 25 mg IM/IV and repeat in 2h if needed. 6.25-12.5 mg tid; up to 12.5 mg IM/IV.	◉C ✿v Potential for total respiratory depression in patients <2 yrs.

COLD AND COUGH COMBINATIONS

DRUG	DEA CLASS	ANTIHISTAMINE	DECONGESTANT	COUGH SUPPRESSANT	OTHER CONTENT	DOSE
Atuss DS	RX	Chlorpheniramine Maleate, 4 mg/5 ml	Pseudoephedrine HCl, 30 mg/5 ml	Dextromethorphan HBr, 30 mg/5 ml		**>12 yo:** 1-2 tsps q12h. **6-12 yo:** 1/2-1 tsp q12h. **2-6 yo:** 1/2 tsp q12h. **<2 yo:** As directed by a physician.
Cheratussin AC	CV			Codeine Phosphate, 10 mg/5 ml	Guaifenesin, 100 mg/5 ml	**≥12 yo:** 2 tsp q4h. **Max:** 6 doses/24h. **6-12 yo:** 1 tsp q4h. **Max:** 6 doses/24h.
Cheratussin DAC	CV		Pseudoephedrine HCl 30 mg/5 ml	Codeine Phosphate, 10 mg/5 ml	Guaifenesin, 100 mg/5 ml	**≥12 yo:** 2 tsp q4h. **Max:** 4 doses/24h. **6-12 yo:** 1 tsp q4h. **Max:** 4 doses/24h.
Hydrocodone Bitartrate/ Homatropine Methylbromide Syrup	CIII			Hydrocodone Bitartrate, 5 mg/5 ml	Homatropine Methylbromide, 1.5 mg/5 ml	**Adults:** 1 tsp q4-6h. **Max:** 6 tsps/24h. **6-12 yo:** 1/2 tsp q4-6h. **Max:** 3 tsps/24h.

Promethazine DM	RX	Promethazine HCl, 6.25 mg/5 ml		Dextromethorphan HBr, 15 mg/5 ml	≥**12 yo:** 1 tsp q4-6h. **Max:** 30 ml/24h. **6-11 yo:** 1/2-1 tsp q4-6h. **Max:** 20 ml/24h. **2-5 yo:** 1/4-1/2 tsp q4-6h. **Max:** 10 ml/24h.
Promethazine VC	RX	Promethazine HCl, 6.25 mg/5 ml	Phenylephrine HCl, 5 mg/5 ml		≥**12 yo:** 1 tsp q4-6h. **Max:** 30 ml/24h. **6-11 yo:** 1/2-1 tsp q4-6h. **Max:** 30 ml/24h. **2-5 yo:** 1/4-1/2 tsp q4-6h.
Promethazine VC/ Codeine	CV	Promethazine HCl, 6.25 mg/5 ml	Phenylephrine HCl, 5 mg/5 ml	Codeine Phosphate, 10 mg/5 ml	≥**12 yo:** 1 tsp q4-6h. **Max:** 30 ml/24h. **6-11 yo:** 1/2-1 tsp q4-6h. **Max:** 30 ml/24h.
Promethazine w/ Codeine	CV	Promethazine HCl, 6.25 mg/5 ml		Codeine Phosphate, 10 mg/5 ml	≥**12 yo:** 1 tsp q4-6h. **Max:** 30 ml/24h. **6-11 yo:** 1/2-1 tsp q4-6h. **Max:** 30 ml/24h.

DRUG	DEA CLASS	ANTIHISTAMINE	DECONGESTANT	COUGH SUPPRESSANT	OTHER CONTENT	DOSE
Rezira	CIII		Pseudoephedrine HCl, 60 mg/5 ml	Hydrocodone Bitartrate, 5 mg/5 ml		**≥18 yo:** 5 ml q4-6h. **Max:** 4 doses/24h.
R-Tanna	RX	Chlorpheniramine Tannate, 9 mg	Phenylephrine Tannate, 25 mg			**Adults:** 1-2 tabs q12h.
R-Tanna Pediatric Suspension	RX	Chlorpheniramine Tannate, 4.5 mg/5 ml	Phenylephrine Tannate, 5 mg/5 ml			**>6 yo:** 1-2 tsps q12h. **2-6 yo:** 1/2-1 tsp q12h. **<2 yo:** Titrate dose individually.
Semprex-D	RX	Acrivastine, 8 mg	Pseudoephedrine HCl, 60 mg			**≥12 yo:** 1 cap q4-6h qid.
Tessalon	RX			Benzonatate, 200 mg (cap), 100 mg (perles)		**>10 yo:** 1 cap tid. **Max:** 600 mg/24h.
Tussicaps	CIII	Chlorpheniramine Polistirex, 8 mg (FS); 4 mg (HS)		Hydrocodone Polistirex, 10 mg (FS); 5 mg (HS)		**≥12 yo:** 1 full strength cap q12h. **Max:** 2 doses/24h. **6-11 yo:** 1 half strength cap q12h. **Max:** 2 doses/24h.

Tussigon	CIII			Hydrocodone Bitartrate, 5 mg	Homatropine Methylbromide, 1.5 mg	**Adults:** 1 tab q4-6h. **Max:** 6 tabs/24h. **6-12 yo:** 1/2 tab q4-6h. **Max:** 3 tabs/24h.
Tussionex Pennkinetic	CIII	Chlorpheniramine Polistirex, 8 mg/5 ml		Hydrocodone Polistirex, 10 mg/5 ml		**≥12 yo:** 1 tsp q12h. **Max:** 2 doses/24h. **6-11 yo:** 1/2 tsp q12h. **Max:** 2 doses/24h.
Zonatuss	RX			Benzonatate, 150 mg		**>10 yo:** 1 cap tid. **Max:** 600 mg/24h.
Zutripro	CIII	Chlorpheniramine Maleate, 4 mg/5 ml	Pseudoephedrine HCl, 60 mg/5 ml	Hydrocodone Bitartrate, 5 mg/5 ml		**≥18 yo:** 5 ml q4-6h. **Max:** 4 doses/24h.

IMMUNIZATIONS

RECOMMENDED IMMUNIZATION SCHEDULE FOR PERSONS AGED 0–6 YEARS • UNITED STATES, 2012

Vaccine ▼ Age ►	Birth	1 month	2 months	4 months	6 months	9 months	12 months	15 months	18 months	19–23 months	2–3 years	4–6 years
Hepatitis B[1]	Hep B	HepB					HepB					
Rotavirus[2]			RV	RV	RV[2]							
Diphtheria, tetanus, pertussis[3]			DTaP	DTaP	DTaP		see footnote[3]	DTaP				DTaP
Haemophilus influenzae type b[4]			Hib	Hib	Hib[4]		Hib					
Pneumococcal[5]			PCV	PCV	PCV		PCV					PPSV
Inactivated poliovirus[6]			IPV	IPV			IPV					IPV
Influenza[7]							Influenza (Yearly)					
Measles, mumps, rubella[8]							MMR		see footnote[8]			MMR
Varicella[9]							Varicella		see footnote[9]			Varicella
Hepatitis A[10]							Dose 1[10]				HepA Series	
Meningococcal[11]							MCV4 — see footnote [11]					

Range of recommended ages for all children   Range of recommended ages for certain high-risk groups   ///// Range of recommended ages for all children and certain high-risk groups

This schedule includes recommendations in effect as of December 23, 2011. Any dose not administered at the recommended age should be administered at a subsequent visit, when indicated and feasible. The use of a combination vaccine generally is preferred over separate injections of its equivalent component vaccines. Vaccination providers should consult the relevant Advisory Committee on Immunization Practices (ACIP) statement for detailed recommendations, available online at http://www.cdc.gov/vaccines/pubs/acip-list.htm. Clinically significant adverse events that follow vaccination should be reported to the Vaccine Adverse Event Reporting System (VAERS) online (http://www.vaers.hhs.gov) or by telephone (800-822-7967).

1. **Hepatitis B (HepB) vaccine.** (Minimum age: birth)

   At birth:
   - Administer monovalent HepB vaccine to all newborns before hospital discharge.
   - For infants born to hepatitis B surface antigen (HBsAg)–positive mothers, administer HepB vaccine and 0.5 mL of hepatitis B immune globulin (HBIG) within 12 hours of birth. These infants should be tested for HBsAg and antibody to HBsAg (anti-HBs) 1 to 2 months after receiving the last dose of the series.
   - If mother's HBsAg status is unknown, within 12 hours of birth administer HepB vaccine for infants weighing ≥2000 grams, and HepB vaccine plus HBIG for infants weighing <2000 grams. Determine mother's HBsAg status as soon as possible and, if she is HBsAg-positive, administer HBIG for infants weighing ≥2000 grams (no later than age 1 week).

   Doses after the birth dose:
   - The second dose should be administered at age 1 to 2 months. Monovalent HepB vaccine should be used for doses administered before age 6 months.
   - Administration of a total of 4 doses of HepB vaccine is permissible when a combination vaccine containing HepB is administered after the birth dose.
   - Infants who did not receive a birth dose should receive 3 doses of a HepB-containing vaccine starting as soon as feasible (see the *Catch-Up Immunization Schedule*).
   - The minimum interval between dose 1 and dose 2 is 4 weeks, and between dose 2 and 3 is 8 weeks. The final (third or fourth) dose in the HepB vaccine series should be administered no earlier than age 24 weeks and at least 16 weeks after the first dose.

2. **Rotavirus (RV) vaccines.** (Minimum age: 6 weeks for both RV-1 [Rotarix] and RV-5 [Rota Teq])
   - The maximum age for the first dose in the series is 14 weeks, 6 days; and 8 months, 0 days for the final dose in the series. Vaccination should not be initiated for infants aged 15 weeks, 0 days or older.
   - If RV-1 (Rotarix) is administered at ages 2 and 4 months, a dose at 6 months is not indicated.

3. **Diphtheria and tetanus toxoids and acellular pertussis (DTaP) vaccine.** (Minimum age: 6 weeks)
   - The fourth dose may be administered as early as age 12 months, provided at least 6 months have elapsed since the third dose.

4. ***Haemophilus influenzae* type b (Hib) conjugate vaccine.** (Minimum age: 6 weeks)
   - If PRP-OMP (PedvaxHIB or Comvax [HepB-Hib]) is administered at ages 2 and 4 months, a dose at age 6 months is not indicated.
   - Hiberix should only be used for the booster (final) dose in children aged 12 months through 4 years.

5. Pneumococcal vaccines. (Minimum age: 6 weeks for pneumococcal conjugate vaccine [PCV]; 2 years for pneumococcal polysaccharide vaccine [PPSV])
- Administer 1 dose of PCV to all healthy children aged 24 through 59 months who are not completely vaccinated for their age.
- For children who have received an age-appropriate series of 7-valent PCV (PCV7), a single supplemental dose of 13-valent PCV (PCV13) is recommended for:
  — All children aged 14 through 59 months
  — Children aged 60 through 71 months with underlying medical conditions.
- Administer PPSV at least 8 weeks after last dose of PCV to children aged 2 years or older with certain underlying medical conditions, including a cochlear implant. See MMWR 2010:59(No. RR-11), available at http://www.cdc.gov/mmwr/pdf/rr/rr5911.pdf.

6. Inactivated poliovirus vaccine (IPV). (Minimum age: 6 weeks)
- If 4 or more doses are administered before age 4 years, an additional dose should be administered at age 4 through 6 years.
- The final dose in the series should be administered on or after the fourth birthday and at least 6 months after the previous dose.

7. Influenza vaccines. (Minimum age: 6 months for trivalent inactivated influenza vaccine [TIV]; 2 years for live, attenuated influenza vaccine [LAIV])
- For most healthy children aged 2 years and older, either LAIV or TIV may be used. However, LAIV should not be administered to some children, including 1) children with asthma, 2) children 2 through 4 years who had wheezing in the past 12 months, or 3) children who have any other underlying medical conditions that predispose them to influenza complications. For all other contraindications to use of LAIV, see MMWR 2010;59(No. RR-8), available at http://www.cdc.gov/mmwr/pdf/rr/rr5908.pdf.
- For children aged 6 months through 8 years:
  — For the 2011–12 season, administer 2 doses (separated by at least 4 weeks) to those who did not receive at least 1 dose of the 2010–11 vaccine. Those who received at least 1 dose of the 2010–11 vaccine require 1 dose for the 2011–12 season.
  — For the 2012–13 season, follow dosing guidelines in the 2012 ACIP influenza vaccine recommendations.

8. Measles, mumps, and rubella (MMR) vaccine. (Minimum age: 12 months)
- The second dose may be administered before age 4 years, provided at least 4 weeks have elapsed since the first dose.
- Administer MMR vaccine to infants aged 6 through 11 months who are traveling internationally. These children should be revaccinated with 2 doses of MMR vaccine, the first at ages 12 through 15 months and at least 4 weeks after the previous dose, and the second at ages 4 through 6 years.

9. **Varicella (VAR) vaccine.** (Minimum age: 12 months)
   - The second dose may be administered before age 4 years, provided at least 3 months have elapsed since the first dose.
   - For children aged 12 months through 12 years, the recommended minimum interval between doses is 3 months. However, if the second dose was administered at least 4 weeks after the first dose, it can be accepted as valid.

10. **Hepatitis A (HepA) vaccine.** (Minimum age: 12 months)
    - Administer the second (final) dose 6 to 18 months after the first.
    - Unvaccinated children 24 months and older at high risk should be vaccinated. See *MMWR* 2006;55(No. RR-7), available at http://www.cdc.gov/mmwr/pdf/rr/rr5507.pdf.
    - A 2-dose HepA vaccine series is recommended for anyone aged 24 months and older, previously unvaccinated, for whom immunity against hepatitis A virus infection is desired.

11. **Meningococcal conjugate vaccines, quadrivalent (MCV4).** (Minimum age: 9 months for Menactra [MCV4-D], 2 years for Menveo [MCV4-CRM])
    - For children aged 9 through 23 months 1) with persistent complement component deficiency; 2) who are residents of or travelers to countries with hyperendemic or epidemic disease; or 3) who are present during outbreaks caused by a vaccine serogroup, administer 2 primary doses of MCV4-D, ideally at ages 9 months and 12 months or at least 8 weeks apart.
    - For children aged 24 months and older with 1) persistent complement component deficiency who have not been previously vaccinated; or 2) anatomic/functional asplenia, administer 2 primary doses of either MCV4 at least 8 weeks apart.
    - For children with anatomic/functional asplenia, if MCV4-D (Menactra) is used, administer at a minimum age of 2 years and at least 4 weeks after completion of all PCV doses.
    - See *MMWR* 2011;60:72–76, available at http://www.cdc.gov/mmwr/pdf/wk/mm6003. pdf, and Vaccines for Children Program resolution No. 6/11-1, available at http://www. cdc.gov/vaccines/programs/vfc/downloads/resolutions/06-11mening-mcv.pdf, and *MMWR* 2011;60:1391–2, available at http://www.cdc.gov/mmwr/pdf/wk/mm6040. pdf, for further guidance, including revaccination guidelines.

RECOMMENDED IMMUNIZATION SCHEDULE FOR PERSONS AGED 7–18 YEARS • UNITED STATES, 2012

Vaccine ▼ Age ▶	7–10 years	11–12 years	13–18 years
Tetanus, diphtheria, pertussis[1]	1 dose (if indicated)	1 dose	1 dose (if indicated)
Human papillomavirus[2]	see footnote[2]	3 doses	Complete 3-dose series
Meningococcal[3]	See footnote[3]	Dose 1	Booster at 16 years old
Influenza[4]		Influenza (yearly)	
Pneumococcal[5]		See footnote[5]	
Hepatitis A[6]		Complete 2-dose series	
Hepatitis B[7]		Complete 3-dose series	
Inactivated poliovirus[8]		Complete 3-dose series	
Measles, mumps, rubella[9]		Complete 2-dose series	
Varicella[10]		Complete 2-dose series	

Range of recommended ages for all children   Range of recommended ages for catch-up immunization   Range of recommended ages for certain high-risk groups

This schedule includes recommendations in effect as of December 23, 2011. Any dose not administered at the recommended age should be administered at a subsequent visit, when indicated and feasible. The use of a combination vaccine generally is preferred over separate injections of its equivalent component vaccines. Vaccination providers should consult the relevant Advisory Committee on Immunization Practices (ACIP) statement for detailed recommendations, available online at http://www.cdc.gov/vaccines/pubs/acip-list.htm. Clinically significant adverse events that follow vaccination should be reported to the Vaccine Adverse Event Reporting System (VAERS) online (http://www.vaers.hhs.gov) or by telephone (800-822-7967).

1. **Tetanus and diphtheria toxoids and acellular pertussis (Tdap) vaccine.** (Minimum age: 10 years for Boostrix and 11 years for Adacel)
   • Persons aged 11 through 18 years who have not received Tdap vaccine should receive a dose followed by tetanus and diphtheria toxoids (Td) booster doses every 10 years thereafter.
   • Tdap vaccine should be substituted for a single dose of Td in the catch-up series for children aged 7 through 10 years. Refer to the *Catch-Up Schedule* if additional doses of tetanus and diphtheria toxoid–containing vaccine are needed.

- Tdap vaccine can be administered regardless of the interval since the last tetanus and diphtheria toxoid–containing vaccine.

2. Human papillomavirus vaccines (HPV4 [Gardasil] and HPV2 [Cervarix]). (Minimum age: 9 years)
- Either HPV4 or HPV2 is recommended in a 3-dose series for females aged 11 or 12 years. HPV4 is recommended in a 3-dose series for males aged 11 or 12 years.
- The vaccine series can be started beginning at age 9 years.
- Administer the second dose 1 to 2 months after the first dose and the third dose 6 months after the first dose (at least 24 weeks after the first dose).
- See *MMWR* 2010;59:626–632, available at http://www.cdc.gov/mmwr/pdf/wk/mm5920.pdf.

3. Meningococcal conjugate vaccines, quadrivalent (MCV4).
- Administer MCV4 at age 11 through 12 years with a booster dose at age 16 years.
- Administer MCV4 at age 13 through 18 years if patient is not previously vaccinated.
- If the first dose is administered at age 13 through 15 years, a booster dose should be administered at age 16 through 18 years with a minimum interval of at least 8 weeks after the preceding dose.
- If the first dose is administered at age 16 years or older, a booster dose is not needed.
- Administer 2 primary doses at least 8 weeks apart to previously unvaccinated persons with persistent complement component deficiency or anatomic/functional asplenia, and 1 dose every 5 years thereafter.
- Adolescents aged 11 through 18 years with human immunodeficiency virus (HIV) infection should receive a 2-dose primary series of MCV4, at least 8 weeks apart.
- See *MMWR* 2011;60:72–76, available at http://www.cdc.gov/mmwr/pdf/wk/mm6003.pdf, and Vaccines for Children Program resolution No. 6/11-1, available at http://www.cdc.gov/vaccines/programs/vfc/downloads/resolutions/06-11mening-mcv.pdf, for further guidelines.

4. Influenza vaccines (trivalent inactivated influenza vaccine [TIV] and live, attenuated influenza vaccine [LAIV]).
- For most healthy, nonpregnant persons, either LAIV or TIV may be used, except LAIV should not be used for some persons, including those with asthma or any other underlying medical conditions that predispose them to influenza complications. For all other contraindications to use of LAIV, see *MMWR* 2010;59(No.RR-8), available at http://www.cdc.gov/mmwr/pdf/rr/rr5908.pdf.
- Administer 1 dose to persons aged 9 years and older.
- For children aged 6 months through 8 years:
  — For the 2011–12 season, administer 2 doses (separated by at least 4 weeks) to those who did not receive at least 1 dose of the 2010–11 vaccine. Those who received at least 1 dose of the 2010–11 vaccine require 1 dose for the 2011–12 season.
  — For the 2012–13 season, follow dosing guidelines in the 2012 ACIP influenza vaccine recommendations.

5. Pneumococcal vaccines (pneumococcal conjugate vaccine [PCV] and pneumococcal polysaccharide vaccine [PPSV]).
- A single dose of PCV may be administered to children aged 6 through 18 years who have anatomic/functional asplenia, HIV infection or other immunocompromising condition, cochlear implant, or cerebral spinal fluid leak. See *MMWR* 2010:59(No. RR-11), available at http://www.cdc.gov/mmwr/pdf/rr/rr5911.pdf.
- Administer PPSV at least 8 weeks after the last dose of PCV to children aged 2 years or older with certain underlying medical conditions, including a cochlear implant. A single revaccination should be administered after 5 years to children with anatomic/functional asplenia or an immunocompromising condition.

6. Hepatitis A (HepA) vaccine.
- HepA vaccine is recommended for children older than 23 months who live in areas where vaccination programs target older children, who are at increased risk for infection, or for whom immunity against hepatitis A virus infection is desired. See *MMWR* 2006;55 (No. RR-7), available at http://www.cdc.gov/mmwr/pdf/rr/rr5507.pdf.
- Administer 2 doses at least 6 months apart to unvaccinated persons.

7. Hepatitis B (HepB) vaccine.
- Administer the 3-dose series to those not previously vaccinated.
- For those with incomplete vaccination, follow the catch-up recommendations.
- A 2-dose series (doses separated by at least 4 months) of adult formulation Recombivax HB is licensed for use in children aged 11 through 15 years.

8. Inactivated poliovirus vaccine (IPV).
- The final dose in the series should be administered at least 6 months after the previous dose.
- If both OPV and IPV were administered as part of a series, a total of 4 doses should be administered, regardless of the child's current age.
- IPV is not routinely recommended for U.S. residents aged 18 years or older.

9. Measles, mumps, and rubella (MMR) vaccine.
- The minimum interval between the 2 doses of MMR vaccine is 4 weeks.

10. Varicella (VAR) vaccine.
- For persons without evidence of immunity (see *MMWR* 2007;56[No. RR-4], available at http://www.cdc.gov/mmwr/pdf/rr/rr5604.pdf), administer 2 doses if not previously vaccinated or the second dose if only 1 dose has been administered.
- For persons aged 7 through 12 years, the recommended minimum interval between doses is 3 months. However, if the second dose was administered at least 4 weeks after the first dose, it can be accepted as valid.
- For persons aged 13 years and older, the minimum interval between doses is 4 weeks.

CATCH-UP IMMUNIZATION SCHEDULE FOR PERSONS AGED 4 MONTHS–18 YEARS WHO START LATE OR WHO ARE MORE THAN 1 MONTH BEHIND • UNITED STATES, 2012

Vaccine	Minimum Age for Dose 1	Minimum Interval Between Doses			
		Dose 1 to dose 2	Dose 2 to dose 3	Dose 3 to dose 4	Dose 4 to dose 5
Persons aged 4 months through 6 years					
Hepatitis B	Birth	4 weeks	8 weeks and at least 16 weeks after first dose; minimum age for the final dose is 24 weeks		
Rotavirus[1]	6 weeks	4 weeks	4 weeks[2]		
Diphtheria, tetanus, pertussis[3]	6 weeks	4 weeks	4 weeks	6 months	6 months[3]
Haemophilus influenzae type b[4]	6 weeks	4 weeks if first dose administered at younger than age 12 months; 8 weeks (as final dose) if first dose administered at age 12–14 months; No further doses needed if first dose administered at age 15 months or older	4 weeks[4] if current age is younger than 12 months; 8 weeks (as final dose)[4] if current age is 12 months or older and first dose administered at younger than age 12 months and second dose administered at younger than 15 months; No further doses needed if previous dose administered at age 15 months or older	8 weeks (as final dose) This dose only necessary for children aged 12 months through 59 months who received 3 doses before age 12 months	
Pneumococcal[5]	6 weeks	4 weeks if first dose administered at younger than age 12 months; 8 weeks (as final dose for healthy children) if first dose administered at age 12 months or older or current age 24 through 59 months; No further doses needed for healthy children if first dose administered at age 24 months or older	4 weeks if current age is younger than 12 months; 8 weeks (as final dose for healthy children) if current age is 12 months or older; No further doses needed for healthy children if previous dose administered at age 24 months or older	8 weeks (as final dose) This dose only necessary for children aged 12 months through 59 months who received 3 doses before age 12 months or for children at high risk who received 3 doses at any age	
Inactivated poliovirus[6]	6 weeks	4 weeks	4 weeks	6 months[6] minimum age 4 years for final dose	
Meningococcal[7]	9 months	8 weeks[7]			
Measles, mumps, rubella[8]	12 months	4 weeks			
Varicella[9]	12 months	3 months			
Hepatitis A	12 months	6 months			
Persons aged 7 through 18 years					
Tetanus, diphtheria/ tetanus, diphtheria, pertussis[10]	7 years[10]	4 weeks	4 weeks if first dose administered at younger than age 12 months; 6 months if first dose administered at 12 months or older	6 months if first dose administered at younger than age 12 months	

299 KEY: ⊙ PREGNANCY RATING; ✽ BREASTFEEDING SAFETY; H HEPATIC ADJUSTMENT; R RENAL ADJUSTMENT

Human papillomavirus[13]	9 years	Routine dosing intervals are recommended[13]				
Hepatitis A	12 months	6 months				
Hepatitis B	Birth	4 weeks	8 weeks (and at least 16 weeks after first dose)			
Inactivated poliovirus[3]	6 weeks	4 weeks	4 weeks[3]	6 months[3]		
Meningococcal[8]	9 months	8 weeks[8]				
Measles, mumps, rubella[7]	12 months	4 weeks				
Varicella[8]	12 months	3 months if person is younger than age 13 years / 4 weeks if person is aged 13 years or older				

The figure provides catch-up schedules and minimum intervals between doses for children whose vaccinations have been delayed. A vaccine series does not need to be restarted, regardless of the time that has elapsed between doses. Use the section appropriate for the child's age. Always use this table in conjunction with the accompanying childhood and adolescent immunization schedules and their respective footnotes.

1. Rotavirus (RV) vaccines (RV-1 [Rotarix] and RV-5 [Rota Teq]).
- The maximum age for the first dose in the series is 14 weeks, 6 days; and 8 months, 0 days for the final dose in the series. Vaccination should not be initiated for infants aged 15 weeks, 0 days or older.
- If RV-1 was administered for the first and second doses, a third dose is not indicated.

2. Diphtheria and tetanus toxoids and acellular pertussis (DTaP) vaccine.
- The fifth dose is not necessary if the fourth dose was administered at age 4 years or older.

3. *Haemophilus influenzae* type b (Hib) conjugate vaccine.
- Hib vaccine should be considered for unvaccinated persons aged 5 years or older who have sickle cell disease, leukemia, human immunodeficiency virus (HIV) infection, or anatomic/functional asplenia.
- If the first 2 doses were PRP-OMP (PedvaxHIB or Comvax) and were administered at age 11 months or younger, the third (and final) dose should be administered at age 12 through 15 months and at least 8 weeks after the second dose.
- If the first dose was administered at age 7 through 11 months, administer the second dose at least 4 weeks later and a final dose at age 12 through 15 months.

4. Pneumococcal vaccines. (Minimum age: 6 weeks for pneumococcal conjugate vaccine [PCV]; 2 years for pneumococcal polysaccharide vaccine [PPSV])
- For children aged 24 through 71 months with underlying medical conditions, administer 1 dose of PCV if 3 doses of PCV were received previously, or administer 2 doses of PCV at least 8 weeks apart if fewer than 3 doses of PCV were received previously.

- A single dose of PCV may be administered to certain children aged 6 through 18 years with underlying medical conditions. See age-specific schedules for details.
- Administer PPSV to children aged 2 years or older with certain underlying medical conditions. See *MMWR* 2010:59(No. RR-11), available at http://www.cdc.gov/mmwr/pdf/rr/rr5911.pdf.

5. Inactivated poliovirus vaccine (IPV).
- A fourth dose is not necessary if the third dose was administered at age 4 years or older and at least 6 months after the previous dose.
- In the first 6 months of life, minimum age and minimum intervals are only recommended if the person is at risk for imminent exposure to circulating poliovirus (ie, travel to a polio-endemic region or during an outbreak).
- IPV is not routinely recommended for U.S. residents aged 18 years or older.

6. Meningococcal conjugate vaccines, quadrivalent (MCV4). (Minimum age: 9 months for Menactra [MCV4-D]; 2 years for Menveo [MCV4-CRM])
- See *Recommended Immunization Schedule for Persons Aged 0 through 6 Years* and *Recommended Immunization Schedule for Persons Aged 7 through 18 Years* for further guidance.

7. Measles, mumps, and rubella (MMR) vaccine.
- Administer the second dose routinely at age 4 through 6 years.

8. Varicella (VAR) vaccine.
- Administer the second dose routinely at age 4 through 6 years. If the second dose was administered at least 4 weeks after the first dose, it can be accepted as valid.

9. Tetanus and diphtheria toxoids (Td) and tetanus and diphtheria toxoids and acellular pertussis (Tdap) vaccines.
- For children aged 7 through 10 years who are not fully immunized with the childhood DTaP vaccine series, Tdap vaccine should be substituted for a single dose of Td vaccine in the catch-up series; if additional doses are needed, use Td vaccine. For these children, an adolescent Tdap vaccine dose should not be given.
- An inadvertent dose of DTaP vaccine administered to children aged 7 through 10 years can count as part of the catch-up series. This dose can count as the adolescent Tdap dose, or the child can later receive a Tdap booster dose at age 11–12 years.

10. Human papillomavirus (HPV) vaccines (HPV4 [Gardasil] and HPV2 [Cervarix]).
- Administer the vaccine series to females (either HPV2 or HPV4) and males (HPV4) at age 13 through 18 years if patient is not previously vaccinated.
- Use recommended routine dosing intervals for vaccine series catch-up; see *Recommended Immunization Schedule for Persons Aged 7 through 18 Years.*

RECOMMENDED ADULT IMMUNIZATION SCHEDULE
FIGURE 1. RECOMMENDED ADULT IMMUNIZATION SCHEDULE, BY VACCINE AND AGE GROUP[1]
UNITED STATES, 2012

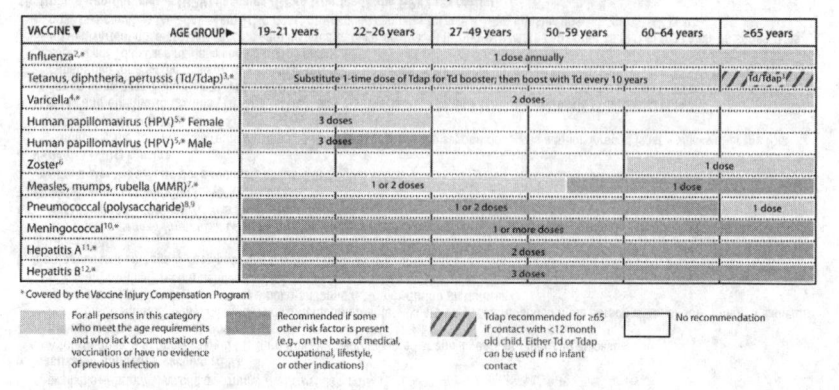

VACCINE ▼ AGE GROUP ►	19–21 years	22–26 years	27–49 years	50–59 years	60–64 years	≥65 years
Influenza[2,*]	1 dose annually					
Tetanus, diphtheria, pertussis (Td/Tdap)[3,*]	Substitute 1-time dose of Tdap for Td booster; then boost with Td every 10 years					/// Td/Tdap[3] ///
Varicella[4,*]	2 doses					
Human papillomavirus (HPV)[5,*] Female	3 doses					
Human papillomavirus (HPV)[5,*] Male	3 doses					
Zoster[6]					1 dose	
Measles, mumps, rubella (MMR)[7,*]	1 or 2 doses				1 dose	
Pneumococcal (polysaccharide)[8,9]	1 or 2 doses					1 dose
Meningococcal[10,*]	1 or more doses					
Hepatitis A[11,*]	2 doses					
Hepatitis B[12,*]	3 doses					

* Covered by the Vaccine Injury Compensation Program

For all persons in this category who meet the age requirements and who lack documentation of vaccination or have no evidence of previous infection	Recommended if some other risk factor is present (e.g., on the basis of medical, occupational, lifestyle, or other indications)	/// Tdap recommended for ≥65 if contact with <12 month old child. Either Td or Tdap can be used if no infant contact No recommendation

FIGURE 2. VACCINES THAT MIGHT BE INDICATED FOR ADULTS, BASED ON MEDICAL AND OTHER INDICATIONS[†]
UNITED STATES, 2012

| INDICATION ► / VACCINE ▼ | Pregnancy | Immunocompromising conditions (excluding human immunodeficiency virus [HIV])[3,6,7,14] | HIV infection[4,5,13,14] CD4+ T lymphocyte count | | Men who have sex with men (MSM) | Heart disease, chronic lung disease, chronic alcoholism | Asplenia[13] (including elective splenectomy and persistent complement component deficiencies) | Chronic liver disease | Diabetes, kidney failure, end-stage renal disease, receipt of hemodialysis | Health-care personnel |
			<200 cells/μL	≥200 cells/μL						
Influenza[2,*]	1 dose TIV annually				1 dose TIV or LAIV annually	1 dose TIV annually				1 dose TIV or LAIV annually
Tetanus, diphtheria, pertussis (Td/Tdap)[3,*]	Substitute 1-time dose of Tdap for Td booster; then boost with Td every 10 years									
Varicella[4,*]	Contraindicated				2 doses					
Human papillomavirus (HPV)[5,*] Female	3 doses through age 26 years					3 doses through age 26 years				
Human papillomavirus (HPV)[5,*] Male	3 doses through age 26 years					3 doses through age 21 years				
Zoster[6]	Contraindicated				1 dose					
Measles, mumps, rubella[7,*]	Contraindicated				1 or 2 doses					
Pneumococcal (polysaccharide)[8,9]					1 or 2 doses					
Meningococcal[10,*]					1 or more doses					
Hepatitis A[11,*]					2 doses					
Hepatitis B[12,*]					3 doses					

* Covered by the Vaccine Injury Compensation Program

For all persons in this category who meet the age requirements and who lack documentation of vaccination or have no evidence of previous infection

Recommended if some other risk factor is present (e.g., on the basis of medical, occupational, lifestyle, or other indications)

Contraindicated

No recommendation

1. Additional information

- Advisory Committee on Immunization Practices (ACIP) vaccine recommendations and additional information are available at: http://www.cdc.gov/vaccines/pubs/acip-list.htm
- Information on travel vaccine requirements and recommendations (eg, for hepatitis A and B, meningococcal, and other vaccines) available at http://wwwnc.cdc.gov/travel/page/vaccinations.htm

2. Influenza vaccination

- Annual vaccination against influenza is recommended for all persons 6 months of age and older.
- Persons 6 months of age and older, including pregnant women, can receive the trivalent inactivated vaccine (TIV).
- Healthy, nonpregnant adults younger than age 50 years without high-risk medical conditions can receive either intranasally administered live, attenuated influenza vaccine (LAIV) (FluMist) or TIV. Healthcare personnel (HCP) who care for severely immunocompromised persons (ie, those who require care in a protected environment) should receive TIV rather than LAIV. Other persons should receive TIV.
- The intramuscular or intradermal administered TIV are options for adults aged 18-64 years.
- Adults aged 65 years and older can receive the standard dose TIV or the high-dose TIV (Fluzone High-Dose).

3. Tetanus, diphtheria, and acellular pertussis (Td/Tdap) vaccination

- Administer a one-time dose of Tdap to adults younger than age 65 years who have not received Tdap previously or for whom vaccine status is unknown to replace one of the 10-year Td boosters.
- Tdap is specifically recommended for the following persons:
  — pregnant women more than 20 weeks' gestation,
  — adults, regardless of age, who are close contacts of infants younger than age 12 months (eg, parents, grandparents, or child care providers), and
  — HCP.
- Tdap can be administered regardless of interval since the most recent tetanus or diphtheria-containing vaccine.
- Pregnant women not vaccinated during pregnancy should receive Tdap immediately postpartum.
- Adults 65 years and older may receive Tdap.
- Adults with unknown or incomplete history of completing a 3-dose primary vaccination series with Td-containing vaccines should begin or complete a primary vaccination series. Tdap should be substituted for a single dose of Td in the vaccination series with Tdap preferred as the first dose.
- For unvaccinated adults, administer the first 2 doses at least 4 weeks apart and the third dose 6-12 months after the second.
- If incompletely vaccinated (ie, less than 3 doses), administer remaining doses. Refer to the ACIP statement for recommendations for administering Td/Tdap as prophylaxis in wound management. *

4. Varicella vaccination

- All adults without evidence of immunity to varicella (as defined below) should receive 2 doses of single-antigen varicella vaccine or a second dose if they have received only 1 dose.
- Special consideration for vaccination should be given to those who
  — have close contact with persons at high risk for severe disease (eg, HCP and family contacts of persons with immunocompromising conditions) or
  — are at high risk for exposure or transmission (eg, teachers; child care employees; residents and staff members of institutional settings, including correctional institutions; college students; military personnel; adolescents and adults living in households with children; nonpregnant women of childbearing age; and international travelers).
- Pregnant women should be assessed for evidence of varicella immunity. Women who do not have evidence of immunity should receive the first dose of varicella vaccine upon completion or termination of pregnancy and before discharge from the healthcare facility. The second dose should be administered 4-8 weeks after the first dose.
- Evidence of immunity to varicella in adults includes any of the following:
  — documentation of 2 doses of varicella vaccine at least 4 weeks apart;
  — U.S.-born before 1980 (although for HCP and pregnant women, birth before 1980 should not be considered evidence of immunity);
  — history of varicella based on diagnosis or verification of varicella by a healthcare provider (for a patient reporting a history of or having an atypical case, a mild case, or both, healthcare providers should seek either an epidemiologic link to a typical varicella case or to a laboratory-confirmed case or evidence of laboratory confirmation, if it was performed at the time of acute disease);
  — history of herpes zoster based on diagnosis or verification of herpes zoster by a healthcare provider; or
  — laboratory evidence of immunity or laboratory confirmation of disease.

5. Human papillomavirus (HPV) vaccination

- Two vaccines are licensed for use in females, bivalent HPV vaccine (HPV2) and quadrivalent HPV vaccine (HPV4), and one HPV vaccine for use in males (HPV4).
- For females, either HPV4 or HPV2 is recommended in a 3-dose series for routine vaccination at 11 or 12 years of age, and for those 13 through 26 years of age, if not previously vaccinated.
- For males, HPV4 is recommended in a 3-dose series for routine vaccination at 11 or 12 years of age, and for those 13 through 21 years of age, if not previously vaccinated. Males 22 through 26 years of age may be vaccinated.
- HPV vaccines are not live vaccines and can be administered to persons who are immunocompromised as a result of infection (including HIV infection), disease, or medications. Vaccine is recommended for immunocompromised persons through age 26 years who did not

get any or all doses when they were younger. The immune response and vaccine efficacy might be less than that in immunocompetent persons.

- Men who have sex with men might especially benefit from vaccination to prevent condyloma and anal cancer. HPV4 is recommended for men who have sex with men through age 26 years who did not get any or all doses when they were younger.
- Ideally, vaccine should be administered before potential exposure to HPV through sexual activity; however, persons who are sexually active should still be vaccinated consistent with age-based recommendations. HPV vaccine can be administered to persons with a history of genital warts, abnormal Papanicolaou test, or positive HPV DNA test.
- A complete series for either HPV4 or HPV2 consists of 3 doses. The second dose should be administered 1-2 months after the first dose; the third dose should be administered 6 months after the first dose (at least 24 weeks after the first dose).
- Although HPV vaccination is not specifically recommended for HCP based on their occupation, HCP should receive the HPV vaccine if they are in the recommended age group.

6. Zoster vaccination

- A single dose of zoster vaccine is recommended for adults 60 years of age and older regardless of whether they report a prior episode of herpes zoster. Although the vaccine is licensed by the Food and Drug Administration (FDA) for use among and can be administered to persons 50 years and older, ACIP recommends that vaccination begins at 60 years of age.
- Persons with chronic medical conditions may be vaccinated unless their condition constitutes a contraindication, such as pregnancy or severe immunodeficiency.
- Although zoster vaccination is not specifically recommended for HCP, HCP should receive the vaccine if they are in the recommended age group.

7. Measles, mumps, rubella (MMR) vaccination

- Adults born before 1957 generally are considered immune to measles and mumps. All adults born in 1957 or later should have documentation of 1 or more doses of MMR vaccine unless they have a medical contraindication to the vaccine, laboratory evidence of immunity to each of the three diseases, or documentation of provider-diagnosed measles or mumps disease. For rubella, documentation of provider-diagnosed disease is not considered acceptable evidence of immunity.

Measles component:

- A routine second dose of MMR vaccine, administered a minimum of 28 days after the first dose, is recommended for adults who
  — are students in postsecondary educational institutions;
  — work in a healthcare facility; or
  — plan to travel internationally.

- Persons who received inactivated (killed) measles vaccine or measles vaccine of unknown type from 1963 to 1967 should be revaccinated with 2 doses of MMR vaccine.

Mumps component:
- A routine second dose of MMR vaccine, administered a minimum of 28 days after the first dose, is recommended for adults who
    — are students in postsecondary educational institutions;
    — work in a healthcare facility; or
    — plan to travel internationally.
- Persons vaccinated before 1979 with either killed mumps vaccine or mumps vaccine of unknown type who are at high risk for mumps infection (eg, persons who are working in a healthcare facility) should be considered for revaccination with 2 doses of MMR vaccine.

Rubella component:
- For women of childbearing age, regardless of birth year, rubella immunity should be determined. If there is no evidence of immunity, women who are not pregnant should be vaccinated. Pregnant women who do not have evidence of immunity should receive MMR vaccine upon completion or termination of pregnancy and before discharge from the healthcare facility.

HCP born before 1957:
- For unvaccinated HCP born before 1957 who lack laboratory evidence of measles, mumps, and/or rubella immunity or laboratory confirmation of disease, healthcare facilities should consider routinely vaccinating personnel with 2 doses of MMR vaccine at the appropriate interval for measles and mumps or 1 dose of MMR vaccine for rubella.

8. Pneumococcal polysaccharide (PPSV) vaccination
- Vaccinate all persons with the following indications:
    — age 65 years and older without a history of PPSV vaccination;
    — adults younger than 65 years with chronic lung disease (including chronic obstructive pulmonary disease, emphysema, and asthma); chronic cardiovascular diseases; diabetes mellitus; chronic liver disease (including cirrhosis); alcoholism; cochlear implants; cerebrospinal fluid leaks; immunocompromising conditions; and functional or anatomic asplenia (eg, sickle cell disease and other hemoglobinopathies, congenital or acquired asplenia, splenic dysfunction, or splenectomy [if elective splenectomy is planned, vaccinate at least 2 weeks before surgery]);
    — residents of nursing homes or long-term care facilities; and
    — adults who smoke cigarettes.
- Persons with asymptomatic or symptomatic HIV infection should be vaccinated as soon as possible after their diagnosis.
- When cancer chemotherapy or other immunosuppressive therapy is being considered, the interval between vaccination and

initiation of immunosuppressive therapy should be at least 2 weeks. Vaccination during chemotherapy or radiation therapy should be avoided.

- Routine use of PPSV is not recommended for American Indians/Alaska Natives or other persons younger than 65 years of age unless they have underlying medical conditions that are PPSV indications. However, public health authorities may consider recommending PPSV for American Indians/Alaska Natives who are living in areas where the risk for invasive pneumococcal disease is increased.

9. Revaccination with PPSV

- One-time revaccination 5 years after the first dose is recommended for persons 19 through 64 years of age with chronic renal failure or nephrotic syndrome; functional or anatomic asplenia (eg, sickle cell disease or splenectomy); and for persons with immunocompromising conditions.
- Persons who received PPSV before age 65 years for any indication should receive another dose of the vaccine at age 65 years or later if at least 5 years have passed since their previous dose.
- No further doses are needed for persons vaccinated with PPSV at or after age 65 years.

10. Meningococcal vaccination

- Administer 2 doses of meningococcal conjugate vaccine quadrivalent (MCV4) at least 2 months apart to adults with functional asplenia or persistent complement component deficiencies.
- HIV-infected persons who are vaccinated should also receive 2 doses.
- Administer a single dose of meningococcal vaccine to microbiologists routinely exposed to isolates of *Neisseria meningitidis*, military recruits, and persons who travel to or live in countries in which meningococcal disease is hyperendemic or epidemic.
- First-year college students up through age 21 years who are living in residence halls should be vaccinated if they have not received a dose on or after their 16th birthday.
- MCV4 is preferred for adults with any of the preceding indications who are 55 years old and younger; meningococcal polysaccharide vaccine (MPSV4) is preferred for adults 56 years and older.
- Revaccination with MCV4 every 5 years is recommended for adults previously vaccinated with MCV4 or MPSV4 who remain at increased risk for infection (eg, adults with anatomic or functional asplenia or persistent complement component deficiencies).

11. Hepatitis A vaccination

- Vaccinate any person seeking protection from hepatitis A virus (HAV) infection and persons with any of the following indications:
  — men who have sex with men and persons who use injection drugs;
  — persons working with HAV-infected primates or with HAV in a research laboratory setting;
  — persons with chronic liver disease and persons who receive clotting factor concentrates;

- persons traveling to or working in countries that have high or intermediate endemicity of hepatitis A; and
- unvaccinated persons who anticipate close personal contact (eg, household or regular babysitting) with an international adoptee during the first 60 days after arrival in the United States from a country with high or intermediate endemicity.* The first dose of the 2-dose hepatitis A vaccine series should be administered as soon as adoption is planned, ideally 2 or more weeks before the arrival of the adoptee.
- Single-antigen vaccine formulations should be administered in a 2-dose schedule at either 0 and 6-12 months (Havrix), or 0 and 6-18 months (Vaqta). If the combined hepatitis A and hepatitis B vaccine (Twinrix) is used, administer 3 doses at 0, 1, and 6 months; alternatively, a 4-dose schedule may be used, administered on days 0, 7, and 21-30 followed by a booster dose at month 12.

12. Hepatitis B vaccination
- Vaccinate persons with any of the following indications and any person seeking protection from hepatitis B virus (HBV) infection:
  - sexually active persons who are not in a long-term, mutually monogamous relationship (eg, persons with more than one sex partner during the previous 6 months); persons seeking evaluation or treatment for a sexually transmitted disease (STD); current or recent injection-drug users; and men who have sex with men;
  - HCP and public safety workers who are exposed to blood or other potentially infectious body fluids;
  - persons with diabetes younger than 60 years as soon as feasible after diagnosis; persons with diabetes who are 60 years or older at the discretion of the treating clinician based on increased need for assisted blood glucose monitoring in long-term care facilities, likelihood of acquiring hepatitis B infection, its complications or chronic sequelae, and likelihood of immune response to vaccination;
  - persons with end-stage renal disease, including patients receiving hemodialysis; persons with HIV infection; and persons with chronic liver disease;
  - household contacts and sex partners of persons with chronic HBV infection; clients and staff members of institutions for persons with developmental disabilities; and international travelers to countries with high or intermediate prevalence of chronic HBV infection; and
  - all adults in the following settings: STD treatment facilities; HIV testing and treatment facilities; facilities providing drug-abuse treatment and prevention services; healthcare settings targeting services to injection-drug users or men who have sex with men; correctional facilities; end-stage renal disease programs and facilities for chronic hemodialysis patients; and institutions and nonresidential daycare facilities for persons with developmental disabilities.
- Administer missing doses to complete a 3-dose series of hepatitis B vaccine to those persons not vaccinated or not completely vaccinated. The second dose should be administered 1 month after the first dose; the third dose should be given at least 2 months after the second dose (and at least 4 months after the first dose). If the combined hepatitis A and hepatitis B vaccine (Twinrix) is used, give 3 doses at 0, 1, and 6 months; alternatively, a 4-dose Twinrix schedule, administered on days 0, 7, and 21-30 followed by a booster dose at month 12 may be used.

• Adult patients receiving hemodialysis or with other immunocompromising conditions should receive 1 dose of 40 µg/mL (Recombivax HB) administered on a 3-dose schedule or 2 doses of 20 µg/mL (Engerix-B) administered simultaneously on a 4-dose schedule at 0, 1, 2, and 6 months.

13. Selected conditions for which *Haemophilus influenzae* type b (Hib) vaccine may be used

• 1 dose of Hib vaccine should be considered for persons who have sickle cell disease, leukemia, or HIV infection, or who have anatomic or functional asplenia if they have not previously received Hib vaccine.

14. Immunocompromising conditions

Inactivated vaccines generally are acceptable (eg, pneumococcal, meningococcal, and influenza [inactivated influenza vaccine]), and live attenuated vaccines generally are avoided in persons with immune deficiencies or immunocompromising conditions. Information on specific conditions is available at http://www.cdc.gov/vaccines/pubs/acip-list.htm

*These schedules indicate the recommended age groups and medical indications for which administration of currently licensed vaccines is commonly indicated for adults ages 19 years and older, as of January 1, 2012. For all vaccines being recommended on the adult immunization schedule: a vaccine series does not need to be restarted, regardless of the time that has elapsed between doses. Licensed combination vaccines may be used whenever any components of the combination are indicated and when the vaccine's other components are not contraindicated. For detailed recommendations on all vaccines, including those used primarily for travelers or that are issued during the year, consult the manufacturers' package inserts and the complete statements from the Advisory Committee on Immunization Practices (http://www.cdc.gov/vaccines/pubs/acip-list.htm).

Report all clinically significant postvaccination reactions to the Vaccine Adverse Event Reporting System (VAERS). Reporting forms and instructions on filing a VAERS report are available at http://www.vaers.hhs.gov or by telephone, 800-822-7967.

Information on how to file a Vaccine Injury Compensation Program claim is available at http://www.hrsa.gov/vaccinecompensation or by telephone, 800-338-2382. Information about filing a claim for vaccine injury is available through the U.S. Court of Federal Claims, 717 Madison Place, N.W., Washington, D.C. 20005, telephone, 202-357-6400.

Additional information about the vaccines in this schedule, extent of available data, and contraindications for vaccination also is available at http://www.cdc.gov/vaccines or from the CDC-INFO Contact Center at 800-CDC-INFO (800-232-4636) in English and Spanish, 8:00 a.m. to 8:00 p.m., Monday through Friday, excluding holidays.

Use of trade names and commercial sources is for identification only and does not imply endorsement by the U.S. Department of Health and Human Services.

INSULIN FORMULATIONS

TYPE OF INSULIN	BRAND (MANUFACTURER)	ONSET* (HRS)	PEAK* (HRS)	DURATION* (HRS)	COMMON PITFALLS
Rapid-acting					
Glulisine	**Apidra** (Sanofi-Aventis)	<0.25	0.5-1.5	1 to 3	Hypoglycemia occurs if lag time is too long or the patient exercises w/in 1 hr of dose; w/ high-fat meals, the dose should be adjusted downward.
Lispro	**Humalog** (Lilly)	<0.25	0.5 to 1.5	3 to 5	
Aspart	**NovoLog** (Novo Nordisk)	<0.25	0.5 to 1	3 to 5	
Short-acting					
Regular	**Humulin R** † (Lilly)	0.5 to 1	2.5 to 5	4 to 12	Lag time is not used appropriately; the insulin should be given 20 to 30 min before the patient eats.
	Novolin R (Novo Nordisk)	0.5	1.5 to 2.5	up to 8	
Intermediate-acting					
NPH (Isophane)	**Humulin N** (Lilly)	1 to 3	6 to 12	up to 24	In many patients, breakfast injection does not last until the pm meal; administration with the pm meal does not meet insulin needs on awakening.
	Novolin N (Novo Nordisk)	1.5	4 to 12	up to 24	
Long-acting					
Glargine	**Lantus** (Sanofi-Aventis)	3 to 4	Flat	up to 24	Administer once daily at the same time qd.
Detemir	**Levemir** (Novo Nordisk)	3 to 4	6 to 8	up to 24	

TYPE OF INSULIN	BRAND (MANUFACTURER)	ONSET* (HRS)	PEAK* (HRS)	DURATION (HRS)	COMMON PITFALLS
Combinations Isophane susp (70%)/ regular (30%)	**Humulin 70/30** (Lilly)	0.5 to 1	4 to 6	up to 24	See individual comments.
	Novolin 70/30 (Novo Nordisk)	0.5	2 to 12	up to 24	
Lispro protamine (50%)/ lispro (50%)	**Humalog Mix 50/50** (Lilly)	≤0.25	0.75 to 2	up to 24	See individual comments.
Lispro protamine (75%)/ lispro (25%)	**Humalog Mix 75/25** (Lilly)	≤0.25	0.5 to 2.5	up to 24	See individual comments.
Aspart protamine (70%)/ aspart (30%)	**Novolog Mix 70/30** (Novo Nordisk)	≤0.25	1 to 4	up to 24	See individual comments.

*Approximate parameters following SC injection of an average patient dose; insulin concentration: 100 U/ml.

† Also available: 500 U/ml for insulin-resistant patients (rapid onset; up to 24h duration).

ORAL CONTRACEPTIVES

DRUG	ESTROGEN	PROGESTIN	STRENGTH (ESTROGEN-PROGESTIN)
MONOPHASIC			
Altavera, Levora, Marlissa, Nordette, Portia	Ethinyl Estradiol	Levonorgestrel	30 mcg-0.15 mg
Apri, Desogen, Emoquette, Ortho-Cept, Reclipsen, Solia	Ethinyl Estradiol	Desogestrel	30 mcg-0.15 mg
Aviane, Lessina, Lutera, Orsythia, Sronyx	Ethinyl Estradiol	Levonorgestrel	20 mcg-0.1 mg
Balziva, Briellyn, Femcon Fe, Ovcon 35, Zenchent	Ethinyl Estradiol	Norethindrone	35 mcg-0.4 mg
Beyaz*	Ethinyl Estradiol	Drospirenone	20 mcg-3 mg
Brevicon, Modicon 28, Necon 0.5/35, Nortrel 0.5/35, Wera	Ethinyl Estradiol	Norethindrone	35 mcg-0.5 mg
Cryselle, Erinest, Lo/Ovral, Low-Ogestrel	Ethinyl Estradiol	Norgestrel	30 mcg-0.3 mg
Alyacen 1/35, Cyclafem 1/35, Dasetta 1/35, Necon 1/35, Norethin 1/35, Norinyl 1/35, Nortrel 1/35, Ortho-Novum 1/35	Ethinyl Estradiol	Norethindrone	35 mcg-1 mg
Generess Fe	Ethinyl Estradiol	Norethindrone	25 mcg-0.8 mg
Gianvi, Loryna, YAZ	Ethinyl Estradiol	Drospirenone	20 mcg-3 mg
Gildess Fe 1/20, Junel 1/20, Junel Fe 1/20, Loestrin 21 1/20, Loestrin Fe 1/20, Loestrin 24 Fe, Microgestin 1/20, Microgestin Fe 1/20	Ethinyl Estradiol	Norethindrone Acetate	20 mcg-1 mg
Gildess Fe 1.5/30, Junel 1.5/30, Junel Fe 1.5/30, Loestrin 21 1.5/30, Loestrin Fe 1.5/30, Microgestin 1.5/30, Microgestin Fe 1.5/30	Ethinyl Estradiol	Norethindrone Acetate	30 mcg-1.5 mg

DRUG	ESTROGEN	PROGESTIN	STRENGTH (ESTROGEN-PROGESTIN)
Introvale, Jolessa, Quasense, Seasonale	Ethinyl Estradiol	Levonorgestrel	30 mcg-0.15 mg
Kelnor, Zovia 1/35E	Ethinyl Estradiol	Ethynodiol Diacetate	35 mcg-1 mg
Lybrel	Ethinyl Estradiol	Levonorgestrel	20 mcg-0.09 mg
Necon 1/50, Norinyl 1/50	Mestranol	Norethindrone	50 mcg-1 mg
Ocella, Syeda, Yasmin, Zarah	Ethinyl Estradiol	Drospirenone	30 mcg-3 mg
Ogestrel-28	Ethinyl Estradiol	Norgestrel	50 mcg-0.5 mg
MonoNessa, Previfem, Sprintec	Ethinyl Estradiol	Norgestimate	35 mcg-0.25 mg
Ovcon 50	Ethinyl Estradiol	Norethindrone	50 mcg-1 mg
Safyral*	Ethinyl Estradiol	Drospirenone	30 mcg-3 mg
Zovia 1/50E	Ethinyl Estradiol	Ethynodiol Diacetate	50 mcg-1 mg
BIPHASIC			
Kariva, Mircette	Ethinyl Estradiol	Desogestrel	Phase 1: 20 mcg-0.15 mg Phase 2: 10 mcg-NONE
Lo Loestrin Fe	Ethinyl Estradiol	Norethindrone Acetate	Phase 1: 10 mcg-1 mg Phase 2: 10 mcg-NONE
Loseasonique	Ethinyl Estradiol	Levonorgestrel	Phase 1: 20 mcg-0.1 mg Phase 2: 10 mcg-NONE
Necon 10/11	Ethinyl Estradiol	Norethindrone	Phase 1: 35 mcg-0.5 mg Phase 2: 35 mcg-1 mg

Seasonique	Ethinyl Estradiol	Levonorgestrel	**Phase 1**: 30 mcg-0.15 mg **Phase 2**: 10 mcg-NONE

TRIPHASIC

Aranelle, Leena, Tri-Norinyl	Ethinyl Estradiol	Norethindrone	**Phase 1**: 35 mcg-0.5 mg **Phase 2**: 35 mcg-1 mg **Phase 3**: 35 mcg-0.5 mg
Cyclafem 7/7/7, Nortrel 7/7/7, Ortho-Novum 7/7/7	Ethinyl Estradiol	Norethindrone	**Phase 1**: 35 mcg-0.5 mg **Phase 2**: 35 mcg-0.75 mg **Phase 3**: 35 mcg-1 mg
Cyclessa, Velivet	Ethinyl Estradiol	Desogestrel	**Phase 1**: 25 mcg-0.1 mg **Phase 2**: 25 mcg-0.125 mg **Phase 3**: 25 mcg-0.15 mg
Enpresse, Levonest, Trivora	Ethinyl Estradiol	Levonorgestrel	**Phase 1**: 30 mcg-0.05 mg **Phase 2**: 40 mcg-0.075 mg **Phase 3**: 30 mcg-0.125 mg
Estrostep Fe, Tilia Fe, Tri-Legest Fe	Ethinyl Estradiol	Norethindrone Acetate	**Phase 1**: 20 mcg-1 mg **Phase 2**: 30 mcg-1 mg **Phase 3**: 35 mcg-1 mg
Ortho Tri-Cyclen, Trinessa, Tri-Previfem, Tri-Sprintec	Ethinyl Estradiol	Norgestimate	**Phase 1**: 35 mcg-0.18 mg **Phase 2**: 35 mcg-0.215 mg **Phase 3**: 35 mcg-0.25 mg
Ortho Tri-Cyclen Lo, Tri-Lo Sprintec	Ethinyl Estradiol	Norgestimate	**Phase 1**: 25 mcg-0.18 mg **Phase 2**: 25 mcg-0.215 mg **Phase 3**: 25 mcg-0.25 mg

DRUG	ESTROGEN	PROGESTIN	STRENGTH (ESTROGEN-PROGESTIN)
MISCELLANEOUS COMBINATION			
Natazia	Estradiol Valerate	Dienogest	**Phase 1:** 3 mg-NONE **Phase 2:** 2 mg-2 mg **Phase 3:** 2 mg-3 mg **Phase 4:** 1 mg-NONE
PROGESTIN ONLY			
Camila, Errin, Heather, Jolivette, Micronor, Nora-BE, Nor-QD		Norethindrone	0.35 mg
EMERGENCY (Progestin Only)			
Ella		Ulipristal Acetate	30 mg
Next Choice, Plan B		Levonorgestrel	0.75 mg
Plan B One-Step		Levonorgestrel	1.5 mg

*Includes 0.451 mg Levomefolate Calcium.

SYSTEMIC CORTICOSTEROIDS

CORTICOSTEROID	EQUIVALENT POTENCY	MINERALOCORTICOID POTENCY	FORM/STRENGTH	DOSAGE RANGE
Betamethasone (Celestone)	0.75 mg	0	**Syr:** 0.6 mg/5 ml	**Initial:** 0.6-7.2 mg/d PO.
Betamethasone Sodium Phosphate & Betamethasone Acetate (Celestone Soluspan)	0.75 mg	0	**Inj:** 3 mg/ml	**Initial:** 0.25-9 mg/d IM.
Cortisone Acetate	25 mg	2	**Tab:** 25 mg	**Initial:** 25-300 mg/d PO.
Dexamethasone	0.75 mg	0	**Sol:** 0.5 mg/5 ml, 1 mg/1 ml; **Tab:** 0.5 mg, 0.75 mg, 1 mg, 1.5 mg, 2 mg, 4 mg, 6 mg	**Initial:** 0.75-9 mg/d PO.
Dexamethasone Sodium Phosphate	0.75 mg	0	**Inj:** 4 mg/ml, 10 mg/ml	**Initial:** 0.5-9 mg/d IM/IV.
Hydrocortisone (Cortef)	20 mg	2	**Tab:** 5 mg, 10 mg, 20 mg	**Initial:** 20-240 mg/d PO.
Hydrocortisone Sodium Succinate (Solu-Cortef)	20 mg	2	**Inj:** 100 mg, 250 mg, 500 mg, 1000 mg	**Initial:** 100-500 mg IM/IV.
Methylprednisolone (Medrol)	4 mg	0	**Tab:** 4 mg, 8 mg, 16 mg, 32 mg	**Initial:** 4-48 mg/d PO.
Methylprednisolone Acetate (Depo-Medrol)	4 mg	0	**Inj:** 20 mg/ml, 40 mg/ml, 80 mg/ml	**Initial:** 4-120 mg/d IM.
Methylprednisolone Sodium Succinate (Solu-Medrol)	4 mg	0	**Inj:** 40 mg, 125 mg, 500 mg, 1 gm, 2 gm	**Initial:** 10-40 mg IM/IV.
Prednisolone (Prelone)	5 mg	1	**Syr:** 5 mg/5 ml, 15 mg/5 ml	**Initial:** 5-60 mg/d PO.

KEY: ☻ PREGNANCY RATING; ✽ BREASTFEEDING SAFETY; ℍ HEPATIC ADJUSTMENT; ℝ RENAL ADJUSTMENT

DRUG	EQUIVALENT POTENCY	MINERALOCORTICOID POTENCY	FORM/STRENGTH	DOSAGE RANGE
Prednisolone Sodium Phosphate (Orapred, Pediapred)	5 mg	1	**Sol:** 5 mg/5 ml, 10 mg/5 ml, 15 mg/5 ml, 20 mg/5 ml, 25 mg/5 ml; **Tab,Dissolve:** 10 mg, 15 mg, 30 mg	**Initial:** 5-60 mg/d PO.
Prednisone	5 mg	1	**Sol:** 5 mg/ml, 5 mg/5 ml; **Tab:** 1 mg, 2.5 mg, 5 mg, 10 mg, 20 mg, 50 mg	**Initial:** 5-60 mg/d PO.
Triamcinolone Acetonide (Kenalog-10)	4 mg	0	**Inj:** 10 mg/ml	**Initial:** 2.5-20 mg/d intra-articular.
Triamcinolone Acetonide (Kenalog-40)	4 mg	0	**Inj:** 40 mg/ml	**Initial:** 2.5-100 mg/d IM or 2.5-80 mg/d intra-articular.
Triamcinolone Hexacetonide (Aristospan Intra-lesional, Aristospan Intra-articular)	4 mg	0	**Inj:** 5 mg/ml (intra-lesional), 20 mg/ml (intra-articular)	**Intra-articular:** 2-48 mg/d. **Intra-lesional:** Up to 0.5 mg/in^2 of area affected.

TOPICAL CORTICOSTEROIDS – RELATIVE POTENCY AND DOSAGE

DRUG	HOW SUPPLIED	STRENGTH (%)	POTENCY	FREQUENCY
Alclometasone Dipropionate (Aclovate)	Cre, Oint	0.05	Low-Medium	bid/tid
Amcinonide	Cre, Lot, Oint	0.1	High, Medium (Lot)	bid/tid
Augmented Betamethasone Dipropionate (Diprolene, Diprolene AF)	Gel, Lot, Oint	0.05	Very High	qd/bid
	Cre	0.05	High	qd/bid
Betamethasone Dipropionate	Cre, Lot, Oint	0.05	High	qd/bid
Betamethasone Valerate (Luxiq)	Cre, Lot	0.1	Medium	qd/tid, bid (Lot)
	Foam (Luxiq)	0.12	Medium	bid
	Oint	0.1	High	qd/tid
Clobetasol Propionate (Clobex, Cormax, Olux, Olux-E, Temovate, Temovate E)	Cre, Foam, Gel, Lot, Oint, Sol, Spr	0.05	Very High	bid
	Shampoo (Clobex)	0.05	Very High	qd
Clocortolone Pivalate (Cloderm)	Cre	0.1	Medium	tid
Desonide (DesOwen, Desonate, LoKara, Verdeso)	Cre, Foam, Gel, Lot, Oint	0.05	Low-Medium	bid/tid
Desoximetasone (Topicort, Topicort LP)	Cre, Oint	0.05	High	bid
	Gel	0.05	High	bid
	Cre, Oint	0.25	High	bid

KEY: ⊕ PREGNANCY RATING; ✽ BREASTFEEDING SAFETY; H HEPATIC ADJUSTMENT; R RENAL ADJUSTMENT

DRUG	HOW SUPPLIED	STRENGTH (%)	POTENCY	FREQUENCY
Diflorasone Diacetate (ApexiCon, ApexiCon E)	Cre, Oint	0.05	High-Very High	qd/tid
Fluocinolone Acetonide (Capex, Derma-Smoothe/FS)	Cre, Oint	0.025	Medium	tid/qid
	Cre, Sol	0.01	Medium	tid/qid
	Oil	0.01	Low-Medium	qd
	Shampoo (Capex)	0.01	Low-Medium	qd
Fluocinonide (Vanos)	Cre, Gel, Oint, Sol	0.05	High	bid/qid
	Cre (Vanos)	0.1	Very High	qd/bid
Flurandrenolide (Cordran, Cordran SP)	Cre, Oint	0.025, 0.05	Medium	bid/tid
	Lot	0.05	Medium	bid/tid
	Tape	4 mcg/cm²	Medium	qd/bid
Fluticasone Propionate (Cutivate)	Cre, Lot	0.05	Medium	bid
	Oint	0.005	Medium	bid
Halcinonide (Halog)	Cre, Oint	0.1	High	bid/tid
Halobetasol Propionate (Ultravate)	Cre, Oint	0.05	Very High	qd/bid
Hydrocortisone (Ala-Cort, Ala-Scalp HP, Cortaid)	Cre, Oint	0.5	Low	tid/qid
	Cre, Lot, Oint, Sol	1	Low	tid/qid
	Lot	2	Low	bid/qid
	Cre, Lot, Oint, Sol	2.5	Low	bid/qid

Hydrocortisone Butyrate (Locoid)	Cre, Lot, Oint, Sol	0.1	Medium	bid/tid
Hydrocortisone Probutate (Pandel)	Cre	0.1	Medium	qd/bid
Hydrocortisone Valerate (Westcort)	Cre, Oint	0.2	Medium	bid/tid
Mometasone Furoate (Elocon)	Cre, Lot, Oint	0.1	Medium	qd
Prednicarbate (Dermatop)	Cre, Oint	0.1	Medium	bid
Triamcinolone Acetonide (Kenalog, Triderm)	Cre, Lot, Oint	0.025	Medium	bid/qid
	Cre, Lot, Oint	0.1	Medium	bid/tid
	Cre, Oint	0.5	High	bid/tid
	Spr	0.147 mg/gm	Medium	tid/qid

Headings under a generic drug entry include listings for both single and combination forms of the generic product.

INDEX

A

Abacavir	34
Abatacept	16
Abelcet	48
Abilify	
Antipsychotics	259
Bipolar Agents	261
Depression	247
Miscellaneous	270
Abilify Discmelt	270
Acanya	146
Acarbose	168
Accolate	277
AccuNeb	273
Accupril	
Heart Failure	122
HTN	128
Accuretic	130
Acebutolol	106

Acetaminophen
Miscellaneous	29
Narcotics	20
Acetaminophen/Codeine	20
Aciphex	
GERD	198
Ulcer	195
Zollinger-Ellison	204
Aclovate	319
Acne	145–147
Actemra	19
ActHIB	218
Actiq	21
Activella	
Hormone Therapy	210
Osteoporosis	178
Actonel	177
Actoplus Met	172
Actoplus Met XR	172
Actos	172
Acular LS	161

Acular PF	161
Acyclovir	
Systemic	42
Topical	149
Acyclovir Injection	42
Adacel	222
Adalimumab	
Arthritis	16
Crohn's Disease	205
Psoriasis	151
Adapalene	146
Adcirca	144
Adderall	224
Adderall XR	224
Adefovir	39
ADHD/	
Narcolepsy Agents	223–229
Advair	272
Advair HFA	272
Advicor	114
Afinitor	94

Afluria	220
Aggrenox	119
Agrylin	119
AIDS	32–38
Ala-Cort	320
Alamast	162
Ala-Scalp HP	320
Alavert	287
Albuterol	272
Alcaftadine	162
Alclometasone	319
Alcortin-A	149
Aldactazide	
Heart Failure	126
HTN	143
Aldactone	
Heart Failure	125
HTN	143
Aldara	153
Alefacept	150
Alendronate	176

Alfuzosin...................... 279
Alimta.......................... 97
Alinia 185
Aliskiren 145
Allegra 286
Allegra-D 286
Allopurinol
  Gout 175
  Miscellaneous............ 184
Almotriptan.................. 266
Alocril 162
Aloprim 184
Alora 179
Alosetron 205
Aloxi.......................... 188
Alphagan P 161
Alprazolam................... 231
Alrex.......................... 158
Alsuma 267
Altabax....................... 147
Altace
  Heart Failure............. 123
  HTN........................ 129

Altavera...................... 313
Alvesco 276
Alyacen 313
Alzheimer's Therapy .. 229–230
Amantadine.................. 44
Amaryl 171
Ambien....................... 235
Ambien CR 235
AmBisome.................... 48
Amcinonide.................. 319
Amerge 266
Amevive 150
Amikacin
  Bone Infection............ 45
  LRI........................ 52
  Meningitis................. 60
  Septicemia................ 66
Amiodarone.................. 107
Amitiza....................... 205
Amitriptyline................ 249
Amlodipine
  Angina..................... 102
  Antilipidemic Agents 109
  HTN........................ 139
Amnesteem................... 146

Amoxicillin
  LRI........................ 56
  Otitis Media............... 65
  Skin Infection............. 74
  Ulcer 194
  URI........................ 81
  UTI........................ 87
Amphetamine Salt Combo .. 224
Amphotericin B Lipid Complex.................. 48
Amphotericin B Liposome 48
Ampicillin
  LRI........................ 57
  Meningitis................. 62
  Skin Infection............. 74
  URI........................ 81
  UTI........................ 87
Ampicillin Injection
  Meningitis................. 62
  URI........................ 81
Ampicillin Oral
  LRI........................ 57
  URI........................ 81
  UTI........................ 87
Amrix......................... 268
Amturnide.................... 138
Anagrelide.................. 119

Anagrelide...................119
Anakinra 16
Anaprox
  Dysmenorrhea............ 209
  NSAIDs.................... 28
Anaprox DS
  Dysmenorrhea............ 209
  NSAIDs.................... 28
Anastrozole.................. 92
Androderm 163
Androgel...................... 163
Androgens 163–164
Anemia 214–215
Angeliq....................... 210
Angina 101–104
Anidulafungin 49
Antiarrhythmics 104–108
Antibacterial/Steroid Ophtho Combos 157
Antibiotic Agents 156–157
Anticholinergics 154
Anticonvulsants 235–244
Antiemetics............ 186–191
Antihistamine/ Corticosteroid Combinations 154

Anti-Infective Agents..... 147–149, 207–208
Anti-Infective Combos 149–150
Antilipidemic Agents...109–115
Antineoplastics 92–100
Antiparkinson's Agents........... 250–253
Antipsychotics 254–260
Antispasmodics............ 192
Antithyroid Agents........174
Antivert 189
Antivirals.................... 39–44
Anxiety/Hypnotics 231–235
Anzemet 186
Apexicon 320
Apexicon E 320
Apidra.......................... 311
Aplenzin 246
Aprepitant..................... 191
Apri................................ 313
Aptivus........................... 38
Aranelle....................... 315
Aranesp....................... 215

Arava................................ 18
Arcapta Neohaler 275
Aredia................................ 183
Arformoterol.................... 274
Aricept............................. 229
Arimidex............................ 92
Aripiprazole
  Antipsychotics 259
  Bipolar Agents............. 261
  Depression................... 247
  Miscellaneous............. 270
Aristospan..................... 318
Arixtra............................ 120
Armodafinil.................... 228
Armour Thyroid............. 183
Aromasin......................... 95
Arthritis.................... 16–19
Asacol............................ 202
Asacol HD..................... 202
Ascorbic Acid.............. 200
Asenapine 256
Asmanex 277

Aspirin
  Coagulation Modifiers.... 120
  Narcotics...................... 26
Astelin 284
Astepro 284
Asthma/COPD Preps.. 271–278
Atacand
  Heart Failure...............124
  HTN............................. 132
Atazanavir...................... 36
Atelvia.......................... 177
Atenolol
  Angina 101
  HTN............................ 137
Ativan 232
Ativan Injection 235
Atomoxetine................. 223
Atorvastatin
  Angina 101
  Antilipidemic Agents.... 112
  HTN............................ 139
Atovaquone..................... 66
Atripla............................ 33
Atropine
  Antispasmodics........... 192
  Diarrhea..................... 185

Atrovent HFA 271
Atrovent Nasal 154
Atuss DS..................... 288
Augmentin
  LRI................................56
  Otitis Media..................65
  Skin Infection..............74
  URI................................81
  UTI................................87
Augmentin ES-600.......65
Augmentin XR
  LRI................................57
  URI................................82
Auranofin....................... 16
Avalide......................... 135
Avanafil....................... 281
Avandamet 173
Avandaryl...................... 174
Avandia....................... 172
Avapro......................... 132
Avelox
  LRI................................59
  Skin Infection..............75
  URI................................82
Aviane 313

Avinza.................................... 24
Avodart 280
Axert 266
Axid
   GERD 196
   Ulcer 193
Axiron 163
Azactam 68
Azasan 17
Azasite 156
Azathioprine 17
Azelastine
   Antihistamine Chart 284
   Conjunctivitis.............. 162
   Nasal Preps.................. 154
Azilect................................ 253
Azilsartan 135
Azithromycin
   LRI 55
   MAC 62
   Ophtho Preps................ 156
   Otitis Media................... 64
   Skin Infection............... 72
   URI 79
   UTI 86
Azmacort 277

Azopt 159
Azor 141
Aztreonam 68
Azulfidine 202

B

Bacitracin
   Topical.......................... 147
   Topical Ointment.......... 150
Bactroban 147
Bactroban Nasal 147
Balziva 313
Banzel 238
Baraclude.............................. 39
Bayer Aspirin 120
Beclomethasone
   Asthma/COPD Preps..... 275
   Corticosteroids............ 154
   Nasal Preps................. 155
Beconase AQ 155
Benadryl 286
Benadryl-D Allergy and Sinus
   286
Benazepril............................ 129
Benicar................................ 133

Benicar HCT 136
Bentyl 192
Benzonatate 291
Benzoyl Peroxide.................... 145
Benztropine 250
Bepotastine.......................... 162
Bepreve 162
Betagan 159
Betamethasone
   Systemic Steroid Chart... 317
   Topical.......................... 149
   Topical Steroid Chart ... 319
Betapace 108
Betapace AF 108
Betaxolol............................ 158
Betoptic S 158
Beyaz 313
Biaxin
   LRI 55
   MAC 62
   Otitis Media................... 64
   Skin Infection............... 72
   URI 80
Biaxin XL
   LRI 55
   MAC 62

   Otitis Media................... 64
   Skin Infection............... 72
   URI 80
Bicalutamide 92
Bimatoprost 160
Bipolar Agents........ 261–266
Bisacodyl 199
Bisoprolol............................ 137
Blephamide 157
Boceprevir............................ 39
Bone Infection........... 45–48
BPH 279–281
Brevibloc 106
Brevicon 313
Briellyn............................... 313
Brilinta 116
Brimonidine 161
Brinzolamide 159
Bromday 161
Bromfenac 161
Bromocriptine 251
Brompheniramine.................... 284
Brovana................................ 274
Budeprion SR 246

Budeprion XL.................... 246

Budesonide
  Asthma/COPD Preps 276
  Nasal Preps................. 155

Bumetanide.................... 124

Buprenex 19

Buprenorphine 19

Bupropion 246

Buspirone..................... 234

Butenafine 148

Butrans 20

Byetta........................ 169

Bystolic...................... 137

C

Cabazitaxel..................... 92

Caduet
  Angina...................... 101
  Antilipidemic Agents 109
  HTN......................... 139

Calan
  Angina...................... 103
  Antiarrhythmics........... 108
  HTN......................... 141

Calan SR...................... 140

Calcitonin-Salmon 177

Caldolor........................ 28

Camila....................... 316

Candesartan
  Heart Failure............... 124
  HTN......................... 132

Capex 320

Caprelsa 100

Capsaicin 29

Captopril
  Heart Failure............... 121
  HTN......................... 127

Carafate 192

Carbamazepine
  Anticonvulsants........... 238
  Bipolar Agents........... 261

Carbetapentane 291

Carbidopa.................... 253

Carbinoxamine 284

Cardene SR................... 139

Cardizem 102

Cardizem CD
  Angina...................... 102
  HTN......................... 140

Cardizem LA
  Angina...................... 102
  HTN......................... 140

Cardura
  BPH......................... 280
  HTN......................... 131

Cardura XL 279

Carteolol..................... 159

Cartia XT
  Angina...................... 102
  HTN......................... 140

Carvedilol
  Heart Failure............... 123
  HTN......................... 131

Casodex........................ 92

Catapres...................... 131

Catapres-TTS 131

Cefaclor
  LRI.......................... 53
  Otitis Media................. 62
  Skin Infection.............. 70
  URI.......................... 78
  UTI.......................... 84

Cefadroxil
  Skin Infection.............. 70
  URI.......................... 78
  UTI.......................... 84

Cefazolin
  Bone Infection............. 46
  Septicemia................. 67

Cefdinir
  LRI.......................... 53
  Otitis Media................. 63
  Skin Infection.............. 70
  URI.......................... 78

Cefepime
  LRI.......................... 53
  Skin Infection.............. 70
  UTI.......................... 85

Cefixime
  LRI.......................... 53
  Otitis Media................. 63
  URI.......................... 78
  UTI.......................... 85

Cefotaxime
  Bone Infection............. 46
  Meningitis.................. 61
  Septicemia................. 67

Cefoxitin
  Bone Infection............. 46
  Septicemia................. 67

Cefpodoxime
  LRI.......................... 53
  Otitis Media................. 63
  Skin Infection.............. 70

URI................................78
UTI...............................85

Cefprozil
LRI................................53
Otitis Media....................63
Skin Infection.................71
URI................................79

Ceftaroline
LRI................................53
Skin Infection.................71

Ceftazidime
Bone Infection................46
LRI................................54
Meningitis......................61
Septicemia......................68
Skin Infection.................71
UTI...............................85

Ceftin
LRI................................54
Otitis Media....................63
Skin Infection.................71
URI................................79
UTI...............................86

Ceftriaxone
Bone Infection................46
LRI................................54
Meningitis......................61
Otitis Media....................63
Septicemia......................68

Skin Infection.................71
UTI...............................85

Cefuroxime
Bone Infection................46
LRI................................54
Meningitis......................62
Otitis Media....................63
Septicemia......................68
Skin Infection.................71
URI................................79
UTI...............................86

Celebrex
Arthritis.........................17
Dysmenorrhea...............209
NSAIDs...........................27

Celecoxib
Arthritis.........................17
Dysmenorrhea...............209
NSAIDs...........................27

Celestone..................317
Celexa......................248
Celontin...................238
Cenestin...................211

Cephalexin
Bone Infection................47
LRI................................54
Otitis Media....................64
Skin Infection.................72

URI................................79
UTI...............................86

Certolizumab Pegol
Arthritis.........................17
Crohn's Disease.............205
Cervarix.....................219
Cesamet.....................191
Cetirizine...................284
Cetuximab....................92
Cheratussin AC...........288
Cheratussin DAC.........288
Chlordiazepoxide.........192
Chlorothiazide
Heart Failure.................126
HTN..............................144
Chlorpheniramine
Antihistamine Chart.......284
Cough/Cold Chart...........288
Chlorpromazine...........259
Chlorthalidone............138
Chlor-Trimeton............285
Cholecalciferol............176
Cialis
BPH...............................280
ED................................282

Ciclesonide
Asthma/COPD Preps......276
Nasal Preps...................155
Ciclopirox...................148
Cilastatin.....................45
Cilostazol...................119
Ciloxan......................156
Cimetidine
GERD............................196
Ulcer............................193
Zollinger-Ellison.............203
Cimzia
Arthritis.........................17
Crohn's Disease.............205
Cipro IV
Bone Infection................47
LRI................................58
Skin Infection.................75
URI................................82
UTI...............................88
Cipro Oral
Anti-Infective Agents......208
Bone Infection................47
LRI................................58
Misc. Anti-Infectives........91
Skin Infection.................75
URI................................82
UTI...............................87

Cipro XR 88
Ciprofloxacin
  Anti-Infective Agents 208
  Bone Infection............... 47
  LRI.............................. 58
  Misc. Anti-Infectives 91
  Ophtho Preps.............. 156
  Skin Infection................ 75
  URI.............................. 82
  UTI.............................. 87
Cisplatin 93
Citalopram 248
Claforan
  Bone Infection............... 46
  Meningitis.................... 61
  Septicemia.................... 67
Claravis 146
Clarinex 285
Clarinex-D 285
Clarithromycin
  LRI.............................. 55
  MAC............................ 62
  Otitis Media.................. 64
  Skin Infection................ 72
  Ulcer......................... 194
  URI.............................. 80
Claritin 287

Claritin-D 287
Clavulanate
  Bone Infection............... 47
  LRI.............................. 56
  Otitis Media.................. 65
  Septicemia.................... 69
  Skin Infection................ 74
  URI.............................. 81
  UTI.............................. 87
Clemastine................... 285
Cleocin
  Bone Infection............... 48
  LRI.............................. 60
  Septicemia.................... 69
  Skin Infection................ 77
Clidinium 192
Climara
  Hormone Therapy........ 212
  Osteoporosis 179
Climara Pro
  Hormone Therapy........ 210
  Osteoporosis 178
Clindamycin
  Acne 145
  Bone Infection............... 48
  LRI.............................. 60
  Septicemia.................... 69

  Skin Infection................ 77
  Vaginal 207
Clindesse 207
Clobetasol
  Psoriasis 152
  Topical Steroid Chart 319
Clobex
  Psoriasis 152
  Topical Steroid Chart 319
Clocortolone................ 319
Cloderm......................... 319
Clonidine
  ADHD/Narcolepsy
    Agents................... 223
  HTN............................ 131
Clopidogrel 116
Clorazepate 231
Clotrimazole 149
Clozapine 256
Clozaril 256
**Coagulation
Modifiers** 116–121
Codeine
  Cough/Cold Chart 289
  Narcotics...................... 20

Cogentin 250
Colace.......................... 201
Colchicine 176
Colcrys.......................... 175
Colesevelam
  Antilipidemic Agents 109
  Diabetes..................... 165
Colestid......................... 109
Colestipol 109
Combigan 161
Combivent 272
Combivir......................... 35
Complera 34
Comtan 251
Comvax.......................... 37
Concerta 226
Condylox......................... 149
Conjugated Estrogens
  Hormone Therapy........ 211
  Osteoporosis 178
Conjunctivitis 162
Constulose 201
Contraceptives 209

Copegus 40
Cordarone 107
Cordran 320
Cordran SP 320
Coreg
  Heart Failure 123
  HTN 131
Coreg CR
  Heart Failure 123
  HTN 131
Corgard
  Angina 101
  HTN 137
Cormax 319
Cortef 317
Cortaid 320
Corticosteroids... 154–156, 158
Cortisone 317
Cortisporin 150
Cosopt 159
Coumadin 121
Covera-HS
  Angina 103
  HTN 141
Cozaar 132
Crestor 113

Crixivan 37
Cromolyn 278
Cryselle 313
Cubicin
  Misc. Anti-Infectives 91
  Skin Infection 77
Cutivate 320
Cyclafem 1/35 313
Cyclafem 7/7/7 315
Cyclessa 315
Cyclobenzaprine 268
Cyclosporine 151
Cymbalta
  Anxiety/Hypnotics 233
  Depression 247
  Miscellaneous 29
Cyproheptadine 286
Cytomel 182
Cytotec 193

D

Dabigatran etexilate 116
Dalfopristin 75
Daliresp 278
Dalteparin 117

Daptomycin
  Misc. Anti-Infectives 91
  Skin Infection 77
Darbepoetin Alfa 215
Darifenacin 282
Dasatinib 94
Dasetta 1/35 313
Daytrana 226
Degarelix 94
Delavirdine 33
Demadex
  Heart Failure 125
  HTN 143
Demeclocycline 82
Demerol 23
Denavir 149
Denosumab 179
Depacon 236
Depakene 236
Depakote
  Anticonvulsants 239
  Bipolar Agents 261
  Migraine 267
Depakote ER
  Anticonvulsants 239
  Bipolar Agents 261
  Migraine 267

Depakote Sprinkle Capsules
  Bipolar Agents 261
  Migraine 267
Depo-Medrol 317
Depo-Provera
  Contraceptive 209
Depression 245–250
Derma-Smoothe/FS 320
Dermatop 321
Desipramine 249
Desloratadine 285
Desogen 313
Desogestrel 313
Desonate 319
Desonide 319
DesOwen 319
Desoximetasone 319
Desvenlafaxine 247
Detrol 283
Dexamethasone
  Ophtho Preps 157
  Systemic Steroid Chart .. 317
Dexedrine Spansules 225
Dexilant 197

Dexlansoprazole 197
Dexmethylphenidate........ 225
Dextroamphetamine 225
Dextromethorphan
   Cough/Cold Chart........ 289
   Miscellaneous 270
DiaBeta 171
Diabetes................ 164–174
Diarrhea.................... 185
Diazepam
   Anticonvulsants........... 235
   Anxiety/Hypnotics 232
Dibasic Sodium Phosphate . 199
Diclofenac 27
Dicyclomine 192
Didanosine 34
Dienogest.................... 317
Differin 146
Dificid 91
Diflorasone 320
Diflucan
   Systemic 49
   Vaginal 208

Dilacor XR
   Angina 103
   HTN...................... 140
Dilantin 237
Dilatrate-SR 103
Dilaudid 23
Diltia XT
   Angina 103
   HTN...................... 140
Diltiazem
   Angina 102
   HTN...................... 140
Diovan
   Heart Failure.............. 124
   HTN...................... 133
Diovan HCT................. 136
Diphenhydramine 286
Diphenoxylate............... 185
Diphtheria Toxoid 218
Diphtheria Toxoid,
   Reduced................. 222
Dipivefrin 158
Diprolene 319
Dipyridamole 119
Disopyramide 104

Diuril
   Heart Failure.............. 126
   HTN...................... 144
Divalproex
   Anticonvulsants........... 239
   Bipolar Agents............ 261
   Migraine................. 267
Divigel 212
Docusate................... 201
Dofetilide 107
Dolasetron 186
Donepezil 229
Donnatal 192
Donnatal Extentabs 192
Doribax
   Misc. Anti-Infectives 91
   UTI...................... 84
Doripenem
   Misc. Anti-Infectives 91
   UTI...................... 84
Doryx
   LRI....................... 59
   Skin Infection............. 76
   URI....................... 83
   UTI...................... 89
Dorzolamide................ 159

Doxazosin
   BPH...................... 280
   HTN...................... 131
Doxepin
   Anxiety/Hypnotics 234
   Pruritus/Inflammation ... 150
Doxycycline
   Anti-Infective Agents 149
   LRI....................... 59
   Skin Infection............. 76
   URI....................... 83
   UTI...................... 90
Dronabinol................. 191
Dronedarone............... 107
Drospirenone
   Hormone Therapy........ 210
   Oral Contraceptives
   Chart................... 313
Duac 145
Duetact 173
Dulera 273
Duloxetine
   Anxiety/Hypnotics 233
   Depression................ 247
   Miscellaneous............. 29
Duoneb 272

Duragesic................................ 20
Dutasteride 280
Dyazide 126
Dymista 154
Dynacin
   LRI...................................... 59
   Skin Infection................... 76
   URI...................................... 83
   UTI...................................... 90
DynaCirc CR......................... 139
Dyrenium
   Heart Failure.................... 125
   HTN................................... 143
Dysmenorrhea 209

E

E.E.S.
   LRI...................................... 55
   Skin Infection................... 72
   URI...................................... 80
EC-Naprosyn
   Dysmenorrhea................. 209
   NSAIDs............................... 28
ED 281–282
Edarbi.................................. 132

Edarbyclor.......................... 135
Edurant.................................. 34
Efavirenz 33
Effexor XR
   Anxiety/Hypnotics 233
   Depression..................... 247
Effient................................. 116
Egrifta.............................. 184
Eldepryl.............................. 253
Elestat................................ 162
Eletriptan.......................... 266
Elidel................................. 150
Elitek.................................. 185
Ella.................................... 316
Elocon................................ 321
Eltrombopag...................... 216
Emend................................ 191
Emoquette........................... 313
Emtricitabine....................... 34
Emtriva................................ 35
Enablex............................... 282
Enalapril
   Heart Failure.................... 122
   HTN................................... 129

Enalapril/HCTZ................... 129
Enalaprilat 127
Enbrel
   Arthritis............................ 18
   Psoriasis......................... 153
Endocet................................ 25
Endodan.............................. 26
Enfuvirtide 32
Engerix-B........................... 219
Enjuvia............................... 211
Enoxaparin........................ 118
Enpresse............................ 315
Entacapone........................ 253
Entacavir............................ 39
Enulose.............................. 201
Ephedrine 291
Epiduo............................... 145
Epinastine 162
Epinephrine
   Antiarrhythmics............. 105
   Miscellaneous............... 279
EpiPen............................... 279
EpiPen Jr............................ 279

Epitol................................ 238
Epivir................................. 35
Epivir-HBV.......................... 39
Eplerenone
   Heart Failure.................... 123
   HTN................................... 130
Epoetin Alfa....................... 216
Epogen............................... 216
Eprosartan........................ 132
Epzicom............................... 34
Equetro.............................. 261
Eraxis................................. 49
Erbitux............................... 92
Erlotinib............................ 94
Erinest............................... 313
Errin.................................. 316
Ertaczo............................... 148
Ertapenem
   LRI...................................... 52
   Skin Infection................... 69
   UTI...................................... 84
EryPed
   LRI...................................... 55
   Skin Infection................... 72
   URI...................................... 80

Ery-Tab
  LRI.....................................56
  Skin Infection.................73
  URI....................................80

Erythrocin
  LRI.....................................55
  Skin Infection.................73
  URI....................................80

Erythromycin
  LRI.....................................55
  Otitis Media.....................64
  Skin Infection.................72
  URI....................................80

Erythromycin Base
  Skin Infection.................72
  URI....................................80

Erythromycin Ethylsuccinate
and Sulfisoxazole Acetyl ...64

Escitalopram
  Anxiety/Hypnotics 233
  Depression.................... 248

Esmolol 106

Esomeprazole
  GERD 197
  NSAIDs........................... 27
  Ulcer 194
  Zollinger-Ellison........... 204

Estrace................................ 179

Estradiol
  Hormone Therapy........ 210
  Oral Contraceptives
  Chart........................... 313
  Osteoporosis 178

Estropipate 179

Estrostep Fe........................ 315

Eszopiclone..................... 234

Etanercept
  Arthritis 18
  Psoriasis 153

Ethinyl Estradiol
  Hormone Therapy........ 210
  Oral Contraceptives
  Chart........................... 313
  Osteoporosis 178

Ethosuximide.................... 237

Ethynodiol Diacetate........ 315

Etravirine......................... 33

Evamist 212

Everolimus..................... 94

Evista
  Antineoplastics.............. 97
  Osteoporosis 180

Evoclin 146

Exelon
  Alzheimer's Therapy...... 230
  Antiparkinson's Agents .. 251

Exemestane.................... 95

Exenatide 169

Exforge 142

Exforge HCT....................... 134

Extina 148

Ezetimibe..................... 110

Ezogabine..................... 239

F

Factive 58

Famciclovir 43

Famotidine
  GERD 196
  Ulcer 193
  Zollinger-Ellison........... 203

Famvir.............................. 43

Fanapt............................... 254

Fazaclo............................. 257

Febuxostat 175

Femara.............................. 96

Femcon Fe.......................... 313

femhrt
  Hormone Therapy........ 210
  Osteoporosis 178

Femtrace.......................211

Fenofibrate......................111

Fentanyl............................ 20

Fentora.............................. 21

Feosol 214

Ferrlecit............................ 215

Ferrous 214

Fesoterodine.................... 283

Fexofenadine................... 286

Fidaxomicin..................... 91

Filgrastim........................ 217

Finasteride
  Alopecia 153
  BPH 280

Firmagon 94

Flagyl
  Bone Infection.............. 48
  Vaginal 207

Flagyl ER........................ 207

Flagyl IV........................ 48

Flecainide 105
Flector 27
Fleet Glycerin Laxatives 202
Flexeril 268
Flomax 280
Flonase 155
Flovent HFA.................. 276
Fluconazole
  Systemic 49
  Vaginal 208
FluLaval 221
Flumadine 44
FluMist 220
Fluocinolone................. 321
Fluocinonide
  Psoriasis 153
  Topical Steroid Chart 319
Fluoxetine
  Anxiety/Hypnotics 233
  Depression................ 248
  OCD 269
  PMDD 212
Fluphenazine 260
Flurandrenolide 320
Flurbiprofen................. 161

Fluticasone
  Asthma/COPD Preps 272
  Nasal Preps............... 155
  Topical Steroid Chart 319
Fluvastatin 112
Fluvirin...................... 220
Fluvoxamine................. 269
Fluzone...................... 220
Fluzone High-Dose 220
Fluzone Intradermal 220
Focalin 225
Focalin XR 224
Folic Acid 214
Fondaparinux............... 120
Foradil 274
Formoterol.................. 274
Fortamet 165
Fortaz
  Bone Infection............ 46
  LRI 54
  Meningitis................. 61
  Septicemia................ 68
  Skin Infection............ 71
  UTI 85
Fortesta Gel 164

Fortical...................... 177
Fosamax 176
Fosamax Plus D............ 176
Fosamprenavir 37
Fosinopril
  Heart Failure.............. 122
  HTN 128
Fragmin 117
Frova 266
Frovatriptan 266
Fungal Infection.... 48–51, 158
Furadantin 91
Furosemide
  Heart Failure.............. 125
  HTN 143
Fuzeon 32

G
Gabapentin
  Anticonvulsants 240
  Miscellaneous............. 29
  Neuralgia................. 30
Galantamine 229
Gardasil 219
Gatifloxacin................. 156

Gelnique 283
Gemfibrozil 111
Gemifloxacin 58
Generess Fe 313
Generlac 201
Gentamicin
  Bone Infection............ 45
  LRI 52
  Meningitis................. 60
  Septicemia................ 67
  Topical 147
Gentamicin Sulfate Injection
  Bone Infection............ 45
  LRI 52
  Meningitis................. 60
  Septicemia................ 67
Geodon
  Antipsychotics 256
  Bipolar Agents............ 266
GERD.................. 195–199
Gianvi 313
Gildess Fe 1.5/30 313
Gildess Fe 1/20 313
Glaucoma................ 158–161
Gleevec 95
Glimepiride 171

Glipizide.................... 171
Glipizide ER 171
Glipizide/Metformin........ 170
Glucophage.................. 165
Glucophage XR 165
Glucotrol XL 171
Glucovance 170
Glumetza 165
Glyburide 170
Glycerin 202
Glynase PresTab 171
Glyset 169
Golimumab 18
GoLYTELY 200
Gout 175–176
Gralise 29
Granisetron 186
Granisol 186
Guanfacine 228

H

Haemophilus B Conjugate .. 219
Halcinonide................... 320

HalfLytely.................... 199
Halobetasol.................. 320
Halog........................ 320
Heart Failure 121–127
Heather 316
**Hematopoietic
  Agents**................. 215–218
Heparin....................... 117
Heparin Sodium................ 117
Hepatitis A Vaccine 219
*Hepatitis A Vaccine
  (Inactivated)* 218
Hepatitis B (Recombinant).. 219
Hepsera 39
Homatropine 289
Hormone Therapy..... 210–212
HTN 127–145
Humalog...................... 311
Humalog Mix 50/50 312
Humalog Mix 75/25 312
*Human Papillomavirus
  Recombinant Vaccine,
  Bivalent*.................... 219

*Human Papillomavirus
  Recombinant Vaccine,
  Quadrivalent* 219
Humira
  Arthritis 16
  Crohn's Disease 205
  Psoriasis 151
Humulin 70/30 312
Humulin N 311
Humulin R 311
Hycet 22
Hydrochlorothiazide
  Heart Failure 126
  HTN 135
Hydrocodone
  Cough/Cold Chart 288
  Narcotics.................... 23
Hydrocortisone
  Systemic Steroid Chart.... 317
  Topical..................... 149
  Topical Ointment 150
  Topical Steroid Chart 319
Hydromorphone................ 23
Hydroxychloroquine 18
Hydroxyprogesterone........ 213

Hydroxyzine
  Antiemetics.................. 189
  Antihistamine Chart 284
Hyoscyamine 192
Hyzaar 135

I

Ibuprofen
  Narcotics.................... 23
  NSAIDs....................... 28
Iloperidone 254
Imatinib 95
Imipenem 45
Imipramine 250
Imiquimod 153
Imitrex 267
Immunization Chart ... 292
Incivek 42
Indacaterol 275
Indinavir 37
Infanrix 218
INFeD 214
Infliximab
  Arthritis 18
  Crohn's Disease 205
  Psoriasis 151

Influenza Virus Vaccine...... 220
Innohep 119
Inspra
  Heart Failure............... 123
  HTN 130
Insulin Formulation Chart 311
Insulin Aspart Protamine/
Aspart 312
Insulin, Aspart..............311
Insulin, Detemir............311
Insulin, Glargine 311
Insulin, Glulisine...........311
Insulin, Lispro..............311
Insulin, Lispro Protamine/
Lispro...................... 312
Insulin, NPH.................311
Insulin, NPH/Regular........ 312
Insulin, Regular.............311
Intelence...................... 33
Intermezzo 235
Introvale 314
Intuniv 228
Invanz
  LRI 52
  Skin Infection............... 69
  UTI 84

Invega........................ 254
Invega Sustenna 254
Invirase...................... 38
Iodoquinol 149
Ipratropium
  Asthma/COPD Preps 271
  Nasal Preps............... 154
Iquix......................... 157
Irbesartan.................. 135
Iron........................ 214
Iron Dextran 214
Isentress..................... 32
Isopto Carpine 160
Isosorbide Mononitrate....... 103
Isotretinoin 146
Isradipine 139
Ixabepilone 95
Ixempra....................... 95

J

Jakafi........................ 98
Jalyn........................ 281
Jantoven 121
Janumet 168

Janumet XR 168
Januvia 166
Jentadueto 167
Jevtana 92
Jolessa 314
Jolivette 316
Junel 1.5/30 313
Junel 1/20 313
Junel Fe 1.5/30 313
Junel Fe 1/20 313
Juvisync
  Antilipidemic Agents 111
  Diabetes................... 166

K

Kadian 24
Kaletra 37
Kapvay ER 223
Kariva 314
Keflex
  Bone Infection............. 47
  LRI 54
  Otitis Media................ 64
  Skin Infection............. 72
  URI 79
  UTI 86

Kelnor....................... 314
Kenalog 321
Kenalog-10 318
Kenalog-40 318
Keppra 242
Keppra XR 242
Ketek 54
Ketoconazole 148
Ketorolac.................. 161
Kineret 16
Kombiglyze XR................ 167
Krystexxa 176

L

Labetalol.................. 131
Lacosamide................. 237
Lactulose 201
Lamictal
  Anticonvulsants........... 240
  Bipolar Agents............ 262
Lamictal XR 241
Lamisil 50
Lamivudine
  AIDS......................... 35
  Antivirals.................. 39

Lamotrigine
  Anticonvulsants............ 241
  Bipolar Agents............. 262
Lansoprazole
  GERD 198
  Ulcer 194
  Zollinger-Ellison......... 204
Lantus 311
Lapatinib......................96
Lasix
  Heart Failure 125
  HTN 143
Lastacaft 162
Latanoprost.................. 160
Latuda 256
Laxatives............. 199–202
Lazanda...................... 21
Leena........................ 315
Leflunomide 18
Lenalidomide..................96
Lescol.......................112
Lescol XL 112
Lessina 313
Letrozole.....................96

Levalbuterol 275
Levaquin
  LRI........................58
  Skin Infection............. 75
  URI........................82
  UTI........................88
Levbid....................... 192
Levemir......................311
Levetiracetam 242
Levitra 282
Levobunolol 159
Levocetirizine............... 287
Levodopa 253
Levofloxacin
  LRI........................58
  Ophtho Preps.............. 157
  Skin Infection............. 75
  URI........................82
  UTI........................88
Levonest 315
Levonorgestrel
  Contraceptives 209
  Hormone Therapy 210
  Oral Contraceptives
    Chart................... 313
  Osteoporosis 178

Levora....................... 313
Levothroid................... 182
Levothyroxine 182
Levoxyl 180
Lexapro
  Anxiety/Hypnotics 233
  Depression................ 248
Lexiva 37
Lialda 202
Librax 192
Lidocaine
  Antiarrhythmics........... 105
  Miscellaneous..............30
Lidoderm Patch................30
Linagliptin 167
Linezolid
  LRI........................56
  Skin Infection............. 73
Liothyronine 182
Lipitor......................112
Liraglutide (rDNA Origin) ... 169
Lisdexamfetamine 226
Lisinopril
  Heart Failure 122
  HTN 130

Lithium...................... 263
Lithobid..................... 263
Livalo 113
Lo Loestrin Fe............... 314
Lo/Ovral 313
Locoid....................... 320
Lodrane-D 284
Loestrin 21 1.5/30........... 313
Loestrin 21 1/20 313
Loestrin 24 Fe 313
Loestrin Fe 1.5/30 313
Loestrin Fe 1/20 313
Lokara 319
Lomotil...................... 185
Lopid 111
Lopinavir..................... 37
Lopressor
  Angina 101
  HTN 137
Loprox 148
Loratadine 287
Lorazepam
  Anticonvulsants........... 235
  Anxiety/Hypnotics 232

Lortab............................ 22
Loryna 314
Losartan 135
Loseasonique 314
Lotensin 127
Loteprednol.................... 158
Lotrel........................... 129
Lotrisone 149
Lotronex 205
Lovastatin...................... 112
Lovaza.......................... 115
Lovenox......................... 118
Low-Ogestrel................... 313
LRI 52–60
Lubiprostone 205
Lumigan 160
Lunesta 234
Lurasidone 256
Lutera 313
Luvox CR 269
Luxiq 319
Lybrel 314

Lyrica
  Anticonvulsants........... 243
  Miscellaneous.............. 30
Lysteda 213

M

MAC 62
Macrobid 90
Macrodantin 90
Magnesium...................... 201
Makena 213
Maraviroc 32
Marinol 191
Marlissa 313
Mavik 123
Maxalt.......................... 267
Maxzide
  Heart Failure............. 126
  HTN....................... 143
Measles Vaccine Live........ 221
Meclizine....................... 189
Medrol 317
Medroxyprogesterone
  Contraceptives 209
  Hormone Therapy 210
  Osteoporosis 178

Meloxicam
  Arthritis 18
  NSAIDs 28
Memantine...................... 230
Menactra 221
Meningitis 60–62
Meningococcal
  (groups A, C, Y and
  W-135) Oligosaccharide
  Diphtheria CRM 197
  Conjugate 221
Meningococcal
  Polysaccharide
  A/C/Y/W-135 221
Meningococcal
  Polysaccharide
  Diphtheria Toxoid
  Conjugate Vaccine 221
Menomune A/C/Y/W-135... 221
Menostar 179
Mentax.......................... 148
Menveo 221
Meperidine...................... 23
Mepron 66
Meropenem
  Meningitis................. 61
  Skin Infection............ 70

Merrem
  Meningitis................. 61
  Skin Infection............ 70
Mesalamine 202
Mestranol 315
Metadate CD 227
Metadate ER.................... 227
Metaxalone 268
Metformin 165
Methimazole.................... 174
Methotrexate 19
Methoxsalen 152
Methsuximide 238
Methylin 227
Methylnaltrexone 206
Methylphenidate 227
Methylprednisolone 317
Methyltestosterone 163
Metipranolol 159
Metoclopramide
  Antiemetics 190
  GERD 195
  Miscellaneous............ 206
Metolazone 144

Metoprolol
Angina...................... 101
Heart Failure.............. 124
HTN......................... 137

Metozolv ODT
GERD...................... 195
Miscellaneous........... 206

MetroGel.................... 147

MetroGel-Vaginal......... 207

Metronidazole
Bone Infection............. 48
Topical.................... 147
Vaginal.................... 207

Metronidazole Gel........ 147

Mevacor 112

Mexiletine................. 105

Miacalcin 177

Micafungin 50

Micardis 133

Micardis HCT.............. 136

Miconazole 50

Microgestin 1.5/30........ 313

Microgestin 1/20.......... 313

Microgestin Fe 1.5/30..... 313

Microgestin Fe 1/20....... 313

Micronor.................... 316

Midazolam................ 232

Midazolam Syrup.......... 232

Miglitol.................... 169

Miglustat.................. 184

Migraine........ 266–268

Milnacipran.................30

Minocin
LRI.......................... 59
Skin Infection............. 77
URI.......................... 83
UTI.......................... 90

Minocycline
Acne....................... 146
LRI.......................... 59
Skin Infection............. 77
URI.......................... 83
UTI.......................... 90

MiraLax 201

Mirapex
Antiparkinson's Agents .. 251
Restless Legs Syndrome .. 270

Mirapex ER 251

Mircette 314

Mirena 209

Mirtazapine.............. 249

Miscellaneous........... 29

Miscellaneous Anti-Infectives........91

Misoprostol.............. 193

M-M-R II................... 221

Mobic
Arthritis..................... 18
NSAIDs..................... 28

Modafinil.................. 229

Modicon 28................ 313

Mometasone
Asthma/COPD Preps 277
Nasal Preps.............. 156
Topical Steroid Chart..... 319

Monobasic Sodium Phosphate.................. 199

Monodox
LRI.......................... 59
Skin Infection............. 76
URI.......................... 83
UTI.......................... 89

MonoNessa................ 314

Montelukast
Asthma/COPD Preps 277
Rhinitis.................... 279

Morphine 24

Motrin IB Tablets and Caplets 28

MoviPrep 200

Moxeza..................... 157

Moxifloxacin
Antibiotic Agents......... 157
LRI.......................... 59
Skin Infection............. 75
URI.......................... 82

MS Contin 25

Multaq 107

Mumps Vaccine Live....... 221

Mupirocin................... 147

Muscle Relaxants...... 268

Mycamine................... 50

Mycobutin.................. 62

Mysoline.................. 243

N

Nabilone 191

Nadolol
Angina..................... 101
HTN......................... 137

Naftifine	148
Naftin	148
Namenda	230
Namenda XR	230
Naprosyn	
Dysmenorrhea	209
NSAIDs	28
Naproxen	
Dysmenorrhea	209
Migraine	266
NSAIDs	28
Naratriptan	266
Narcotics	19–26
Nasacort AQ	156
Nasonex	156
Natacyn	158
Natalizumab	206
Natamycin	158
Natazia	316
Nateglinide	169
Natrecor	127
Navane	260
Nebivolol	137

Necon 0.5/35	313
Necon 1/35	313
Necon 1/50	314
Necon 10/11	314
Nedocromil	162
Nelfinavir	38
Neomycin	
Topical	147
Topical Ointment	150
Neoral	151
Neosporin Ointment	147
Nepafenac	161
Nesiritide	127
Neulasta	218
Neumega	217
Neupogen	217
Neurontin	
Anticonvulsants	240
Neuralgia	30
Nevanac	161
Nevirapine	33
Nexavar	99
Nexium	
GERD	197
Ulcer	194

Zollinger-Ellison	204
Nexium IV	197
Next Choice	316
Niacin	115
Niaspan	115
Nicardipine	
Angina	102
HTN	139
Nifedical XL	
Angina	102
HTN	139
Nifedipine	
Angina	102
HTN	139
Nilotinib	96
Niravam	231
Nitazoxanide	185
Nitro-Bid	104
Nitrofurantoin	90
Nitroglycerin	104
Nitrostat	104
Nizatidine	
GERD	196
Ulcer	193
Nora-BE	316

Nordette	313
Norethin 1/35	313
Norethindrone	
Hormone Therapy	210
Oral Contraceptives Chart	313
Osteoporosis	178
Norfloxacin	
Anti-Infective Agents	208
UTI	88
Norgestimate	
Hormone Therapy	210
Oral Contraceptives Chart	313
Norgestrel	313
Norinyl 1/35	313
Norinyl 1/50	314
Noroxin	
Anti-Infective Agents	208
UTI	88
Norpace	104
Norpace CR	104
Norpramin	249
Nor-QD	316
Nortrel 0.5/35	313
Nortrel 1/35	313
Nortrel 7/7/7	315

Nortriptyline 250
Norvasc
  Angina 102
  HTN 139
Norvir 38
Novolin 70/30 313
Novolin N 311
Novolin R 311
Novolog 311
Novolog Mix 70/30 312
Noxafil 50
NSAIDs 27–28, 161
Nucynta 26
Nuedexta 270
NuLYTELY 200
Nuvigil 228

O

OCD 269–270
Ocella 314
Ocufen 161
Ocupress 159
Ofirmev 29

Ofloxacin
  Anti-Infective Agents 208
  LRI 59
  Skin Infection 75
  UTI 88
Ogestrel-28 314
Olanzapine
  Antipsychotics 257
  Bipolar Agents 263
  Depression 248
Oleptro 250
Olmesartan 133
Olopatadine 287
Olux 319
Omega-3-Acid Ethyl Esters... 115
Omeprazole
  GERD 198
  Ulcer 195
  Zollinger-Ellison 204
Omnaris 155
Ondansetron 187
Onglyza 166
Onsolis 122
Opana 26
Opana ER 26
Oprelvekin 217

OptiPranolol 159
Optivar 162
Oracea 149
**Oral Contraceptives
Chart** 313
Orapred 318
Oravig 50
Orencia 16
Ortho Tri-Cyclen 315
Ortho Tri-Cyclen Lo 315
Ortho-Cept 313
Ortho-Novum 1/35 313
Ortho-Novum 7/7/7 315
Orysthia 313
Oseltamivir 44
Osmoprep 200
Osteoporosis 176–180
Otitis Media 62–66
Ovcon-35 313
Ovcon-50 314
Oxcarbazepine 242
Oxiconazole 148
Oxistat 148
Oxsoralen-Ultra 152

Oxybutynin 283
Oxycodone 26
OxyContin 25
Oxymorphone 26
Oxytrol 283

P

Paclitaxel 96
Palgic 285
Paliperidone 254
Palonosetron 188
Pamelor 250
Pamidronate 183
Pancrelipase 206
Pandel 321
Pantoprazole
  GERD 198
  Zollinger-Ellison 204
Parlodel 251
Paroxetine
  Anxiety/Hypnotics 234
  Depression 249
  OCD 269
  PMDD 212
Pataday 287
Patanol 287

Paxil
  Anxiety/Hypnotics 234
  Depression................. 249
  OCD....................... 269

Paxil CR
  Anxiety/Hypnotics 233
  Depression................. 248
  PMDD 212

PCE
  LRI........................ 56
  Skin Infection.............. 73
  URI........................ 80

PCP....................... 66

Pediapred................... 318

Pegasys..................... 40

Pegfilgrastim............... 218

Peginterferon alfa-2a 40

Peginterferon alfa-2b 40

PEG-Intron 40

Pegloticase 176

Pemetrexed................. 97

Pemirolast 162

Penciclovir................. 149

Penicillin VK
  LRI........................ 57
  Skin Infection.............. 74
  URI........................ 82

Pentasa..................... 203

Pepcid
  GERD...................... 196
  Ulcer...................... 193
  Zollinger-Ellison.......... 203

Percocet 25

Percodan 26

Perforomist 275

Perphenazine 260

Pertussis Vaccine
  Acellular, Adsorbed 222

Pertussis Vaccine,
  Acellular.................. 218

Pexeva
  Anxiety/Hypnotics 234
  Depression................. 249
  OCD....................... 269

Phenadoz 190

Phenobarbital.............. 192

Phenylephrine.............. 290

Phenytoin.................. 237

Pilocarpine................. 160

Pilopine HS................ 160

Pimecrolimus 150

Pioglitazone 172

Piperacillin
  LRI........................ 57
  Skin Infection............. 74

Pitavastatin 113

Plan B 316

Plan B One-Step 316

Plaquenil 18

Plavix 116

Pletal 119

PMDD 212–213

Pneumococcal Vaccine
  Polyvalent................. 221

Pneumococcal Vaccine,
  Diphtheria Conjugate...... 222

Pneumovax 23 221

Podofilox.................. 149

Polyethylene Glycol 3350 ... 201

Polymyxin B
  Topical.................... 147
  Topical Ointment.......... 150

Portia 313

Posaconazole............... 50

Potassium 201

Potassium Chloride 199

Potiga 239

Pradaxa....................116

Pramipexole
  Antiparkinson's Agents .. 251
  Restless Legs Syndrome.. 270

Prandimet 164

Prandin 170

Prasugrel..................116

Pravachol..................113

Pravastatin................113

Precose 168

Pred Forte 158

Pred Mild 158

Prednicarbate.............. 321

Prednisolone
  Ophtho Preps............. 157
  Systemic Steroid Chart... 317

Prednisone 319

Prefest 210

Pregabalin
  Anticonvulsants........... 243
  Miscellaneous............. 30

Prelone................... 317

Premarin Tablets
  Hormone Therapy.........211
  Osteoporosis 178

Premarin Vaginal 211
Premphase
  Hormone Therapy........ 210
  Osteoporosis 178
Prempro
  Hormone Therapy........ 210
  Osteoporosis 178
Prevacid
  GERD 198
  Ulcer 194
  Zollinger-Ellison........... 204
Prevacid Solutab
  GERD 198
  Ulcer 194
  Zollinger-Ellison........... 204
Previfem 314
Prevpac 194
Prilosec
  GERD 198
  Ulcer 194
  Zollinger-Ellison........... 204
Primaxin I.V. 45
Primidone...................... 243
Prinivil
  Heart Failure.............. 122
  HTN....................... 128

Prinzide 130
Pristiq...................... 247
ProAir HFA................... 273
Probenecid 176
Probenecid/Colchicine... 176
Procardia XL
  Angina.................... 102
  HTN....................... 139
Procentra................... 225
Prochlorperazine........... 189
Procrit..................... 217
Prolia...................... 179
Promacta................... 216
Promethazine
  Antiemetics 190
  Antihistamine Chart 284
  Cough/Cold Chart........ 288
Promethazine DM 289
Promethazine VC 289
Promethazine VC/Codeine.. 289
Promethazine w/Codeine.. 289
Promethegan............... 190
Propafenone................. 106
Propecia.................... 153

Propine 158
Propranolol
  Angina.................... 101
  Antiarrhythmics.......... 106
  HTN....................... 137
Propylthiouracil 174
Proquin XR 88
Proscar 280
Protonix
  GERD 198
  Zollinger-Ellison........... 204
Protonix IV
  GERD 198
  Zollinger-Ellison........... 204
Protopic 150
Provenge 99
Proventil HFA................274
Provigil 229
Prozac
  Anxiety/Hypnotics 233
  Depression................ 248
  OCD 269
Pruritus/Inflammation .. 150
Pseudoephedrine
  Antihistamine Chart 284
  Cough/Cold Chart........ 288

Psoriasis................ 150–153
Pulmicort................... 276

Q

Qnasl...................... 154
Quasense 314
Quetiapine
  Antipsychotics 258
  Bipolar Agents.......... 264
  Depression................ 245
Quinapril
  Heart Failure............ 122
  HTN....................... 130
Quinidine
  Antiarrhythmics.......... 105
  Miscellaneous............ 270
Quinupristin................ 75
Quixin 157
Qutenza.................... 29
Qvar...................... 275

R

Rabeprazole
  GERD 198
  Ulcer 195
  Zollinger-Ellison........... 204

Raloxifene
  Antineoplastics............... 97
  Osteoporosis 180
Raltegravir............................ 32
Ramelteon 235
Ramipril
  Heart Failure............... 123
  HTN............................ 129
Ranexa 104
Ranitidine
  GERD 196
  Ulcer 193
  Zollinger-Ellison............ 203
Ranolazine........................... 104
Rapaflo 280
Rasagiline 253
Rasburicase 185
Razadyne 229
Razadyne ER 229
Rebetol................................. 41
Reclast 184
Reclipsen 313
Reglan Tablets
  Antiemetics 190
  GERD 195
Relistor 206

Relpax 266
Remeron 249
RemeronSolTab.................... 249
Remicade
  Arthritis 18
  Crohn's Disease............ 205
  Psoriasis.................... 151
Repaglinide.......................... 170
Reprexain............................. 23
Requip
  Antiparkinson's Agents .. 252
  Restless Legs Syndrome.. 271
Rescriptor 33
Restoril 232
Retapamulin 147
Retin-A................................ 147
Retin-A Micro 147
Retrovir................................ 35
Revlimid 96
Reyataz 36
Rezira 290
R-Tanna 290
Rhinocort Aqua 155
Ribavirin 41
Ridaura 16

Rifabutin.............................. 62
Rifaximin
  Diarrhea 185
  Miscellaneous.............. 207
Rilpivirine............................. 34
Rimantadine......................... 44
Risedronate......................... 177
Risperdal
  Antipsychotics 255
  Bipolar Agents............. 265
  Miscellaneous.............. 271
Risperdal Consta 265
Risperdal M-Tab 265
Risperidone
  Antipsychotics 255
  Bipolar Agents............. 265
  Miscellaneous.............. 271
Ritalin 228
Ritalin LA 228
Ritalin SR 228
Ritonavir.............................. 38
Rituxan
  Antineoplastics.............. 98
  Arthritis 19
Rituximab
  Antineoplastics.............. 98
  Arthritis 19

Rivaroxaban 120
Rivastigmine
  Alzheimer's Therapy...... 230
  Antiparkinson's Agents .. 251
Rizatriptan 267
Rocephin
  Bone Infection.............. 46
  LRI........................... 54
  Meningitis................... 61
  Otitis Media................. 63
  Septicemia 68
  Skin Infection.............. 71
  UTI........................... 85
Roflumilast 278
Ropinirole
  Antiparkinson's Agents .. 252
  Restless Legs Syndrome.. 271
Rosiglitazone....................... 172
Rosuvastatin 113
Rozerem 235
Rubella Vaccine Live............ 221
Rufinamide 238
Ruxolitinib 98
Rybix ODT 31
Rynatan 291

Rynatan Pediatric............ 291
Rynatuss 291
Rythmol SR 106
Ryzolt 31

S

Sabril............................ 244
Safyral.......................... 314
Salmeterol.................... 275
Sanctura 283
Sancuso 186
Saphris 256
Saquinavir...................... 38
Sarafem........................ 212
Savella 30
Saxagliptin..................... 167
Scopolamine
  Antiemetics 189
  Antispasmodics 192
Seasonale 314
Seasonique................... 314
Sectral 106
Selegiline 253
Selzentry 32

Semprex-D 290
Septicemia............. 66–69
Septra
  Otitis Media............... 66
  PCP........................... 66
  UTI............................ 89
Septra DS...................... 66
Serevent 275
Seroquel
  Antipsychotics 258
  Bipolar Agents.......... 264
Seroquel XR
  Antipsychotics 258
  Bipolar Agents.......... 264
  Depression................ 245
Sertaconazole 148
Sertraline
  Anxiety/Hypnotics 234
  Depression................ 249
  OCD.......................... 270
  PMDD....................... 213
Sildenafil...................... 281
Silenor 234
Silodosin...................... 280
Simcor......................... 115

Simponi........................... 18
Simvastatin
  Antilipidemic Agents 114
  Diabetes................... 166
Sinemet 252
Sinemet CR 252
Singulair
  Asthma/COPD Preps ... 277
  Rhinitis.................... 279
Sipuleucel-T.................... 99
Sitagliptin
  Antilipidemic Agents 111
  Diabetes................... 168
Skelaxin....................... 268
Skin Infection....... 69–77
Sodium
  GERD....................... 199
  Ulcer....................... 195
Sodium Ascorbate 200
Sodium Bicarbonate 199
Sodium Chloride 199
Sodium Diuril
  Heart Failure............ 126
  HTN.......................... 144

Sodium Ferric Gluconate
  Complex.................... 215
Sodium Sulfate.............. 200
Solia............................ 313
Solifenacin.................... 283
Solodyn........................ 146
Solu-Cortef................... 317
Solu-Medrol.................. 317
Sonata 235
Sorafenib........................ 99
Sotalol 108
Sotret 146
Spiriva 271
Spironolactone
  Heart Failure............ 125
  HTN.......................... 143
Sprintec....................... 314
Sprycel.......................... 94
Sronyx 313
Stalevo......................... 253
Starlix.......................... 169
Stavzor
  Anticonvulsants........ 236
  Bipolar Agents.......... 266
  Migraine................... 268

Staxyn 282
Stelara 151
Stendra 281
Strattera 223
Striant 163
Subsys 22
Sucralfate 192
Sudafed PE Sinus and
  Allergy Tablets 285
Sulbactam 74
Sulfacetamide 157
Sulfamethoxazole
  Otitis Media 66
  PCP 66
  UTI 89
Sulfasalazine 202
Sulfatrim Pediatric
  Otitis Media 66
  PCP 66
  UTI 89
Sulfisoxazole 64
Sumatriptan 267
Sumycin
  Acne 146
  LRI 60
  URI 84
  UTI 90

Sunitinib 99
Suprax
  LRI 53
  Otitis Media 63
  URI 78
  UTI 85
Suprep 201
Sustiva 33
Sutent 99
Syeda 314
Symbicort 272
Symbyax 248
Synercid 75
Synthroid 181
Systemic Corticosteroids
  Chart 317

T

Tacrolimus 150
Tadalafil
  BPH 280
  ED 282
  HTN 144
Tambocor 105
Tamiflu 44
Tamsulosin 280

Tapazole 174
Tapentadol 26
Tarceva 94
Tasigna 96
Tazarotene 152
Tazicef
  Bone Infection 46
  LRI 54
  Meningitis 61
  Septicemia 68
  Skin Infection 71
  UTI 85
Tazobactam
  LRI 57
  Skin Infection 74
Tazorac 152
Taztia XT
  Angina 103
  HTN 140
Teflaro
  LRI 53
  Skin Infection 71
Tegretol 238
Tegretol-XR 238
Tekamlo 138
Tekturna 145
Tekturna HCT 145

Telaprevir 42
Telavancin 77
Telbivudine 42
Telithromycin 54
Telmisartan 133
Temazepam 232
Temodar 100
Temovate 319
Temozolomide 100
Tenofovir Disoproxil
  AIDS 36
  Antivirals 42
Tenoretic 138
Tenormin
  Angina 101
  HTN 137
Terazol 3 208
Terazol 7 208
Terazosin
  BPH 280
  HTN 131
Terbinafine 50
Terconazole 208
Tesamorelin 184
Tessalon 290

Testosterone................ 163
Testred..................... 163
Tetanus Toxoid............ 222
Tetracycline
  Acne 146
  LRI........................ 60
  URI........................ 84
  UTI........................ 90
Teveten..................... 132
Theo-24.................... 278
Theophylline............... 278
Thioridazine 260
Thiothixene 260
Thyroid..................... 183
Thyroid Agents 180–183
Tiazac
  Angina.................... 103
  HTN....................... 140
Ticagrelor.................. 116
Ticarcillin
  Bone Infection........... 47
  Septicemia............... 69
Tigecycline
  LRI........................ 60
  Skin Infection............ 77

Tikosyn 107
Tilia Fe 315
Timentin
  Bone Infection........... 47
  Septicemia............... 69
Timolol..................... 159
Timoptic................... 159
Timoptic in Ocudose ... 159
Tindamax.................. 91
Tinidazole................. 91
Tinzaparin................. 119
Tiotropium................ 271
Tipranavir................. 38
Tizanidine................. 268
TobraDex.................. 157
TobraDex ST.............. 157
Tobramycin
  Bone Infection........... 45
  LRI........................ 52
  Meningitis................ 61
  Ophtho Preps............ 157
  Septicemia............... 67
Tobrex...................... 157
Tocilizumab................ 19
Tofranil.................... 250

Tolterodine................ 283
Topical Corticosteroid
  Chart..................... 319
Topamax
  Anticonvulsants.......... 244
  Migraine.................. 268
Topamax Sprinkle
  Anticonvulsants.......... 244
  Migraine.................. 268
Topicort................... 319
Topiramate
  Anticonvulsants.......... 244
  Migraine.................. 268
Toprol-XL
  Angina.................... 101
  Heart Failure............. 124
  HTN....................... 137
Torsemide
  Heart Failure............. 125
  HTN....................... 143
Toviaz...................... 283
Tradjenta.................. 166
Tramadol.................. 31
Trandolapril............... 123
Tranexamic................ 213
Transderm Scop 189
Tranxene T-Tab 231

Travatan Z 161
Travoprost................ 161
Trazodone................. 250
Tretinoin 147
Treximet 266
Triamcinolone
  Asthma/COPD Preps ... 277
  Nasal Preps.............. 156
  Systemic Steroid Chart... 317
  Topical Corticosteroid
  Chart..................... 319
Triamterene
  Heart Failure............. 125
  HTN....................... 143
Tribenzor.................. 134
Tricor...................... 111
Triderm 321
Trifluoperazine 260
Tri-Legest Fe 315
Trileptal................... 242
Trilyte..................... 200
Trimethoprim
  Otitis Media.............. 66
  PCP....................... 66
  UTI........................ 89
Trinessa................... 315

Tri-Lo Sprintec 315
Tri-Norinyl 315
Tripedia 218
Tri-Previfem 315
Tri-Sprintec 315
Trivora 315
Trizivir 34
Trospium 283
Trusopt 159
Truvada 35
Tussi-12 291
Tussicaps 290
Tussigon 291
Tussionex Pennkinetic ... 291
Twinject 279
Twinrix 219
Twynsta 142
Tygacil
  LRI 60
  Skin Infection 77
Tykerb 96
Tylenol with Codeine 20
Tysabri 206
Tyzeka 42

U

Ulcer 192–195
Ulcerative Colitis 202–203
Ulipristal 317
Uloric 175
Ultram 31
Ultram ER 31
Ultravate 320
Unasyn 74
URI 78–84
Urinary Tract 282–283
Uroxatral 279
Ustekinumab 151
UTI 84–91

V

Vaccines/
  Immunoglobulins ... 218–222
Valacyclovir 43
Valium
  Anticonvulsants 235
  Anxiety/Hypnotics 232
Valproate 236

Valproic Acid
  Anticonvulsants 236
  Bipolar Agents 266
  Migraine 268
Valsartan
  Heart Failure 124
  HTN 133
Valtrex 43
Vancomycin 69
Vancomycin HCl 69
Vandazole 208
Vandetanib 100
Vanos
  Psoriasis 153
  Topical Corticosteroid
  Chart 319
Vaqta 218
Vardenafil 282
Varicella Virus Vaccine Live.. 222
Varivax 222
Vasotec
  Heart Failure 122
  HTN 127
Velivet 315

Venlafaxine
  Anxiety/Hypnotics 233
  Depression 247
Venofer 214
Ventolin HFA 274
Veramyst 155
Verapamil
  Angina 103
  Antiarrhythmics 108
  HTN 140
Verdeso 319
Verelan 141
Verelan PM 141
VESIcare 283
Vfend 51
Viagra 281
Vibativ 77
Vibramycin
  Skin Infection 76
  URI 83
  UTI 90
Vibra-Tabs
  Skin Infection 76
  URI 83
  UTI 90
Vicodin 23

Vicodin ES...................... 23
Vicodin HP...................... 23
Vicoprofen...................... 23
Victoza........................ 169
Victrelis....................... 39
Videx.......................... 34
Videx EC....................... 34
Vigabatrin................... 244
Vigamox....................... 157
Viibryd........................ 245
Vilazodone................... 245
Vimovo......................... 27
Vimpat........................ 237
Viracept....................... 38
Viramune....................... 33
Viramune XR.................... 33
Viread
  AIDS........................ 36
  Antivirals.................. 42
Visicol........................ 199
Vistaril....................... 286
Voltaren-XR.................... 27

Voriconazole................. 51
Vorinostat................... 100
VoSpire ER.................... 274
Vytorin....................... 110
Vyvanse....................... 226

W

Warfarin.................... 121
WelChol
  Antilipidemic Agents... 109
  Diabetes.................. 165
Wellbutrin.................... 246
Wellbutrin SR................. 246
Wellbutrin XL................. 246
Wera.......................... 313
Westcort...................... 321

X

Xalatan....................... 160
Xanax......................... 231
Xanax XR...................... 231
Xarelto....................... 120
Xifaxan
  Diarrhea.................. 185
  Miscellaneous............. 207

Xopenex HFA.................. 275
Xylocaine-MPF................ 105
Xyzal......................... 287

Y

Yasmin........................ 314
YAZ........................... 313

Z

Zafirlukast................. 277
Zaleplon.................... 235
Zanaflex...................... 268
Zantac
  GERD...................... 196
  Ulcer..................... 193
  Zollinger-Ellison......... 203
Zarah......................... 314
Zarontin...................... 237
Zaroxolyn..................... 144
Zavesca....................... 184
Zebeta........................ 137
Zegerid
  GERD...................... 199
  Ulcer..................... 195
Zenchent...................... 313

Zenpep........................ 206
Zentrip....................... 189
Zestoretic.................... 130
Zestril
  Heart Failure............. 122
  HTN....................... 128
Zetia......................... 110
Ziagen........................ 34
Ziana......................... 146
Zidovudine.................. 35
Zinacef
  Bone Infection............ 46
  Meningitis................ 62
  Septicemia................ 68
  UTI....................... 85
Ziprasidone
  Antipsychotics............ 256
  Bipolar Agents............ 266
Zipsor........................ 27
Zithromax
  LRI....................... 55
  MAC....................... 62
  Otitis Media.............. 64
  Skin Infection............ 72
  URI....................... 79
  UTI....................... 86

Zmax
    LRI 55
    URI 79
Zocor 114
Zofran 187
Zofran Injection 187
Zoledronic Acid 184
Zolinza 100
Zollinger-Ellison 203–204
Zolmitriptan 267
Zoloft
    Anxiety/Hypnotics 234
    Depression 249

OCD 270
PMDD 213
Zolpidem 235
Zometa 184
Zomig 267
Zomig Nasal Spray 267
Zonalon 150
Zonatuss 291
Zonegran 238
Zonisamide 238
Zostavax 222
Zoster Vaccine Live 222

Zosyn
    LRI 57
    Skin Infection 74
Zovia 1/50E 314
Zovirax Cream 149
Zovirax Ointment 149
Zovirax Oral 43
Zuplenz 188
Zutripro 291
Zyloprim
    Gout 175
    Miscellaneous 185
Zymar 156

Zymaxid 157
Zyprexa
    Antipsychotics 257
    Bipolar Agents 263
    Depression 245
Zyprexa Relprevv 258
Zyprexa Zydis 263
Zyrtec 284
Zyrtec-D 284
Zyvox
    LRI 56
    Skin Infection 73

2013 PDR® Reference Library ORDER FORM

QTY	TITLE	PRICE	S&H	
—	2013 Physicians' Desk Reference® (PDR), 67th edition	$97.95	$12.95	$ —
—	2013 PDR® for Nonprescription Drugs	$59.95	$9.95	$ —
—	2013 PDR® Nurse's Drug Handbook	$43.95	$7.95	$ —
—	2013 PDR® Pharmacopoeia Pocket Dosing Guide	$11.95	$1.95	$ —
—	2011 NeoFax®, 24th Edition	$41.95	$7.95	$ —
—	PDR® for Nutritional Supplements, 2nd Edition	$59.95	$9.95	$ —
—	Contraceptive Technology, 19th Edition	$79.95	$9.95	$ —
—	PDR® for Herbal Medicines, 4th Edition	$59.95	$9.95	$ —
		Add S&H Per Book		$ —
		Sales Tax (CA, IL, IN, MD, NC, NJ, NY, PA, WA)		$ —
		TOTAL AMOUNT OF ORDER		$ —

Indicate Method of Payment:

☐ **PAYMENT ENCLOSED:**

☐ Check payable to PDR   Charge: ☐ VISA ☐ MasterCard ☐ Amex

ACCOUNT # _____ EXP. DATE _____

SIGNATURE _____ TEL. NO. _____

☐ **BILL ME LATER:**

NAME _____

COMPANY NAME _____

ADDRESS _____

CITY _____ STATE _____ ZIP _____

Order Online at www.PDRbooks.com

Mail to: PDR Distribution, PO Box 824683, Philadelphia, PA 19182-4683
For faster service call **TOLL-FREE 1-800-678-5689** or **FAX** your order to
1-800-294-4146. Please do not mail a confirmation order in addition to your fax.

K9001PH01